T0385028

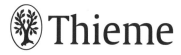

Dedicated to my children, grandchildren, and great-grandchildren

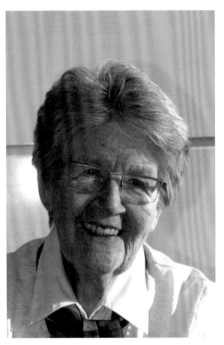

Hanne Marquardt, registered nurse and naturopath, is a pioneer in teaching and practicing RTF. For almost 60 years she has trained around 80,000 therapists and set up 18 training centers around the globe. The founding school is situated in Königsfeld-Burgberg, Germany

Reflexotherapy of the Feet

Second Edition

Hanne Marquardt
International School of Reflexotherapy of the Feet
Königsfeld-Burgberg, Germany

88 illustrations

Thieme
Stuttgart · New York · Delhi · Rio de Janeiro

Library of Congress Cataloging-in-Publication Data
is available from the publisher.

This book is an authorized translation of the 7th German edition published and copyrighted 2012 by Karl F. Haug Verlag, Stuttgart. Title of the German edition: Praktisches Lehrbuch der Reflexzonentherapie am Fuß

Translator: Angela Trowell, Radstock, UK
Illustrator: Christiane Schott, Rottweil, Germany

2nd Czech edition 2016
1st Danish edition 2001
1st French edition 2004
1st Greek edition 2004
3rd Italian edition 2016
1st Japanese edition 2007
1st Korean edition 2010
1st Lithuanian edition 2006
1st Polish edition 2012
1st Portuguese (Brazil) edition 2005
2nd Russian edition 2016
3rd Spanish edition 2015
1st Swedish edition 2004

© 2000, 2017 Georg Thieme Verlag KG
Thieme Publishers Stuttgart
Rüdigerstrasse 14, 70469 Stuttgart, Germany
+49 [0]711 8931 421, customerservice@thieme.de

Thieme Publishers New York
333 Seventh Avenue, New York, NY 10001, USA
+1-800-782-3488, customerservice@thieme.com

Thieme Publishers Delhi
A-12, Second Floor, Sector-2, Noida-201301
Uttar Pradesh, India
+91 120 45 566 00, customerservice@thieme.in

Thieme Publishers Rio, Thieme Publicações Ltda.
Edifício Rodolpho de Paoli, 25° andar
Av. Nilo Peçanha, 50 – Sala 2508
Rio de Janeiro 20020-906 Brasil
+55 21 3172 2297 / +55 21 3172 1896

Cover design: Thieme Publishing Group
Typesetting by DiTech Process Solutions
    Pvt. Ltd., India
Printed in Germany by   5 4 3 2 1
Grafisches Centrum Cuno GmbH & Co. KG, Calbe

ISBN 978-3-13-125242-5
Also available as an e-book:
eISBN 978-3-13-203832-5

Important note: Medicine is an ever-changing science undergoing continual development. Research and clinical experience are continually expanding our knowledge, in particular our knowledge of proper treatment and drug therapy. Insofar as this book mentions any dosage or application, readers may rest assured that the authors, editors, and publishers have made every effort to ensure that such references are in accordance with **the state of knowledge at the time of production of the book**.

Nevertheless, this does not involve, imply, or express any guarantee or responsibility on the part of the publishers in respect to any dosage instructions and forms of applications stated in the book. **Every user is requested to examine carefully** the manufacturers' leaflets accompanying each drug and to check, if necessary in consultation with a physician or specialist, whether the dosage schedules mentioned therein or the contraindications stated by the manufacturers differ from the statements made in the present book. Such examination is particularly important with drugs that are either rarely used or have been newly released on the market. Every dosage schedule or every form of application used is entirely at the user's own risk and responsibility. The authors and publishers request every user to report to the publishers any discrepancies or inaccuracies noticed. If errors in this work are found after publication, errata will be posted at www.thieme.com on the product description page.

Some of the product names, patents, and registered designs referred to in this book are in fact registered trademarks or proprietary names even though specific reference to this fact is not always made in the text. Therefore, the appearance of a name without designation as proprietary is not to be construed as a representation by the publisher that it is in the public domain.

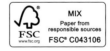

Contents

Part I

Part II

Part III

Part IV

Foreword to the First Edition

I gladly accepted the offer of writing the foreword to this book for two reasons. First, as a professional physician and acupuncturist, I have for years been working on the phenomenon of projections of the whole body into various microsystems; second, I have known Hanne Marquardt for a long time and have myself experienced the profound and convincing effect of RTF on my own feet.

The projection of the organism to clearly circumscribed parts of the body is a known phenomenon. Many new holographic fields, such as ear, skull, nose, hand, and oral cavity have been described during the past decades. Microsystems are used by a large number of therapists all over the world to treat patients, but treatment based on the "microsystem of the foot" can rightly be called the oldest and most widespread method. As a great deal of therapeutic experience exists over a number of decades, RTF does not require much further recommendation.

However, from a strictly scientific point of view a number of questions remain open as the results achieved in everyday work on this microsystem reach beyond that which can be explained by known neural reflex mechanisms.

None of the microsystems can be understood or classified without considering their basic phenomenological character. According to their essence and functions, microsystems are self-reflections of the whole—the macrosystem—each in their own individual and specific way. Their significance lies in the correlation between themselves and the whole: autonomous control systems that strive for homeostasis and harmonization. In modern physics, professionals are beginning to orient themselves in a holistic universe (David Bohm). Chaos and fractal research offers an insight into the openness of non-linear, unrestricted systems, which ultimately suggest a transparent view within the constant repetition of reflections of the whole. A new theory explaining the holistic phenomena of the development of plants, animals, and human beings at the embryonic stage originates from China, the motherland of acupuncture, and is leading to astonishing practical results in agriculture and medicine. In this context, the following remark by Goethe seems appropriate: "No phenomenon is self-explanatory; only many together in methodical order bring about what can be called a 'theory'." More important than the effect of a quantitative summary is the qualitative aspect, which alone leads to the unification of all parts. The parts can guarantee the whole as they carry its information as an intrinsic memory in themselves.

The fear that the basic understanding of our human nature could fail due to the recognition of similarities and self-reflections, originates from the old perception of the world and human nature. But time goes on and it leaves us behind if we don't have the courage to accept and recognize the many changes in our environment that are already obvious.

For 58 years Hanne Marquardt has been working with this method. Her name is closely connected with it and she is rightly acknowledged to be the person responsible for developing reflexotherapy of the feet into a convincing method accepted by medical professionals. She developed it from a basic knowledge to a professional level in Germany and in a number of other countries. The reliability of this therapy has been proved not only by Hanne Marquardt, but by many other therapists besides and after her. They have all worked with these zones in their everyday practice and found them effective. This English edition by Hanne Marquardt is written completely anew and covers her whole professional life's work and conclusions in this field.

To deal with phenomena and similarities demands a clear working concept: Hanne Marquardt is not only gifted with intuition and sensitivity, but also with a remarkable ability to define her thoughts precisely. These professional skills and personal qualities made it possible to teach this method.

Her special charisma shows in her devotion to people: she convincingly teaches her pupils that through an empathic touch the patient can confidently open up and the therapist will be able to increase his/her inner respect for each patient's individual course of life.

Many practical references as to how therapists can accompany their patients through their specific times of suffering add weight to the book and make it stand out against the average professional literature.

Jochen Gleditsch, MD
Honorary President of the German Medical Society
For Acupuncture (DÄGfA),
Specialist in otorhinolaryngology and dentistry,
Lecturer in acupuncture, University of Munich,
Germany

Tao Te Ching, 11th Verse

We join spokes together in a wheel, but it is the center hole that makes the wagon move.

We shape clay into a pot, but it is the emptiness inside that holds whatever we want.

We hammer wood for a house, but it is the inner space that makes it livable.

We work with being, but non-being is what we use.

Laotzu
Translator: Stephen Mitchell

Preface to the Second Edition

With this new English edition of the textbook *Reflexotherapy of the Feet*, all the latest developments of this treatment method are now also available to the English-speaking world. Thieme Publishers and Haug Verlag have loyally covered the subject of feet for more than forty years, highlighting our mutual appreciation of it. This is also reflected in the translation of my books into a further 14 languages. My heartfelt thanks go to all those concerned.

The significantly expanded textbook is the culmination of almost 60 years of professional "foot work." The people from then have undergone major changes over this long period, and the method has been constantly adapted in various ways to meet their particular requirements.

This is reflected in the book by many new insights into therapeutic connections and possibilities.

The following is new to this edition:

- An in-depth examination of the question: What are the reflex zones of the foot?
- Development of the lymphatic zones as an important, contemporary supplement to traditional treatment of the feet.
- New facial zones and their therapeutic benefits.
- A detailed explanation of the therapeutic key to similarity in shape.
- Use of the zones of the pelvic ligaments.
- Assignment of the "tooth microsystem" to the zones of the feet and its practical use.

- The therapeutic "bridge" between the zones of the feet and the meridians.
- New grips to stabilize the autonomic nervous system, e.g., use of the zones of the sphincters, work with the sign of infinity.
- Connection between tonus regulation (Eutonia) in the person in situ and the zones of the feet.
- Development of new grips for ergonomic use of the therapist's hands
- An extensive collection of therapists' experiences "From Practical Experience – For Practical Application" from 25 therapeutic areas
- Studies and publications involving Reflexotherapy of the Feet.

Special thanks are due to all the teaching therapists at our professional schools who for decades have had a significant involvement in the development of reflexotherapy in Europe and beyond. I would also like to thank the countless patients from whom we have been able to gather all our experiences.

I hope that this new English edition will contribute to the further appreciation of this extraordinary and contemporary form of therapy. Holistic manual methods such as working with the feet are of particular value today: they quite literally touch the whole person and help them "onto their feet," thus providing an urgently needed supplement to modern medicine.

Hanne Marquardt

Preface to the First Edition

Two years prior to publication of this book, I spent a few hours every day throughout an entire summer with a young Armenian interpreter working on the translation into English of my textbook. Several years previously she had helped us when we were establishing the School of Reflexotherapy of the Feet in Yerevan, Armenia, by impressively interpreting in many of our practical courses from English into Russian and Armenian. The work we did together on that project was also the basis for a translation of the English manuscript into Russian. I would like to express my special thanks to Ms. Anahit Badalian in recognition of this exceptional accomplishment.

Ms. Joanne Stead also deserves my sincere thanks for her very sensitive editing, proofreading, and amending of the original translation of the book.

My particular thanks go to those responsible at Thieme International Publishers for including my book in their series. "Reflexotherapy of the Feet" is thus one of the first English-language textbooks available on the market for health professionals. It offers a necessary and comprehensive survey of the developments in the treatment of feet over the last 40 years. It is my sincere wish that the findings and collected experiences may meet the needs of today's therapists and patients.

Hanne Marquardt
March 2000

Part I
General Principles

1 Historical Development of Foot Treatments

First Historical References

Development of reflexotherapy of the feet (RTF) from its earliest beginnings to today probably followed a path similar to many other forms of treatment which are now generally accepted. There have always been people with special abilities whose instinct and intuition have told them what is needed for particular illnesses, because they are far more in touch with natural connections and cosmic laws.

Over the centuries ancient knowledge regarding the healing powers of herbs, for example, developed into phytotherapy, while piercing certain points on the body with simple, pointed objects (already historically documented in ancient times) became acupuncture, and sharpened stones and metals used to perform internal procedures on people in earlier times marked the beginnings of surgery.

The beginnings of foot treatments that are now practiced in the Middle East have already been substantiated by millennia-old **Egyptian pictographs** (**Fig. 1.1**), showing that the feet—as well as the hands—are well suited to treatment. In this regard the words of a high official may be approximately rendered as, "Cause me no pain!"—with the response, "I will conduct myself in such a way that you will praise me."

There are also records from the **Far East** of marks on the feet as a result of ancient ritual practices. These are frequently found on the soles of the feet of Buddhist statues, and it is likely that they were for the purposes of religious worship. For decades, however, a simple (and often very painful) treatment of the feet was performed as

a folk remedy in various countries of the Far East, and this was probably the result of more recent Western principles.

Since the last century evidence has also emerged from the **Western world** that the indigenous peoples of Central and North America treated their sick using points on the foot. **Christine Issel** (USA) researched the topic in depth, and in 1990 she compiled interesting evidence in her book *Reflexology: Art, Science and History*. The Cherokee Indians appear to be the only tribe for which there is evidence that they have continued using foot therapy until modern times. It is supposed that they acquired their knowledge from the Incas of South America.

According to ancient sources, various physicians in **Europe** were already performing a kind of zone therapy in the Middle Ages. At the beginning of the last century, in a book **Henry B. Bressler** refers to a document in which around 1,582 physicians described treatment of areas of the hand and foot and the astonishing results they obtained in people who were sick.

All this goes to show that from time immemorial the feet have been ascribed a major, multidimensional significance in many human cultures.

Developments in Modern Times

In the first instance, anyone performing foot treatments today refers to **Dr. William FitzGerald**, an American ENT physician (1872–1942), who in 1917 published the book *Zone Therapy* with **Dr. Edwin Bowers**. No explicit reference is made, either in his literature or in former colleagues' accounts, to the sources from which he developed his most important "tool," viz. the division of the human body into 10 longitudinal zones. As FitzGerald also worked in London, Paris, and Vienna for several years, it is supposed that there he came across old European literature that accorded with this view. Another assumption is that he acquainted himself with the general principles of acupuncture while living in Europe and possibly stylized the 12 familiar main meridians to form 10 longitudinal zones.

The **basic concept** of his work, which he discovered empirically through many years of private practice, was that all the strains and disorders of organs and tissues found in any 1 of the

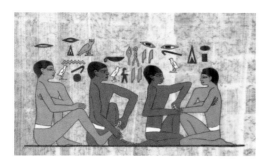

Fig. 1.1 Egyptian pictography (approx. 4,500 years old).

10 longitudinal zones can be therapeutically influenced from the head downward to the hands and feet within this longitudinal zone. Regardless of where FitzGerald obtained his information and notwithstanding that his proposed treatments sometimes appeared bizarre (among other things, he used metal combs, clothes pegs, and thin wooden sticks), this 10-zone grid (**Fig. 2.1**) has continued to provide a reliable working model for our foot treatments up to the present day. It was also in FitzGerald's book of 1917 that I found the first representation of organ zones on the foot.

The historical literature reveals that in spite of a number of detractors, FitzGerald not only treated his own patients highly successfully in accordance with this tried and tested grid pattern, but he also provided practical training for physicians and therapists from different fields for many years. In a later document, one of his closest colleagues, **Dr. George Starr White**, describes how zone therapy was one of the best-known forms of therapy in the United States in 1925.

The American masseuse **Eunice Ingham** (1888–1974) drew on these experiences in the early 1930s. Unlike FitzGerald, however, she did not treat various points on the human body but focused on the feet, through which the 10 body zones also pass. She developed a special treatment technique which she initially called "The Ingham Method of Compression Massage." In 1938 she published the first written synopsis of her experiences under the title *Stories the Feet Can Tell*, and this was followed by her second book, *Stories the Feet Have Told*.

Her work generated widespread interest under the term "Reflexology," especially among lay people. Both her books were published in the United States as well as in many other countries, and her knowledge continues to be used as the basis for self-help and health maintenance by many health-conscious groups to this day.

1.3

The Path from Reflexology to Reflexotherapy of the Feet

In **1958**, as a 25-year-old nurse and therapeutic masseuse, I first read about foot treatment in E. Ingham's book (see above). Since I had trained as a State Registered Nurse in England, the subject was of interest to me, not least because of the language, although its content initially seemed very strange. Above all, I found it implausible that improvements in a person's condition could be achieved at far removed locations just by "applying pressure" to special points on the foot. However, therapeutic curiosity impelled me to examine the specified areas corresponding respectively to the patient's symptoms. To my surprise, not only were they painful but treating them resulted in significant alleviation of the patient's symptoms.

Soon I was employing this new method almost exclusively. Owing to the fact that from the outset I was working with **patients**—and not, as occurs in the United States and other countries, with **clients**—the transition from well-being and prevention to therapy occurred almost of its own accord.

In **1967** I began offering courses for specialists and regarded this training as supplementary for

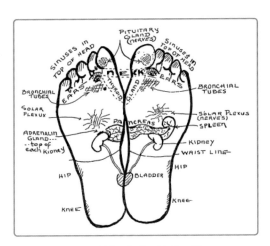

Fig. 1.2 Foot zones 1917; FitzGerald: *Zone Therapy*.

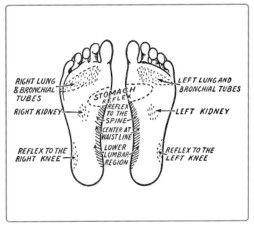

Fig. 1.3 Foot zones 1938; Ingham: *Stories the Feet Can Tell*.

medical therapists with an interest in this area. Not until later did I realize that distinguishing RTF from the lay method made it relatively easy to employ RTF professionally in physical therapy practices, hospitals, and rehabilitation centers.

From **1973** onward, a series of further education and training centers were set up at home and abroad thanks to the high level of demand from therapists and patients.

In **1975** my first book *Reflexzonenarbeit am Fuß* (Reflex Zone Therapy of the Feet. A Comprehensive Guide for Health Professionals) was published. It is still of interest as an introduction to the subject and has now reached 25 editions. At the time, new zones on the foot had already arisen out of practical experience, which refined the anatomical location of traditional zones.

In **1993** the publisher Hippokrates brought out the professionally oriented *Praktisches Lehrbuch der Reflexzonentherapie am Fuß* (Reflexotherapy of the Feet), which has been translated into 14 languages to date.

In **2008** we celebrated 50 years of reflexotherapy of the feet with a large and festive party for professionals at which we presented our work and its many developmental stages.

More about the way in which RTF has developed can be found in my autobiography *Unterm Dach der Füße*.

1.4

What are Reflex Zones of the Feet? An Examination Based on Current Understanding of Vital Processes

As new schools of thought have also emerged in medicine in recent decades, an examination of this question is now more feasible. Above all, the findings of neurobiology and brain research have contributed to a greater acceptance of therapies collectively referred to as Complementary and Integrative Medicine.

The designation "reflex," formerly only used in a neural sense, has been expanded and is now frequently used in connection with fields where empirical evidence exists to demonstrate the functional connections between the part and the whole in the sense of "reflection."

The following list of interactions between the person and the foot cites the anatomical factors known in orthodox medicine first, followed by a larger section given over to methods dealing with the many research projects and discoveries of recent times and on which our many years of practical experience with RTF can also be based.

1.4.1 Known Relationships in Conventional Medicine

Differentiated relationships exist between the feet and the whole person.

- The foot is pervaded by far greater numbers of receptors than other parts of the body. Among other things, this might suggest its special role as a "microsystem" (connection and interaction between the part and the whole). These receptors can be accessed by all kinds of stimuli. They are forwarded to the spinal cord via afferent nerve fibers and either connected in segments or forwarded to the brain.
- Vegetative receptors and nerve fibers of the skin and tissue of the foot are addressed by manual and other stimuli and connected to the pre- and postganglionic synapses.
- The fasciae which run through the whole body—and thus the foot too—are in constant communication with each other. Their information exchange can be activated by corresponding therapies, as well as by RTF.
- The potential of the whole person for development is present in every individual cell at the outset. Each cell interacts with all the others as an organ of perception and an information carrier. This knowledge is confirmed by recent research by Professor **Y. Zhang** *Embryo Containing Information of the Whole Organism*.

1.4.2 New Approaches in Research and Science—General

Western science has been lopsidedly homing in on detail at the expense of fundamental interconnections for a long time. To offset this, developments have been underway since the last century in many areas of research dealing with the interaction between the greater whole and its parts: Niels Bohr, Fritjof Capra, Benoit Mandelbrot, and Bruce Lipton are some of the pioneers of this more diversified, open-minded and lively approach.

Rupert Sheldrake, for example, has been researching "morphogenetic fields" (intangible shape and form developments) for decades and presumes that shapes are produced by oscillatory processes. **David Bohm** has been exploring the perpetual developments and interactions of life from which he has derived a holographic view of the world. Through his detailed explorations of the phenomena of chaos and time, **Ilya Prigogine** has made a significant contribution to a new understanding of the laws of nature and the interconnectedness of all biological systems. **Masuru Emoto** devotes himself to the sensitive qualities of water as a multi-faceted information carrier of major significance for the future of mankind.

1.4.3 New Approaches in the Field of Medical Therapy

To name but a few: in the 1970s **Alfred Pischinger** stated in *The Extracellular Matrix and Ground Regulation* that living systems are highly interconnected and "openly exchange energy with their surroundings." His *matrix* research is of great significance for the understanding of microsystems (see below). Meanwhile, more than 200 years ago, and far in advance of his time, **Samuel Hahnemann** was already speaking of the intangible transfer of information in the field of homeopathy. **Reinhold Voll** succeeded in demonstrating the invisible flow force in meridians using electroacupuncture measurements. **Bernard Bricot** and others have developed dynamic new forms of movement and studies of the human postural system in which the feet are assigned a leading role. *Soma* and *Psyche* are also being reunited in a great variety of treatment methods today.

1.4.4 Reflex Zones as Microsystems and Information Carriers

Small "screenlike self-images" which communicate with the macrosystem, the whole, in the sense of "networks resembling control circuits" are today described as microsystems. Recent studies have confirmed that the possibilities of resonance between the macrosystem and microsystems are always present neutrally and can be activated by corresponding treatments.

Since the last century the last century, physicians and therapists with their spirit of discovery uncovered a number of microsystems and reflex zones and developed these into innovative treatment methods. The most well-known are as follows:

Eye (I. v. Peczely), Nose (W. Fliess, N. Krack) Ear (P. Nogier), Teeth (R. Voll, inter alia), Oral Cavity (J. Gleditsch), Tongue (TCM, inter alia), Skull (T. Yamamoto), Hand and Foot (W. FitzGerald, E. Ingham), Lower Leg (R. Siener), and so on.

However, with its clear similarity to the shape of a seated person, the foot is the microsystem which most accurately reflects the relationship of the part to the whole.

1.4.5 Information about the Existence and Effect of the Reflex Zones of the Feet

Clinical Studies and Publications

- Headache study 1990 Universitat Autonoma de Barcelona
- Sports study 1998 Johannes Gutenberg University Mainz
- Renal perfusion study 1999 Innsbruck University Hospital
- Bowel perfusion study 2001 Innsbruck University Hospital
- Study of patients with gonarthrosis 2006 Friedrich Schiller University Jena

Empirical Experience

- **Sick persons** experience sensations of pain of various kinds and/or symptoms of the autonomic nervous system in associated zones of the feet which do not occur in treatment of **healthy individuals**.
- Acute and chronic painful conditions, functional diseases of the musculoskeletal system, the internal organs, the motor and autonomic nervous systems, the immune and endocrine systems, and emotional disorders can be improved or cured by RTF, within the regenerative capabilities of the individual patient.
- RTF influences basic functions in people who cannot express themselves verbally; for example, infants, those who are unconscious, the severely disabled, or those with multiple disabilities. Among other things, the following may be observed: better intestinal and renal function, improved respiration and cardiovascular activity (observable on the monitor!), stabilization of restlessness—always within the limits of the existing disorder. RTF is also effective for animals.
- The basic matrix information (see above) is also effective for tetraplegics and paraplegics as well as long-term diabetics. We can therefore also obtain some improvements in various organ functions of these patients, although the effects cannot be directly demonstrated by the autonomic nervous system.

Additional Features and Observations

- As a therapy of self-regulation, RTF supports an individual's own healing powers and acts at both tangible and intangible levels. It provides the most important remedy for people, namely **touch** (Paracelsus).
- With RTF it must also be borne in mind that evidence and treatment outcomes can never be completely objective regardless of the manner in which they are obtained and by whom because, as an individual, a person is more than an "object." In recent times it has been confirmed through the discovery of mirror neurons that the thoughts and feelings of both the therapist and the patient alter the respective measurement values (**G. Rizzolatti**).
- Touching one part of a person, such as the foot, always acts as an instrument of communication with the whole body and can trigger targeted responses and changes at remote, functionally and/or energetically associated points.

1.4.6 Practical Working Models for Locating the Zones of the Feet

1. The **10-zone grid** with which W. FitzGerald divided the human being into uniform vertical fields running from the head to the feet. In this way he was able to empirically substantiate the interrelationship between the "macrosystem" (the whole) and the "microsystem" (the part).
2. The principle of **the similarity in shape** between a seated person and his or her feet. In its brilliant simplicity, this serves as the key to the largely exact localization of the individual zones of the feet.

1.4.7 Summary

In therapeutic circles the term "foot reflex" has become established as an abbreviation for the method. For a better understanding of the fact that this does not mean reflexes in the neural sense, the term reflex zones can be seen as an image of a whole in a small area, as one finds in the "reflex" camera, for example. In routine practice reflex zones are usually referred to simply as zones.

We anticipate that current information about the subject will be supplemented by additional and differentiated findings in future. However, the general principles of today can already contribute to a deeper understanding of vital processes—in general medicine and manual treatments as well. The observation that an increasing number of doctors are also open to the inclusion of evidence-based (based on experience) treatment methods when caring for patients is encouraging.

With all the understandable necessity to prove the effects of RTF from our side too, our patients continue to be the most significant advocates of the method because they provide daily confirmation that it works, and how!

1.4.8 Abbreviated Form for Daily Practice

What is "Reflexotherapy of the Feet (RTF)"?

In the reflex zones of the feet we work in a so-called microsystem, a "screenlike self-image" in miniature, which is in an interactive relationship with the macrosystem, the whole person. RTF belongs to the group of complementary treatment methods which address and re-orient the person at all levels, always within the context of their regenerative capabilities, as a regulation therapy. It does not combat or suppress symptoms but supports the patient's self-healing powers, their "inner doctor."

Although the areas of the feet are not reflexes in the neural sense, the use of the term "reflex" has become more widespread in therapeutic language in recent decades. It may be understood as the reflection of the large image on the small surface of a "reflex" camera.

As a manual form of therapy, RTF conveys the important medicine of touch. The different responses of the patient to the therapeutic impulse make individual treatment of individual pathologies possible.

Dividing the human being into 10 imaginary longitudinal zones which extend as far as the feet (W. FitzGerald), and the similarity in shape between a seated person and a foot (our logo), are proven working models and aids to orientation for reliable location of the individual zones.

There are clinical studies and further publications regarding decades of empirical experience.

2   Two Working Models for a Practical Approach to Reflexotherapy of the Feet

2.1

The Grid Pattern according to William FitzGerald

W. FitzGerald proceeded on the simple working model that the human body can be divided into 10 equal segments, from the head down to the feet, which he called **body zones** (**Fig. 2.1**, Chapter 1.2).

2.1.1   Vertical Division into 10 Longitudinal Zones

The longitudinal body zones appear as approximately equal vertical fields, lined up in a medial to lateral direction from zone 1 to 5, respectively. Thereby, **W. FitzGerald** discovered a useful key for showing the correlations between the whole person and the foot in a pictorial and practically understandable manner:

The organs, tissues, and systems through which a longitudinal zone passes in the body are represented in the **same longitudinal zone** on the feet, reduced in proportion. The following examples illustrate this:

- The eyes are in body zones 2 and 3 with their related zones on the second and third toes.
- The hip joints belong to body zone 4 and are in the same longitudinal body zone on the feet, that is, close to the lateral malleolus.

All **bilateral** organs and joints (e.g. kidneys, ears, and shoulders) are represented on the right **and** left foot.

The zones of **unilateral** organs are on the **same** side as in the body (e.g., the zone of the spleen is on the left foot while the zones of the appendix and gall bladder are on the right foot).

Organs located in the **center of the body** have their corresponding zone in the center of the pair of feet, that is, in the respectively assigned longitudinal zone on the right and left foot (e.g., heart, stomach, and bladder).

2.1.2   Horizontal Division

In addition to the vertical 10-zone division, from 1967 onward a further distinction was made possible by three horizontal lines:

- The first horizontal line passes in situ to the right and left of the sternum over the clavicle at shoulder height and demarcates the areas

of the **head and neck.** Transferred to the foot, this line passes through the 10 metatarsophalangeal joints and thus identifies the toes as being assigned to the head and neck.

- The second horizontal line roughly corresponds in situ to the waistline, is found at the base of the metatarsal bones in the feet and is known as the **Lisfranc line**. The organs of the **thorax** and **upper abdomen** are arranged between the first and second horizontal line in both the body and the feet.
- A third horizontal line corresponds in situ to the demarcation of the trunk from the lower extremities and is shown on the feet by a connecting line between the outer and inner malleoli. The reflex zones of the **stomach** and **pelvic organs** are found in the resulting area.

With this reciprocal assignment of the macrosystem to the person and microsystem to the foot, like placing a piece in a mosaic, it is easy to find the location or projection of the individual organs with the help of the longitudinal and horizontal grid.

> Notional classification into linear fields should not be viewed as a narrowly focused, rigid division either in the body or on the feet because the human being represents a system of flowing vital energy in which all processes are interconnected.

The longitudinal and horizontal zones are literally used as auxiliary lines in practical tuition: they help in the transition from an abstract, model-oriented approach to an individual, animated consideration of the human being.

2.2

Macrosystem of the Human Body as Recognized in Various Microsystems

In observing life processes, throughout the ages philosophers have realized that the information contained in the part is included in the whole, and vice versa. This is also known in medicine through the omnipotence of the first human cells which are initially capable of differentiating and developing into any organ, tissue, or system.

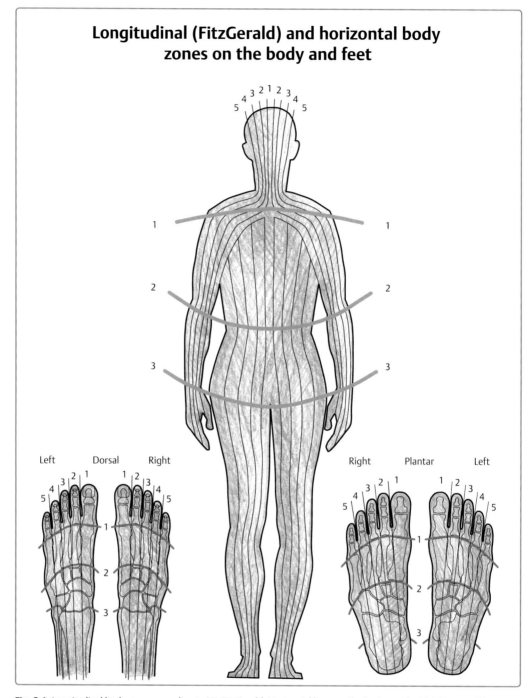

Fig. 2.1 Longitudinal body zones according to W. FitzGerald. Horizontal lines on the body and feet (H. Marquardt).

After a one-sided era of scientific philosophy in medicine and therapy, in recent decades the pendulum has swung back somewhat. Many therapists have realized that:

> "The form of medicine prevalent today has plenty in the way of technology but little in the way of images."

This more open-minded attitude is reflected in the justification or rediscovery of various methods used in **complementary medicine** in which functional and therapeutic relationships are overridingly appreciated as a necessary addition to hitherto overestimated analytical thinking.

The application of the term "reflex zones," which was previously used in a strictly medical sense, has been opened up as a result of the development and reinvigoration of various diagnostic and therapeutic methods which cannot solely be explained in terms of anatomical structure and function of the nervous system. The term "somatotopy" commonly used for the phenomenon of whole body projections in the past is now frequently replaced by the term "microsystem"; these terms are synonyms.

Like others methods employed in complementary medicine, increasingly it has been possible to verify reflexotherapy of the feet (RTF) by means of experimental studies in recent years. Being receptive to a way of thinking involving analogy (similarity) presupposes taking seriously the "as well as" ambivalence of phenomenological features and relinquishing a purely linear and causal way of thinking when assessing living processes in the human body.

Similarities in shape, in other words, comparable anatomical structures inside the human body, irrespective of their distance from each other, often indicate internal and functional correlations because "it is the spirit that creates form" (Carl Huter). They have long been used in different therapies. The best known is **auriculotherapy** according to Nogier, which is based on the similarity in shape of a human embryo and the outer ear.

J. Gleditsch and **J. Bossy** describe tried and tested somatotopies in detail. **L. Mees** demonstrates a multitude of convincing similarities in shape and their therapeutic connections. **A. Pischinger** assumes that biological systems comprise a network, are energetically open, and interact with each other and their environment.

Research of this kind confirms my approach to the subject because it can also serve as a basis for understanding functional processes within RTF.

> **Appropriate qualities** for practicing RTF include:
> - A good measure of physical and emotional stability
> - A sound medical and therapeutic background
> - Open-mindedness to investigate new methods in terms of their practical effect
> - Courage to take unconventional routes in order to unite the qualities of head, heart, and hand during treatment of the feet.

2.2.1 Similarity in Shape between a Seated Person and the Foot

Fig. 2.3 shows the obvious similarity between the shape of the foot and that of a seated person: the simple structure of the upright foot reveals the outline of a seated person, and conversely, the outline of a seated person represents the anatomical shape of the foot.

2.2.2 Anatomical Assignment of the Zones of the Foot

Generally speaking:
- The zones of the front side of a person are represented on the **dorsum** of the foot: the ventral side of the person = the dorsal side of the foot.
- The zones of the rear side of a person are represented on the **soles** of the feet: the dorsal side of the person = the plantar side of the foot.

In the **horizontal plane**, the following assignments apply:
- The zones of the head and neck correspond to the toes.

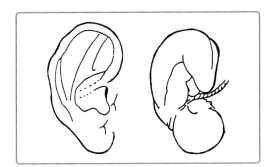

Fig. 2.2 Similarity in shape between the ear and embryo (P. Nogier: *Practical Introduction to Auriculotherapy*).

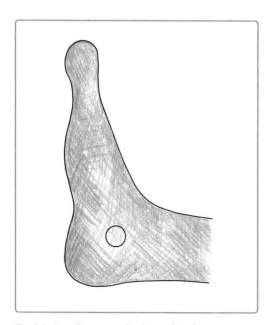

Fig. 2.3 Seated person in the shape of the foot.

- The zones of the thorax and upper abdomen roughly correspond to the metatarsals.
- The zones of the abdomen and pelvis correspond to the tarsal bones up to the malleoli.
- The zones of the thighs correspond to the distal part of the lower legs.

RTF, which we have been performing and teaching for many years, is based on an acceptance of correlations between the foot and a seated person which can be represented pictorially, as demonstrated by the similarity in shape. It has proved its worth as a practical working basis for decades.

For anatomical orientation, the **bones of the feet** are named in English and Latin in dorsal, plantar, medial, and lateral views in **Figs. 2.4** and **2.5**.

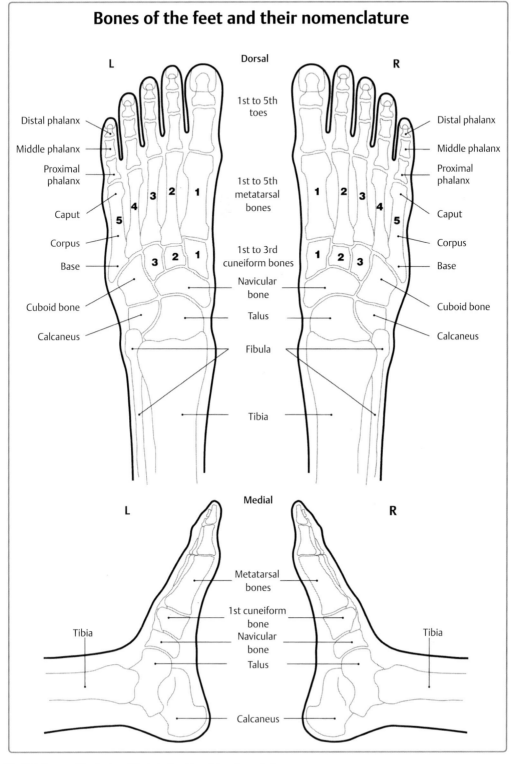

Bones of the feet and their nomenclature

L

Dorsal

R

Distal phalanx

Middle phalanx

Proximal phalanx

Caput

Corpus

Base

Cuboid bone

Calcaneus

1st to 5th toes

1st to 5th metatarsal bones

1st to 3rd cuneiform bones

Navicular bone

Talus

Fibula

Tibia

Distal phalanx

Middle phalanx

Proximal phalanx

Caput

Corpus

Base

Cuboid bone

Calcaneus

Medial

L

R

Tibia

Metatarsal bones

1st cuneiform bone

Navicular bone

Talus

Calcaneus

Tibia

Fig. 2.4 Bones of the feet and their designations (dorsal, medial).

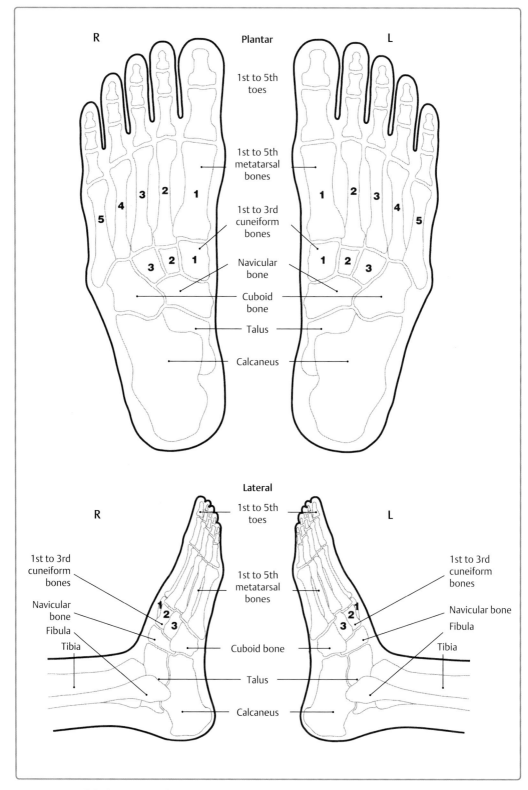

Fig. 2.5 Bones of the feet and their designations (plantar, lateral).

3 Basic Therapeutic Grips: Touching, Treating

3.1

Touch

Although, on a superficial level, it would also be possible to perform reflexotherapy of the feet (RTF) with technical instruments, I have opted for the **manual** approach, because the need for inter-relationships based on the quality of human touch inevitably increases with the mechanization of therapeutic applications. Many people sense the imbalance which arises through lack of physical contact. They sense, usually subconsciously, that the very nature of a treatment, its innermost essence, is related to the secret of touch—in the words of Antoine de Saint-Exupéry: "It is only with the heart that one can see rightly; what is essential is invisible to the eye."

All manual forms of therapy can provide the direct interpersonal knowledge that being touched physically and being moved emotionally are closely interrelated.

As a matter of fact, an electromagnetic energy field of a highly personal nature develops through touch. Two "open force fields" meet and strive for continual homeostasis (maintenance of functions in anatomical control systems). The common understanding of innervation is that a stimulus is conveyed to the receptors of the sensitive nervous system in the foot tissue by means of touch.

In any attempt to explain the principle of "touch," however, it should always be borne in mind that it cannot be described solely theoretically but can only be understood through personal experience.

3.2

Grip Technique

3.2.1 Basic Thumb Grip

(Figs. 3.1–3.3)
As a sensitive and personal instrument, the hand is best able to "understand" the foot when it is used in accordance with its anatomical structure.

> In this way, our muscles, joints and tendons are used in accordance with their natural function and without any risk of strain or damage.

To begin with, I advise preferential use of the thumb as it is good at providing therapeutic

stimuli, thanks to its special position and dominance. Although the four fingers, opposed to the thumb, are also in contact with the foot, their involvement is passive while the thumb is being used actively. Above all, the thumb being opposed to the index finger results in a wide, open space resembling a horseshoe or the letter "U" and this permits free and unrestrained movement.

The grip technique employed today has been developed after years of practical experimentation to find the most appropriate manner of using the hand. In the early years, many therapists, including myself, applied excessive mechanical pressure, needlessly triggering complaints such as increased pain in the joints and muscles.

> The therapeutic grip is characterized by a rhythmical up and down movement which allows the hand to work for longer without strain because we employ the dynamic principle of strength and momentum while avoiding mechanical pressure.

The Basic Thumb Grip and its Phases of Movement

The rhythmic movement continues to act on the foot tissue and gives both patient and therapist the sensation that opposing—and yet coordinated—poles of movement and rest are combining to form a harmonious whole.

Each grip therefore consists of an active and passive phase of roughly equal duration.

Active Phase of the Thumb

The active phase consists of the following components:
- After gentle touching of the zone, the first part of the treatment stimulus results from the arm being actively swung forward from the shoulder. This is similar to when a pendulum or a swing begins swinging (without any additional up/down movement of the wrist).
- The forearm, wrist, and hand are in the **mid-position** between supination and pronation and form a natural horizontal line. As a result of the physiological position of the arm and hand thus obtained, the thumb is slightly **pronated** and can be used without strain. When the flat and relaxed, slightly radially positioned thumb pad has established contact

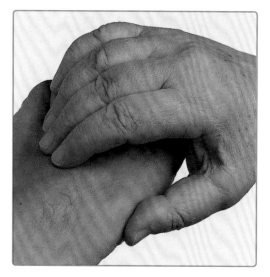

Fig. 3.1 Initial position: touch, **without any** pressure.

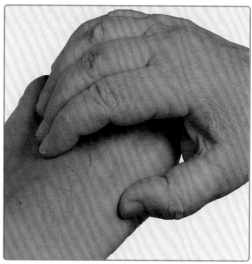

Fig. 3.2 By swinging the arm, the distal phalanx of the thumb is moved passively.

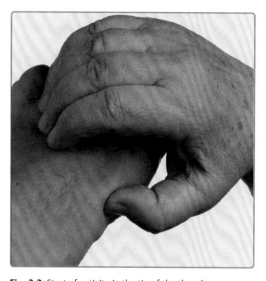

Fig. 3.3 Start of activity in the tip of the thumb.

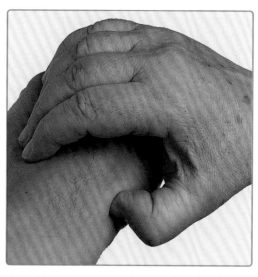

Fig. 3.4 Maximum activity of the tip of the thumb corresponds to conveying the stimulus deep into the tissue. Afterward, the thumb swings back into its passive initial position and begins the next step.

with the foot tissue **without any pressure**, by swinging the arm forward, the distal phalanx of the thumb is gently unrolled passively and flexed significantly. The thenar eminence is completely relaxed until now and the tip of the thumb is still in gentle contact with the foot tissue, with a pressure equivalent to that exerted by the weight of a postage stamp.

● Only now does the tip of the thumb actively assume control, increasing the bend toward

an angle of 90°. At the same time, the muscle tension in the **thenar eminence** also increases and the therapeutic stimulus of the distal phalanx is directed more or less vertically and selectively into the depth of the tissue.

● The distal phalanx of the thumb is now bent as far as it will go, with compressed tension similar to the collective strength of an archer before he releases the arrow. This is the point at which the **therapeutic stimulus** is directed into the tissue.

Passive Phase

By **spontaneously releasing** the tension in the thenar eminence and the tip of the thumb, the arm can swing back passively and return the thumb to its neutral initial position. Again the thumb pad lies relaxed on the tissue and the fingers still support the foot from the opposite side.

The next grip starts with the renewed, active, forward-swinging movement of the arm, leading again into the two phases of movement in the same sequence as before. The continuous alternation between tensed force and released calm produces an undulating rhythm which moves effortlessly, as if by itself, through the tissue of the foot millimeter by millimeter as a result of the impetus of the movement.

3.2.2 Basic Index Finger Grip

(**Figs. 3.5, 3.6**)

It is usually more practical, and less work for the hand, to use the index finger on the **dorsal** parts of the foot. Here too, the approach is rhythmical; but the thumb now provides passive support on the opposite side. However, the swaying rhythm is not reflected in the pendulum movement of the whole arm here, as would occur with the thumb grip, but is transformed into an up-

and-down movement of the **wrist**, similar to the swaying of a suspension bridge when walked across.

Active Phase

The active phase is composed as follows:

- The grip starts with a pronounced extension of the wrist (the back of the hand points to the forearm).
- The entire index fingertip touches the tissue of the foot gently and **without any pressure** and the thumb provides support on the side opposite the fingers.
- The wrist gently swings back into its neutral initial position while the index finger becomes more rounded as a result.
- While the distal phalanx of the index finger gradually transfers the area of contact to the fingertip through the swinging of the wrist, it becomes increasingly active and in a vertical position it applies the stimulus deep into the tissue with increasing intensity.

Passive Phase

In a manner similar to the thumb grip, the built-up tension is then released; the index finger passively returns to its initial position and the wrist gently swings back into an extended position to start the next grip from there.

The following applies to all **fingernail shapes**: Bending with the thumb and index finger grip is restricted to the point at which irritation by the nails causes too much discomfort, even if they are

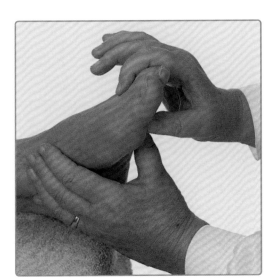

Fig. 3.5 Basic index finger grip in its phases of movement. Initial position.

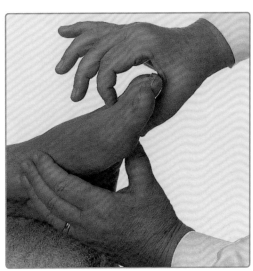

Fig. 3.6 Basic index finger grip in maximum activity.

cut and filed short. Usually though, patients do not experience much pain caused by a fingernail—it is more often the therapist's impression.

3.2.3 Alternating Strokes

(Figs. 3.7, 3.8)

The term relates to the way in which the hands are used:

- The tissue is stroked gently but purposefully in the proposed direction and in an alternating manner, using the **flat** thumb pads or one or two fingertips of both hands. Before one hand finishes the slight pull of the tissue, the other starts stroking along the same line, producing a flowing, continuous movement.
- The length of the individual stroking movements depends on the condition of the tissue: if it feels viscid or tumid, the movements must be shorter; if it feels normal in consistency, the individual movements can be longer.
- While the index fingers are working, the thumbs support the foot on the side opposite the fingers, keeping it in position. If the alternating strokes are performed with the thumb, the fingers support the foot.

These grips are preferable in zones related to the **lymphatic system** so as to avoid excessively forceful specific stimuli, initially in the medial and lateral zones near the Achilles tendon usually. Later, after gaining more experience, it will be possible to treat other lymphatic zones with the same alternating stroking movements.

3.2.4 Stretching Grip

(Fig. 3.9)

Tissue stretching particularly lends itself in the **interdigital spaces**, because it is here that the blood supply can be improved most efficiently:

- The skin folds between the toes are held between thumb pad and index fingertip and are pulled in a distal direction until the thumb pad and fingertip meet.
- During this pulling movement, the hand performs a slightly curved movement in plantar and/or dorsal direction.
- The intensity of the grip remains relatively constant throughout and is adjusted to the patient's breathing (in the inhalation phase the stimulus is usually well assimilated). The other hand supports the foot in a functional and ergonomic position, preferably in the toe joint areas. The grip is repeated several times.

3.2.5 Sedating Grip

The name indicates the function of this grip: the aim is to reduce a patient's acute symptomatic complaints by calmly holding the zone concerned.

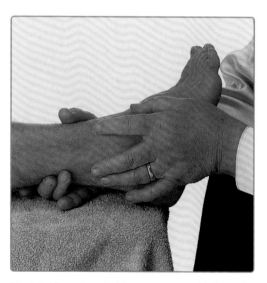

Fig. 3.7 Alternating stroking movements with fingertips 3 and 4.

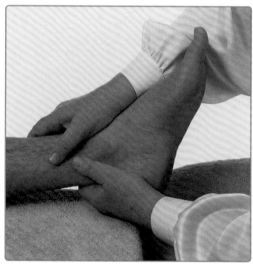

Fig. 3.8 Alternating stroking movements with the thumb.

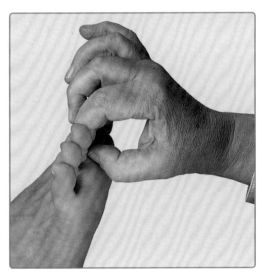

Fig. 3.9 Stretching grip in the interdigital webbing.

The technique is similar to that of the basic grip:
- The strained zone is first touched gently with the thumb pad in a slightly radial position.
- Gently swinging the arm forward moves the distal phalanx of the thumb from a horizontal into a vertical position.
- In this position the therapeutic stimulus is conveyed deep into the tissue, adjusted to the current responsiveness of the patient's autonomous nervous system.
- Unlike the customary basic grip, this thumb position is maintained **without any movement** until the local pain in this zone has significantly decreased.
- Only now does the thumb return to its relaxed initial position and the sedating grip is repeated millimeter by millimeter over the entire zone.

The sedating grip can be performed just as well with the **index finger** at corresponding places on the foot.

Application of the Sedating Grip

The sedating grip is generally used for
- **Treatment of pain** in the symptom zone (Chapter 16) and for
- **RTF scar treatment** (Chapter 25).
- The sedating grip can also be used if a zone **is unexpectedly painful** during treatment (Chapter 12.2.1).

If the patient is especially **irritated** initially, it may suffice to hold the zone concerned calmly, without conveying a clear specific stimulus deep into the tissue.

Practical Advice

In the active phase of the grip, therapists with weak or hypermobile thumb and finger joints should gently lead the distal phalanx quite clearly in a 90° angle direction and take care that the stimulus is only conveyed into the tissue after the vertical position of the distal phalanx of the thumb or finger has been fully reached. This protects the joints from excessive strain and makes them more stable. With the basic thumb grip, it is particularly important that the wrist is not bent upward because this would increase the instability of the metacarpophalangeal joint and lead to its further weakening.

> A few words of encouragement: A delicate touch, performed with inner determination and concentrated empathy can bring about a more effective change in tissue tone than a rougher touch.
> The personal care and concentration with which the therapeutic grip is performed determines its quality and efficacy to a far greater degree than is often assumed.

3.2.6 Rules of Grip Application

Direction of Movement

As a result of the swinging movement produced when working rhythmically, the "forward" working direction is determined by itself, irrespective of the point on the foot where the thumb or finger starts. The more impartially we are able to take the patient's feet in our hands, the faster our hands will decide for themselves whether to start working
- in a distal to proximal direction or vice versa, or
- in a medial to lateral direction or vice versa.

As many of us have long since lost this spontaneous impartiality over time, patience and practice are required before we can rely on our intuitive skills again. **Approved working directions** are indicated by arrows and proposed for trial in the detailed illustrations of the individual zones (Chapter 10ff.).

If a patient is very sensitive, not only should consideration be given to the economical use of our hands but also to their illness and condition when choosing the working direction.

From My Practice

Many years ago I saw a very sensitive 75-year-old patient with mild symptoms of angina pectoris and a heavy cold who was finding it increasingly difficult to expectorate the accumulated phlegm in his respiratory tract. During the first assessment (Chapter 11), in addition to the heart and respiratory zones, I noticed severe strain in the gastrointestinal tract, the inguinal region, and lower spine. I wanted to bring him relief in the expectoration and loosening of phlegm from the bronchial region, and worked in a tonifying manner in the zones of the bronchi in a proximal to distal direction, in other words from "bottom" to "top," in the direction of the zone of the pharyngonasal cavity.

After a few grips, the patient sat up abruptly and showed clear signs of gagging and incipient vomiting. More through instinct than reason, I immediately decided to change the working direction, starting to treat him in a distal to proximal direction. To our mutual astonishment, the gag reflex then ceased as spontaneously as it had started. The patient subsequently told me that he had had a hiatus hernia for decades but had not wanted to have an operation because of his unstable general condition.

As the trachea, bronchi, and esophagus are in part also treated in the same area due to their anatomical proximity within the reflex zones, at the outset I was unable to differentiate in the selection of zones but was guided by the patient's impressive response with regard to which working direction was appropriate for him.

Upon inquiry, the well-known triad of **diaphragmatic, inguinal,** and **umbilical hernia** was confirmed in this patient. After a few treatments, during which I tonified the hernia zones, I was able to vary the working direction in the region of the esophagus and trachea zones without triggering any disturbing reactions because the tonus in the tissues surrounding the diaphragm and hernias had improved. The patient remained stable until his death 12 years later.

Intensity and Speed of the Grip

The therapeutic grip can be varied in **intensity** and in **working rhythm** and **speed,** and is thus adjusted to the patient's respective responsiveness and condition.

This results in a wide range of variations and possible applications:

- The **grip intensity** varies from soft and calm (sedating) to strong and profound (tonifying).
- **The working rhythm** and **speed** vary from slow and deliberate (sedating) to quick and determined (tonifying).

Duration of Therapeutic Stimulus

The duration of the precise stimulus depends on the patient's limits. In the past—even when I myself initially became acquainted with the reflex zones—pain stimuli could in some circumstances be tolerated for minutes. With the sensitivity of patients today, it usually suffices to apply **stimuli lasting seconds,** repeated at the same point some minutes later, and at ongoing intervals until the zone has clearly improved in terms of tissue quality and perception of pain (Chapter 12.2).

Normalization of a zone is recognizable from the following signs:
- The site on the foot is less painful.
- The blood supply to this site has improved.
- The tissue tonus has returned to normal as far as possible.
- The patient displays fewer symptoms of strain involving the autonomous nervous system.

3.2.7 Learning Aids

As the theoretical description of a practical grip is very complicated, I have simplified the approach by using visual comparisons.
- **The trampoline:** The tissue tonus in the foot resembles the tension of a trampoline on which the thumb jumps like a trampolinist (active phase) and is bounced up again (passive phase).
- **The hosepipe:** The very slightly pronated thumb pad resembles the nozzle of a hosepipe. When watering plants, we should take care that the water flows unimpeded to the intended site—that is, we create the stimulus with the tip of the thumb at precisely the corresponding point in the tissue (active phase). Just as the nozzle of the hosepipe is removed from the well-watered plant, after the active phase the thumb returns to its relaxed initial position (passive phase).
- **The pencil tip:** The distal phalanx of the thumb resembles the tip of a well-sharpened pencil, which puts a clear, precise point on the "blank page" deep in the tissue (active) and is gently removed from it (passive).

- **High and low tide:** The thumb is seen as a wave, the foot tissue as the shore on which the active phase acts as the high tide and the passive movement the low tide.
- **The gas pedal:** Lightly touching the gas pedal with the foot corresponds to the beginning of the grip, slowly increasing the amount of "gas" to the maximum (active phase). The foot lets the gas pedal gently return to the initial position (passive phase).
- **The balloon:** At the beginning of the grip, the thenar eminence is as relaxed as an empty balloon, and when bent to the maximum it is as tight as a blown-up balloon. The thumb passively swinging back corresponds to the spontaneous escape of air from the balloon.
- **The stamp:** A stamp is imprinted in a precise location deep in the paper (active) and then, without smudging the printed image, gently removed from the paper again (passive).
- **The ball:** A child taps the ball to the ground (active phase); it bounces back of its own accord (passive phase) due to the resistance of the ground (= tonus in the tissue).

- **The elastic spring:** An elastic spring is compressed (active) and rebounds to its original shape when released (passive).

These examples of visual comparisons illustrate the use of the **thumb** and can also be applied to the **index finger**.

3.3

Summary

Although the technique of RTF with its few basic grips seems simple, it should be borne in mind that so-called "simple" grips demand our full attention and patience when practising. The erroneous impression is frequently given that simple things are easy and quick to learn and they are therefore overlooked.

Any therapist can check for themselves whether the technique works: if joint strains, pain, and muscular tension frequently occur as a result of this work, the grips must be fundamentally rehearsed and rearranged. "Mechanics exhaust while dynamics refresh."

4 Characteristics of Abnormal Zones; Limits of Dosage

4.1

Signs of Abnormal Zones

Everyone has "reflective" zones in the microsystem of their feet which in a **healthy** person, as with healthy organs, display **no abnormalities** but can be discerned when there are **pathological** changes by
- the expression of pain,
- irritation of the autonomic nervous system, and
- palpation findings.

Expression of Pain

Many patients react spontaneously to the therapeutic grip in an abnormal area with verbal remarks or other indications of pain and should be encouraged to express their feelings freely. Thus they can help beginners, in particular, not to exceed their limits regarding the appropriate dosage.

Irritations of the Autonomous Nervous System

Such irritations are triggered by the therapeutic grip being too rough, too quick, or too strong and signal the need for a change of approach in the area, even if these zones **themselves** are not always painful.

Patients who arrive with damp hands or other signs of strain involving the autonomic nervous system should generally be treated gently and with delicate grips. Usually, their responsiveness is significantly improved by stabilizing grips at the start of the respective treatment.

Palpation Findings—Tactile Findings

We can train our tactile qualities in such a way that we can eventually recognize abnormal zones by changes in their temperature and tissue tonus. At this stage we no longer have to depend solely on the patient's reactions to determine the appropriate dosage. To acquire this skill, empathy and an interest in the work are required, as well as a relatively large amount of practice.

4.2

Signs of Dosage Limits

Each course of therapy represents a very personal relationship between two people. Both have their individual approach and their own way of handling it.

The appropriate **dosage** is of crucial significance for the result of the treatment and demands both careful observation of the patient's reactions during treatment and a good deal of sympathetic understanding. In earlier times the pain experienced in a zone was sufficient indication to change a given dosage.

> With the patient of today, who is often more sensitive and more easily irritated, the current responsiveness of their **autonomic nervous system** often determines the dosage more reliably than the pain triggered in the zones on the foot.

Signs Indicating Strain Involving the Autonomous Nervous System

The most common signs indicating that the dosage limit has been reached **during** treatment are:
- Rapid, heavy, and persistent perspiration of the palms
- Perspiration in particular areas of the body; for example, in the segment or dermatome, or affecting the whole body
- Obvious, marked and spontaneous changes in
  - Pulse frequency: usually in the direction of tachycardia
  - Complexion: very pale or very red
  - Body temperature: too warm, too cold, persistent shivering with goose bumps
  - Salivation: usually reduced
  - Respiration rate: too shallow and too fast, sometimes faltering as well
- Nausea, originating from the stomach or cardiovascular system

- Unexpected emotional reactions; for example, signs of anxiety, consternation and fear, apparently unmotivated crying
- A strong sensation of inner coldness and inner trembling, onset of numbness in the fingertips

Audible and Visible Signs

The audible and visible reactions of the patient are easier to perceive and more conspicuous, but on their own they are inconclusive for an assessment of the dosage:

- Audible signs such as frightened exclamations or sighing, faint moaning or embarrassed laughter
- Gestures or facial expressions, such as tightly pressed lips, increased wrinkles on the forehead, restless eyelid movements
- Gestures and signs expressing significant anxiety, severe pain or subjective discontent
- Visible tension in various muscle groups or throughout the whole body

The audible and visual signs **alone** are not stable enough to determine the appropriate dosage for the following reasons. Some people are overanxious and show signs of the excessive strain anticipated **before** they feel any pain; others believe they must suffer stoically whatever the therapist proposes and want to impress us with their "toughness." Usual comments in such situations are: "Do whatever it is you have to do," or "Don't let me get in your way," or "I can stand quite a bit."

How to Deal with Overreactions during Treatment

Above all, at the beginning it is not always easy to find the appropriate grip intensity despite our best efforts. This is part of the hard work involved in anything new and can be improved with patient practice from one treatment to the next. However, we should react spontaneously to **signs of overreaction**

- by reducing the intensity of the grip and the working speed, and/or
- with a stabilizing grip (Chapter 6.2.3), which may also consist of simply holding the irritated site gently and calmly for a short time, which is often sufficient in itself,
- by reestablishing our own composure, posture, and breathing rhythm.

As soon as a patient overreacts to treatment, it is helpful to ensure that we consciously relate to their inner regenerative powers and not to the existing irritation.

If we respond to the momentary irritation of the other with our own, we double it and achieve the opposite of that intended. We can best meet this requirement if we appropriate such experiences with vigilant monitoring and concede that the first attempt does not have to be "perfect."

We achieve sovereignty in our work of our own accord when we constantly face up to and rehearse our own uncertainty patiently and without personal devaluation because this is the way in which we are most likely to overcome it.

General Principles

Topics of the Introductory Course for Professionals

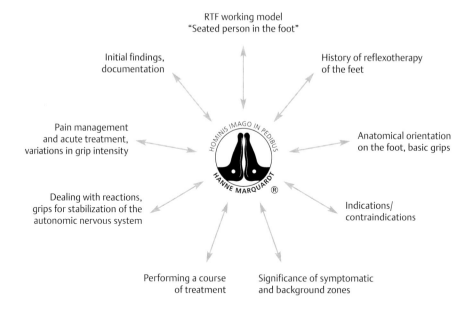

Fig. 4.1 Course Diagram I.

5 Indications and Contraindications

5.1

Reliable Indications for Beginners

Many questions usually arise only when we begin to apply a new method in our daily practice. Therefore, it is worth giving **prior** consideration to how starting to use a new treatment method might look in practical terms.

Patients from the following indication groups have proved effective for this:

- Skeletomuscular disturbances and malfunctions (e.g., cervical or lumbar syndrome, muscular hypertonus, ischialgias, restricted movement of various joints)
- Digestive troubles (e.g., problems in the upper abdomen, meteorism, liver and gall bladder disorders, constipation, hemorrhoids)
- Dysmenorrhea and other functional disturbances of the menstrual cycle
- Chronic or acute cold or sinusitis, susceptibility to colds
- Lymphatic disorders, especially in children, allergies
- Headaches of various kinds and origin

Initially we should not choose the most severely ill patients, but take our time to slowly gain the necessary experience and confidence in reflexotherapy of the feet (RTF). If we can correctly assess our professional and personal possibilities and limitations, we will work with greater certainty and, if applicable, without hesitating to ask for advice or to refer the patient back to the physician.

5.2

Contraindications

As with any effective therapy, there are also contraindications with RTF. We distinguish between absolute and relative contraindications.

5.2.1 Absolute Contraindications

RTF is absolutely contraindicated in the following cases:

- Acute **inflammations** of the **venous and lymphatic systems** (risk of venous thrombosis, thrombophlebitis, and/or spreading the focus of inflammation through the lymphatic system).
- If the patient had phlebitis **previously**, the current condition of their venous system must be checked by a physician **before** commencing RTF.
- If there are **foreign bodies** in close proximity to vital organs and systems (e.g., shell splinters in the upper neck from battlefield injuries).
- **Aneurysms** (bulges in arterial blood vessels, e.g., in the aorta) if known.
- **Transplants**.
- **Melanomas,** in particular on the feet and legs, regardless of whether operated on or not.
- **Psychoses** (e.g., manic–depressive psychosis, schizophrenia). As disorders can occur very abruptly and intermittently, we advise against the use of RTF, even during symptom-**free** periods.

5.2.2 Relative Contraindications

Illnesses Directly Connected with the Feet

Sudeck's atrophy of the foot. Patients with Sudeck's atrophy can be treated with RTF but not on the affected foot, as direct treatment could give rise to increasing strain on the tissue. However, in addition to other measures, such patients can be treated by applying collateral and contralateral therapy, that is, at the assigned points on the other foot and on the hand on the same side (Chapter 18.4.2).

Gangrene of the foot, for example, in diabetic patients or as a consequence of frostbite or severe circulatory disturbances. No direct treatment of the gangrenous foot with RTF. If need be, collateral and contralateral therapy also lends itself here.

Generalized mycosis of the feet (Athlete's foot) or weeping eczema. The skin of the affected areas should not be treated directly. Treatment through fine cotton socks has proved very useful, however. Together with local natural applications, a fundamental change of diet is important here.

Rheumatic diseases, which also affect the feet. In the acute, painful phase, we advise against any treatment of the feet. Even after the acute symptoms have abated, only neutral stabilizing grips should be used initially in order to prevent the symptoms flaring up again. In the **chronic** stage, careful treatment can be provided in the zones of the autonomic nervous system, the vertebral column, and the excretory organs. Here too, de-acidification of the digestive organs through a change of diet is very important.

Diseases Which Do *Not* Affect the Feet

Infectious and highly pyrexic diseases. As a rule, patients with these diseases are taken care of in hospital. When the acute febrile disease abates, RTF therapists with corresponding experience can also be employed in hospital to support metabolic organs, the lymphatic and circulatory system, and the autonomic nervous system.

Experience in various situations, above all involving children, has shown that in a febrile state (e.g., in childhood illnesses) the organism itself activates so many healing impulses that some well-chosen stabilizing grips or holding the feet calmly several times a day will suffice (Chapter 23).

Psychosomatic diseases. Experienced therapists who work in psychosomatic specialist clinics may treat patients with RTF in consultation with the physician in order to favorably influence the physical disorders and symptoms accompanying their current life issues, for example:

- Stimulation of the activity of the excretory organs, intestine, and kidneys
- Stabilization of the circulatory system
- Relief of spinal and joint problems
- Regulation of sleep quantity and quality
- Pain support before and/or during menstruation, etc.

People who are suffering from stress generally appreciate the "medicine of touch" very much—above all, on the feet. As these are the most remote parts of the body, they convey a certain distance from the whole person and permit touch most easily there. In addition, experience from psychosomatic clinics shows that RTF can act as a "door for communication" for psychotherapeutic conversations with patients with neuroses, etc. Good cooperation between therapists and physicians is particularly important here.

With such treatments, it goes without saying that we correctly assess our personal and professional limitations and avoid suggestions or interpretations of certain disease patterns.

If the **leukocyte count** has fallen below 2,500 (e.g., in patients with autoimmune diseases, including AIDS), treatment of the zones of the foot should not be organ-specific. However, neutral stroking and stabilizing grips are useful, quite practical too, because touch is very important for patients in this group as a whole and because they often suffer from cold feet.

If a better result can be expected with certain **operations**, RTF should no longer be performed, for example:

- on patients whose chronically inflamed tonsils can no longer be regenerated with the aid of noninvasive methods such as classical homeopathy, neural therapy, RTF, or manual lymphatic drainage,
- on female patients with large myomas, disturbing the normal function of other organs or causing unexpectedly strong and frequent periods,
- patients with gallstones who suffer from recurrent colic in spite of various treatments or whose gallstones can no longer be excreted in the normal way because of their size, etc.,

However, the aforementioned patients can and should be treated postoperatively to bring about the elimination of narcotic poisons and support the healing process.

High-risk pregnancy. We also include this condition among the relative contraindications as a precautionary measure. As the term "high-risk pregnancy" can be interpreted in various ways, the use of RTF, even if it has been prescribed, must also be discussed with the woman in person. We should not persuade her to have treatment if she has serious misgivings about RTF (or other therapies).

Although pregnancy should not be regarded as an "illness," our general advice is not to start treatment until around the fourth month of pregnancy. Many women are particularly unstable physically and emotionally in the initial months and simply need more rest (Chapter 22).

An important further contraindication exists if the **therapist** has major doubts and **fears about the patient's illness** or about possible **reactions**. Misinterpreted ambitions or excessive personal drive to help can do more harm than good.

6 Stabilization and Harmonization of the Autonomic Nervous System

6.1

Stabilizing Grips for Physical and Psychological Effects

6.1.1 General Information

Increasing use has been made of stabilizing grips in reflexotherapy of the feet (RTF) in recent years as many patients are either already unstable **before** treatment or they react unexpectedly quickly and strongly to therapeutic stimuli. The uses for stabilizing grips vary, for example:

- To get the patient into the right frame of mind at the start of a treatment, and/or
- When symptoms of being overloaded occur during treatment.
- As a harmonizing conclusion to treatment.

The following grips are simple and produce convincing results in daily practice as a result of their spontaneous effect.

As the balance which we want to achieve in our irritated patient as a result of the stabilizing grips originates from ourselves, it is worth checking first our own posture and breathing rhythm for a few seconds. This ensures that the patient is stabilized quickly, without our becoming overwhelmed.

6.1.2 Heel-stretching Grip

(Figs. 6.1, 6.2)

As deficiencies in the autonomic nervous system are often revealed by muscular hypertonus and a change in breathing, the first stabilizing grip involves stretches which start at the heel and have a balancing and relaxing effect on the often-tense musculature and the breathing.

Performance: We place both palms under both of the patient's heels and observe their current respiratory rhythm. It will often differ from how we think it should be. Usually, we would want to change this situation immediately and make an evaluation which is more theoretically based than situation- and people-oriented in deciding between "right" and "wrong," "good" and "bad."

> A conscious acceptance of the particular presumed deficiency in the patient's muscle tone or breathing provides the most appropriate starting point for change and harmonization.

Stretching of the heels therefore starts in the inhalation phase without too much attention to any possible breathing deficiency present. The stimulus of stretching is steadily increased so as to be

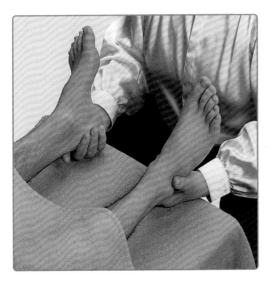

Fig. 6.1 Heel-stretching grip on both feet.

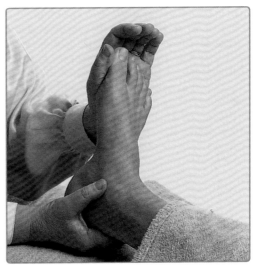

Fig. 6.2 Heel-stretching grip on one foot.

perceptible throughout the patient's body—that is, as far as the spinal column and head. It almost always balances hypertonus in various muscle groups spontaneously. As a result, the next breath is usually already somewhat calmer and deeper.

If the patient's breathing is very short and fast, the following modifications may be made:

- Either only **one** stretch is performed within a few breaths, or
- the stretch is extended slightly at the end of the inhalation phase as a nonverbal invitation to breathe more deeply.

Working with a patient's breathing in a differentiated manner also protects those involved against individual manipulation of these very intimate processes. To quote the Bible, (John 3:8): "The wind blows wherever it pleases. You hear its sound, but you cannot tell where it comes from or where it is going. So it is with everyone born of the Spirit." (The synonym for "breath" is "spirit" in Aramaic.)

It is worth ensuring that we maintain our own breathing rhythm while employing the stabilizing grips to avoid unnecessary fluctuations in our own vitality. If we adjust ourselves—usually subconsciously—to the breathing rhythm of the patient, we cannot really offer improvement of their condition and, in addition, we irritate and weaken ourselves.

6.1.3 "Energy Cap"

Performance: We select the area of our hands that represents a personal energy field, namely the center of the palms, and place it very **gently** on the medial side of both the metatarsophalangeal joints in a concave shape for about 20 to 30 seconds.

By doing so, we touch reflex zones that are particularly closely connected to life-regulating processes: the cerebellum, thyroid, heart, and neck. Patients usually respond very quickly to this contact by the center of the palm with increased well-being and inner peace.

When performing this grip, our sitting posture should above all ensure the stabilization of the spine between the shoulder blades so as to convey the central strength of the spine to the shoulders, arms, and hands. The freedom this produces in our posture avoids putting pressure and weight on the patient's feet.

As it is ineffective to try to illustrate this grip, I have limited myself to a textual description.

6.1.4 **Respiration-regulating Grip**
(Fig. 6.3)

Performance: We hold the feet on the medial side, again with both hands, and bending the end phalanges of our thumbs, we move with caution and determination toward the center of the upper margin of the zone of the diaphragm, that is, the center of the proximal margin of the transverse arch of the foot. On the patient's next inhalation, using the tip of the thumb we gently move the feet so far into dorsal flexion that the ankle joint is also moved into a slight dorsal flexion.

In the exhalation phase, the tension which has built up in the ankles is gently released back into the normal position. Here too, we adjust ourselves to the patient's existing breathing first, without controlling it arbitrarily.

If the respiration is quick and shallow during the initial inhalation phase, this grip can also be held for two or three breaths and only released again during a subsequent exhalation. Thus, the movement of the diaphragm between the thoracic and abdominal cavities gradually becomes deeper and calmer. As the diaphragm is partially enervated by a branch of the solar plexus, the stabilizing effects of this point are reinforced and include the regulation of the autonomous nervous system.

If we perform this grip in an upright seating position, gently swaying backward and forward from the pelvis, it hardly requires any effort, as during the forward movement the weight of the trunk is transferred to the hands and arms, which move both feet at the same time without any trouble.

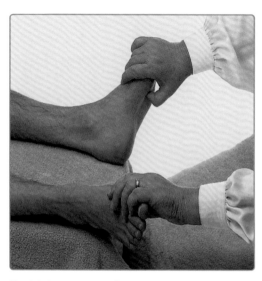

Fig. 6.3 Respiratory regulation grip.

6.1.5 Palms-to-Soles Grip

(Fig. 6.4)
We adopt a sitting posture at a corresponding distance from which the whole trunk is moved forward from the groin (the back is not hunched). Depending on the proportion of our trunk to the arms, the elbows can be supported near the knees or held freely between the well-separated knees and legs.

Performance: Both palms are placed on both soles of the feet **without any pressure**. If the soles are much larger than our hands, we check where the feet feel coldest or most in need of touch. There the hands rest quietly until the patient's irritation has subsided.

As palms and soles have a highly personal aura, we should also be careful with our own energies, that is, maintaining our breathing rhythm while performing this grip, clearly limiting its duration or selecting another if we are not currently able to withstand much stress.

Placing the **dorsal part of the hands** on the soles of the feet is recommended as a gentler **alternative**. For this variant, we revert to the usual working distance from the feet.

6.1.6 Yin-Yang Grip

(Figs. 6.5, 6.6)
The name for this stabilizing grip originates from acupuncture. According to Eastern philosophy, the universe is understood to be the interaction of two interrelated polarities which complement each other, of Yin (the earthly, feminine, receptive principle) and Yang (the cosmic, masculine, pro-creating principle).

In the so-called meridians, "invisible, symmetrical lines which connect points with a similar therapeutic effect" according to Hartmut Heine, both forms of differently poled energy flow through the body as Yin and Yang.

Performance: This stabilizing grip is performed in the flow direction of meridian energy. It begins or ends on the inside and/or outside of the knee. One

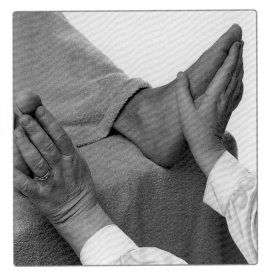

Fig. 6.4 Palms-to-soles grip.

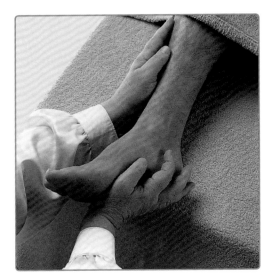

Fig. 6.5 Yin-Yang stroking, start.

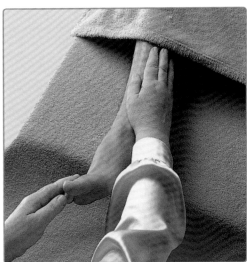

Fig. 6.6 Yin-Yang stroking, finish.

hand smoothly strokes the outside of the lower leg, medially margined by the rim of the tibia. It continues over the dorsum of the foot, ending beyond the second to fifth toes (Yang meridians). At the same time, proximal of the metatarsophalangeal joints, the other hand strokes the sole of the foot along its medial side and lower leg to the inside of the knee (Yin meridians). For each new stroke both hands return to their initial position.

This quiet, calm stroking is performed several times in succession on each foot and lower leg. It has proven to be of particularly value for patients who are very **ticklish** or display **instability of the autonomic nervous system**.

If the patient's feet and/or the therapist's hands perspire, stroking is performed with the feet covered.

Variation

The Yin-Yang strokes can also be performed on **both feet** simultaneously. As the wrists need a far larger radius of movement to perform an inward rotation with bilateral stroking, we must sit further away from the patient's feet than usual.
With the trunk bent well forward, we begin stroking the outside of both knees simultaneously (Yang area up to the tibia margin) and continue while slowly moving into the upright seating position until we reach the second to fifth toes.

Without losing contact with the skin of the tips of the toes, we continue stroking on the plantar part of the feet while distinctly rotating our wrists inward. It should be ensured that it is really the plantar part—not only the medial side of the foot—that is touched. Both hands calmly stroke the Yin area on the insides of the heels up as far as the insides of both knees.

To bridge the distance between the inner (Yin) and outer (Yang) sides at the level of the knee, at the end of the Yin stroke we now raise the hands so that only the fingertips are lightly in contact with the skin, creating the medial to lateral connection with the Yang side. At this point, the palms are applied gently to the skin once more on the outside for the new Yang stroke.

6.1.7 Solar Plexus Grip

The Solar Plexus Zone (see **Fig. 10.31**) is particularly well-suited to balancing the autonomic nervous system in the event of overreactions during or after RTF treatment.

Performance: We place both thumb pads in the respective plantar area between the base of the first metatarsal and first sphenoid bone.

In the event of a **stronger sympathicotonic** reaction by the patient (e.g., severe pain, spasms, stress, raised blood pressure, tachycardia, lightly or heavily perspiring hands and feet), the **sedating grip** is used. Its intensity may vary from gentle to strong.

For **vagotonic** conditions (e.g., slower pulse, a fall in blood pressure) the zone is **tonified** more vigorously or gently depending on the patient's current needs (see Chapter 10.8.4, under "Solar Plexus").

6.1.8 "Small Energy Cycle"

(Fig. 6.7)
Like the Yin-Yang grip, this stabilizing grip is based on meridian teachings. I learned it in 1970s, performed in situ, in courses run by Willy Penzel (acupoint massage). In accordance with the basic principle "Seated person in the foot," I transferred it to the zones on the foot.

Effect: This grip is particularly effective for physical and mental imbalance, as it is employed in the zones of the center of the body. At the same time it connects
- ventral and dorsal,
- cranial and caudal, and
- right and left.

Performance: With this gentle grip, the zones of the central meridian "conception" and "governor vessel" are connected to each other. They are both located in the FitzGerald longitudinal body zone I, both in situ and in the zones on the feet. This ellipse can be performed simultaneously with both hands on both feet with thumbs, index or middle fingers. Practice and keen observation help in deciding where the grip begins and ends.

As shown in **Fig. 6.7**, the path from the pelvic floor to the lower lip is indicated as the "conception

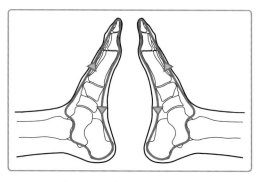

Fig. 6.7 Small energy cycle.

vessel" (dorsal on the foot, arrow), from there the flow direction of the "governor vessel" is medial/plantar from the head to the pelvic floor and changes back into the "conception vessel" without interruption.

The grip is performed approximately 10 to 15 times, with greater or lesser frequency depending on the patient's needs. For the sake of the patient's back, the therapist may sway backward and forward gently. Over time the therapist's sensitivity is developed to such an extent that the fingers sense where there are particular areas of congestion in the "small energy cycle." Often they can be found in the lower part of the longitudinal arch, in other words, in the lumbar region. In these sections the grip can be repeated several times in the strained section until the tissue feels "more permeable."

If the aforementioned flow direction of the grip does not suit the patient, variations can be offered, and they can usually determine spontaneously which is the more effective in the current treatment. Three further options:
1. Thumbs and fingers start bimanually in the pelvic floor at the same time and cover the different ventral and dorsal paths back to the lips. Or:
2. Thumbs and fingers select the reverse direction: start at the lips, at the same time they are led ventrally and dorsally to the pelvic floor. Or:
3. The bimanual grip is performed in the reverse direction: at the front (= dorsal on the foot) down to the pelvic floor, at the back (= medial-plantar on the foot) up to the lips.

In particular, the "small energy cycle" has proved valuable for pregnant women with fetuses in the breech position. Together with the zones of the pelvic ligaments (Chapter 27), it can support turning of the child into normal presentation.

As many patients have scars on the front of the trunk, this central connection of the meridian energy fields is also well suited to RTF scar treatment (Chapter 25).

6.1.9 The Lemniscate—the Symbol for Infinity

(Fig. 6.8)
The horizontal eight is well known as a mathematical sign and the symbol for infinity. It is also used in anthroposophical medicine and in methods which strengthen the fine motor skills and coordination of children and adults.

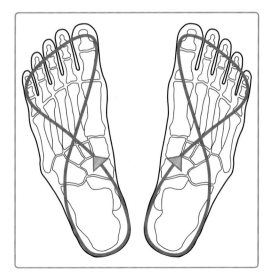

Fig. 6.8 Lemniscate (symbol for infinity).

Effect: The gentle, bimanual grip on the plantar side of the feet has a balancing effect in all situations in which the focus is on transition and stressful conditions, such as starting school (for children), moving house, emotionally difficult stages of life, situations involving shock, familial and professional changes.

It has a special place in **terminal care,** when people have to cope with the transition from finite earthly life to infinity (Chapter 24.2).

Performance: The patient's heels should project approximately two to three centimeters beyond the lower end of the treatment table. The **backs** of both the therapist's hands lie flat with the fingers pointing in a medial direction toward the heels in the zones of the lumbar spine. The upper circle of the eight starts there. It first moves in a distal to lateral direction toward the fifth toe, then in a medial direction toward the two big toes and then to the intersection of the eight.

Here the transition to the lower circle takes place. It moves around the heel and closes at approximately the level of the Lisfranc joint line. There the new figure of eight begins. The lemniscate can be repeated 10, 12, or even more times. The therapist sways back and forth gently as a result of the dynamic movement of the hands and consequently can also move his or her own spine gently and rhythmically in time.

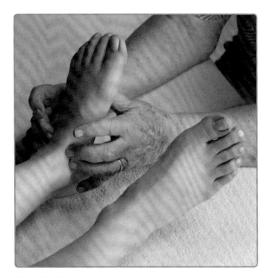

Fig. 6.9 "Groin opener."

6.1.10 "Groin opener"

(Fig. 6.9)

Effect: As the transition from the trunk into the lower extremities is often congested, the grip can support

- organs located in the small pelvis
- bones, muscles, and nerves
- the lymph, the arterial and venous blood, and
- the energy paths of the meridians

in their function and flow force, because it moves the ankle joint which corresponds to the zone of the groin. As a result, the entire small pelvis area becomes more mobile and better supplied with blood. This benefits both the local tissue around the malleoli and the "reflective" zones.

Performance: Both thumbs support the zone of the shoulder girdle distinctly from the plantar side. Two fingers on each side simultaneously start close to the inner and outer malleoli and work their way through the entire zone of the groin from both sides with swaying grips until all four fingers are next to each other. After the active phase deep in the tissue, each of the fingers returns to its starting position neutrally and starts the next grip.

With each active movement of the fingers, the thumbs push the forefoot cranially and release the tension again in the passive phase. As there is a lot of lymph tissue in these zones, the fingers work gently. However, the thumbs can forcefully push the forefoot into dorsal flexion. A rhythmic

movement is thus produced which can be felt as far as the head.

The grip is repeated until the joint can be moved backward and forward more smoothly. However, in doing so the patient's limits must always be observed, because not everyone is happy to be moved by someone else from the outset, even if it is seemingly "only" the small joints which are involved.

The zones of the genital area, the abdominal wall, and the thigh may likewise be treated using this bimanual grip.

6.1.11 Practical Advice

The individual grips for stabilization of the autonomic nervous system are performed or repeated until the patient's condition has normalized. This may vary between 10 seconds and 1 to 2 minutes.

- When choosing these grips, we should not be guided by personal preference for one grip or another, but by the patient's individual requirements. Sensitivity in making this decision may be obtained through practice and inner awareness. It is closely related to our ability to deal with sensitive issues, that is, to our intuitive skills.
- Usually, one of the grips described is sufficient when repeated several times to counteract the temporary irritation. In addition, we can also choose a second grip which we alternate with the first grip we have chosen.
- Beware of the unplanned application of various stabilizing grips. This would only convey restlessness and uncertainty.
- So that patients remain "focused" during the performance of stabilizing grips, their inner awareness may be invoked, for instance by asking the question: "How does that feel?"
- As a precaution when dealing with contact-shy or particularly agitated patients, or for those who already have damp or wet feet at the start of the treatment, we should perform the grips through a light blanket or sheet or with the feet clothed (no artificial fibers, if possible). People who are irritated in this way are particularly grateful when we avoid getting too close too early on through direct skin contact.
- When we are not feeling well ourselves, we should opt for flowing, animated grips:
  - Heel stretching
  - Respiratory regulation
  - Yin-Yang

- Small energy cycle
- Lemniscate
- Groin opener
- After selecting the right stabilizing grip, we will often find that we feel better again ourselves because a well-chosen grip not only revitalizes the patient but the therapist as well.

We do not have to learn the most natural and obvious grip for the harmonization of health because our hands have already employed it in many situations. We simply take the restless feet or individual painful areas between our warm hands and let the patient feel our compassion.

6.2

Eutonic Grips for Harmonization

6.2.1 "Webbed Toe" Grip

(Fig. 6.10)

Effect: The grip at the connecting point of the zones of the head, neck, and shoulder girdle creates more space between the individual toes. It thus stimulates the resolution of Hypertonicity and "opens" the energy flow of the corresponding organ zones. It is particularly effective in children and adults with the following:

- Shoulder and neck problems
- Headaches, hypotension, and hypertension
- Chronic respiratory problems, including asthma
- Frontal and maxillary sinus stresses
- Eye and ear problems
- Lymphatic stresses and teething problems
- Emotional stresses and distress

Performance: The therapist's fingers are carefully threaded into the interstices of the patient's toes as far as the individual skin folds. The thumb of the free hand provides support at the soles. Then the toes are moved in all directions and their interstices gently expanded.

In the same way, the patient's toes can **actively** move the therapist's fingers, also with plantar thumb support. After approximately 20 to 30 seconds the fingers are slowly withdrawn. The patient can then compare the treated foot with the other one to consciously appreciate and describe the change.

Another stabilizing grip is selected for **athlete's foot** and where the interstices of the toes are too narrow.

6.2.2 Shoulder–Arm Grip

Effect: The shoulder girdle and thorax expand so that the cardiovascular system and respiration are harmonized and stabilized. The tone in the musculature and joints of the shoulder through the arms and hands is regulated. The excessive tension in the segmental zones, above all of the upper back, in which there are connections to the organs of the upper abdomen, is normalized.

Performance: The right **and** left sides are always treated, even if the complaints are unilateral. It usually makes sense to start with the side under less strain. The therapist remains seated to one side of the patient while the grip is performed. One palm raises the patient's shoulder slightly so that the other can push underneath the long sacrospinalis muscle between the inner shoulder blade margin and the medial thoracic spine.

The therapist's fingers move from being flat into a raised position and palpate the tone of the back musculature. Intermittent tensions can often be found here, including on the subjectively complaint-free side. The raised fingers are held on the painful site until the patient's nervous system has adjusted to the stimulus. This can be recognized by the fact that the back tissue can slowly "sink" into the therapist's fingers. When the tissue tone has been regulated in this way, the pain can no longer be felt and the fingers return to the flat starting position.

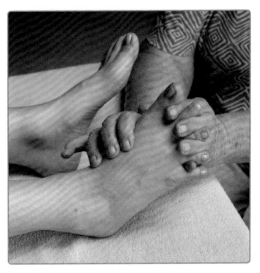

Fig. 6.10 Toe web grip.

The free hand gently raises the patient's shoulder again and places itself in the vicinity of the working hand. From there, over the dorsal shoulder girdle, both hands start stroking the back of the arms as far as the hands simultaneously. After performing the grip, a brief "creative pause" of approximately 20 to 40 seconds is important so that the patient can experience and convey the change consciously. Comparison with the other side, as yet untreated, provides spontaneous proof that the tone has been regulated.

After this, the shoulder-arm grip is repeated on the other side, followed in turn by a brief pause for observation. If necessary, the grip is repeated several times during the treatment. The fingers of **both** hands can also be placed under the patient's shoulder girdle **at the same time**. The **connective tissue zones** of the liver/gall bladder (right side) and stomach (left side) in the back can therefore also be targeted in this way.

Variation: The fingers make contact from the long sacrospinalis muscle as far as the spinous processes of the thoracic spine and apply the therapeutic stimulus there in the same manner.

6.2.3 Pelvis–Leg Grip

Effect: This grip relieves the lower spine, above all, the sacrum, sacroiliac joint, and gluteal muscles. The frequently blocked transition from the trunk to the legs becomes freer. The movement in the flow systems of the legs (venous and arterial blood, lymph, nerves, meridian energy) is stimulated. Contact with "Mother Earth" is perceived with greater awareness.

Whether the effect of stroking is explained by
- the flow direction of the Yang meridians,
- the improvement in innervation from the lower spine, or simply
- the regulation of tone,

the outcome is the same. It is presumably a case of interaction at all these levels.

Performance: Like the shoulder–arm grip, this grip is performed through the clothing (preferably a pair of trousers). Here too, treatment can begin on the complaint-**free** side. The therapist stands next to the patient's knees with one leg lunging forward on one side of the treatment table while the other foot is positioned at the foot end parallel to the bench.

One hand gently supports the longitudinal arch of the sole of the foot. The other hand laterally reaches under the back at the level of the lower margin of the ribcage and iliac crest. It strokes under the gluteal region of that side and along the dorsal area of the leg.

Note: The hand should cover the entire popliteal space. In the lower third of the calf stroking is continued in a dorsal to lateral direction as far as the back of the feet and toes.

The grip may be repeated three to four times on each leg. With this grip too, there is a brief creative pause for self-awareness before changing to the other side.

Variation: When one hand has started stroking from the back and buttocks, the other is added medially at mid-thigh level. Both hands stroke along the dorsal part of the leg and finish at the sole and back of the foot. Getting up from the treatment table should take place slowly and carefully in order to feel and convey the change which has occurred.

Caution
This grip is contraindicated for patients at risk of a prolapsed disk or with very severe, medically unexplained pain in the lower back, as the complaints may intensify as a result of the temporary right–left imbalance.

6.2.4 Sacrum Grip

Effect: As this grip is applied in the dorsal center of the body, it has a **centering** effect both at a physical and emotional level. It relieves the lower spine, including the sacrum and coccyx, and gives the sensation of a good, stable base. This grip is experienced deep in the pelvis by pregnant women as a loosening and expanding sensation. However, caution should be employed in the case of pregnant women with **inferior vena cava syndrome** (supine hypotensive syndrome, in which the lower vena cava is compressed).

Some patients put it aptly without realizing when they describe being upset as "not being themselves," "not being completely with it," or "being out of it."

Performance: The grip is rightly also called the "Pizza or Baker's Grip," as one after the other, the therapist's flat hands push underneath the patient's sacrum. The therapist should sit to one side of the table at an appropriate distance to avoid strain on back when bending forward. Depending on the length of the therapist's forearms, these lie wholly or partially on the treatment table.

The hands are so far under the sacrum that both the **eminences** of the hand near the **wrist** are in the vertical median line of the sacrum and the fingers touch the other half of the gluteal region without any pressure. The eminences of the hand can lie there quietly or are slowly raised to the sacrum so that it is somewhat elevated. This position is held in order for the patient to slowly be able to release hypertonus in the sacrum. As soon as the patient is able to "sink" into the therapist's hands, the pain usually subsides significantly because the tissue tone has normalized.

The feeling of release is reinforced when the therapist slowly starts to withdraw his or her hands from underneath the patient's back and finally their entire pelvic region "sinks" into the treatment table in a relaxed state. A brief pause for self-awareness and description of the change from "before" to "after" is also important with this grip.

If **overweight**, the patient can first turn on one side to enable the therapist's hands to comfortably get into the right position before the patient moves back into a supine position.

Caution should also be exercised with this grip in patients with a prolapsed disk in the lower spine or with medically unexplained severe pain.

6.3

Sphincter Treatment for Harmonization of the Autonomic Nervous System

As most sphincters are innervated by the autonomic nervous system, treating them can also be used to stabilize and harmonize the patient's physical and mental state. The effect is similar to treatment with stabilizing grips.

Although the cardia, Bauhin (ileocaecal) valve, and mouth of the uterus (uterine cervix) are not "traditional" sphincters, they are included in treatment. Practical work has shown that these organ transitions can likewise be used to regulate muscle tone.

Indications

- Spasms (e.g., pyloric spasm in infants, vesical spasm after operations)
- Sphincter deficiencies (e.g., the bladder)
- Pains of any kind, including of an emotional nature

- Problems falling asleep and staying asleep
- Burn-out syndrome
- Attention deficit and hyperactivity disorder (ADHD) and lapses in concentration
- Shock situations, states of anxiety.

6.3.1 Practical Application

All eight specified zones are held gently in a distal to proximal direction for approximately 8 seconds. After 4 seconds the other hand starts to reach into the next zone, while the first hand completes the 8 seconds with the same intensity. The eight zones are:

- Lips (right and left)
- Cardia (entrance to the stomach)
- Pylorus (gastric outlet)
- Sphincter of Oddi (introduction of gall and pancreatic juices into the duodenum)
- Bauhin's (ileocecal) valve
- Bladder sphincter
- Cervix
- Anus

This procedure is repeated several times. The intensity of the grips depends on the overall condition of the patient. An extensive period of rest subsequently stabilizes the result.

6.3.2 Additional Possibilities

Time and again it is also useful to treat zones of sphincters individually. The therapist and patient can work together here to achieve the best possible regulation of tone. The zone in question is first sedated for a few seconds and after a brief pause tonified and/or first tonified and then sedated. As most patients provide very clear feedback about the effect, the choice can be made in keeping with the individual circumstances, and this is an exciting experience which reinforces the patient's trust in their own perceptions.

Examples for Treating Sphincters Individually

- Cardia for hiatus hernia, irritated stomach
- Pylorus for pylorospasm. Although infants cannot express themselves verbally, the spontaneous change in their voice and facial expression clearly indicates which type of treatment of the pylorus suits them better.
- Bauhin (ileocaecal) valve for Crohn's disease, among other things, as well as for severe emotional stress

- Bladder sphincter for spasms or weakness
- Uterine cervix (together with pelvic floor and bladder) to support the involution of the pelvic tissue after childbirth
- Anus for hemorrhoids, including pre- and postoperative.

6.3.3 Sedate or Tonify?

Experience shows that the decision as to whether sphincter treatment is sedating or tonifying does not only depend on anatomical and physiological circumstances. We can also rely on the patient's spontaneous awareness and the strength of their inner self-regulation. The fact that we do treat them for the specified indications is, in my opinion, more important than the consideration as to which technique we employ.

The "partner patient" with careful observation of the effect often provides the best guidance: sometimes they sense that after a few minutes of sedating a zone, gentle, swaying tonification rounds off the effect of the treatment; sometimes they find that quiet holding of the zone after tonifying results in stabilization and harmonization of the condition.

6.4

Summary

Although grips to stabilize the autonomic nervous system do not require much physical strength, they can have a weakening effect on us if we fail to take enough care of ourselves. Working with such subtle forces means dealing with imponderable qualities which are directly related to our vitality. The more aware we are of this, the better we learn to deal with our forces and to strike a healthy balance between giving and receiving.

Incidentally, the grips are far less complicated than might appear from the theoretical description. We can simply trust our hands' own intelligence as they "know" instinctively how to "handle" something.

7 Preparation for Treatment

7.1

The Relationship between Patient and Therapist

Applying manual methods provides us with a good opportunity to build up a genuine partnership with our patients.

By demonstrating calm and concentration during treatment, we can usually put a stop to some patients' desire to talk too much. Now and then, however, it is more important to lend a compassionate ear to listen to their sorrows than to actively treat certain points on the feet.

Our task is to make patients realize that during the treatment it is more important to monitor their own reactions carefully, to trace even subtle changes, and to express them clearly than to demand too much theoretical information, such as the nomination of certain zones.

7.2

Instructions for the Patient

Method. Clear information on the main principles of reflexotherapy of the feet (RTF) *before* the first treatment helps both sides and provides a sound introduction to the therapy. For many years I have used an illustration showing a seated person in the shape of the foot as a practical working model (see **Fig. 2.3**). I have observed that this simple and graphic comparison offers people of all ages and educational levels the easiest access to this method because it addresses people's imagination directly, bypassing their intellect.

Attempts to describe RTF in words will not lead to much because confidence in a therapy and a therapist grows best through personal experience.

The significance of pain. Patients should be informed about the **significance and purpose** of pain at the start of a series of treatments. According to R. Voll, pain is "the cry of the tissue for flowing energy." Pain convinces patients, often surprisingly quickly, that it is time to get the necessary treatment. The local pain released by the grips in certain areas of the foot should therefore be regarded by the therapist as an important indicator that treatment is required.

However, a painful area on the foot does not initially provide any diagnostic or therapeutic information about the type, cause, and duration of the patient's illness.

When the patient realizes that there is no need to passively surrender to the pain caused by the treatment and that their **personal pain threshold** is acknowledged and respected, they will find it easier to accept the pain as a warning and not simply regard it as the enemy (see Chapter 8).

Resting phase after treatment. *Before* their first appointment, we should inform our patients about the importance and necessity of the resting phase following treatment, to avoid unnecessary time pressure. The resting phase is important because the first phase of regeneration takes place during this period. Patients who do not rest deprive themselves of a significant amount of recuperation and improvement.

7.3

Preparing for the First Treatment

Before the initial assessment (visual and palpatory) a brief overview of the patient's history is compiled. This can shed light on the circumstances which have resulted in the current illness. In addition, it enables a more differentiated decision to be made regarding whether RTF might perhaps be contraindicated. It includes the following questions:

- Which problems or symptoms, chronic or acute, are paramount at the start of treatment?
- How long have they been present and what triggered them (e.g., an accident, inflammation, stress, etc.)?
- How are the excretory organs, the intestine, kidneys, and skin functioning?
- What kind of treatment has already been employed for these symptoms and/or is the patient undergoing other therapies at the same time?
- What is the patient's quality of sleep (dreams) and general emotional state?
- Are varicose veins or phlebitis present, and were they present at any time in the past?

- Does the patient have scars (even small ones) as a result of operations or accidents? Where are they located and how long have they been there?
- What is the condition of the teeth (root treatments, different metals in the mouth, and indications of a possible allergy to silver amalgam)?
- Is the patient taking any medicine which might influence the outcome of treatment, for example, strong sedatives or analgesics, psychotropic drugs, beta blockers, phenprocoumon, etc. or medicine which necessitates particularly careful treatment of the symptom zone, for example, insulin or other hormone preparations, including contraceptives? (Chapter 16.3).
- Eating and drinking habits, abuse of drugs, nicotine or alcohol?

7.4

Patient Positioning during Treatment

7.4.1 General Instructions

The treatment will be more effective if the patient is positioned appropriately. The following conditions are helpful:

- A well-aired, warm, bright, quiet room
- A sufficiently wide, well-padded treatment table at a suitable height
- Neck and knee supports, where appropriate
- A light blanket, preferably made of natural fibers, because heat loss may occur during treatment, even if the ambient temperature is warm. In addition, being covered gives the patient the feeling that their personal space is protected.

Patients will find that they feel better if they remove their watches and jewelry at least temporarily. We advise patients to do so during treatment and also suggest doing so at home now and again, especially at night, and carefully observe the effects. Among other things, this suggestion is based on acupuncture in which metal needles are used in a targeted manner to **change the local energy field**. If meridians come into contact with metals or other materials in an undifferentiated manner, this can lead to more or less clearly appreciable changes in their energy. Congestion

may also arise in the nervous, venous, and lymphatic system as a result.

Being comfortably positioned includes loosening the belt, collar, bra, corset, and skirt or trouser waistband to allow unrestricted breathing movements.

Usually the patient's head and neck need to be supported by a small pillow. This serves the purpose, especially with beginners, of enabling them to have direct eye contact with the patient at all times in order to monitor reactions, and it promotes mutual trust.

7.4.2 Variations

When making a **home visit** to a bed-ridden patient, the location of the bed will influence the position and working posture of the therapist. With some imagination and the aid of pillows, cushions, and footstools, effective treatment is possible in conditions other than those usual for working, perhaps exceptionally even standing up.

It goes without saying that patients in severe pain are involved in deciding how and where it is most comfortable for them to lay. Likewise,

- pregnant women,
- patients suffering from a heart condition or rheumatism, or
- patients with breathing difficulties

need to be positioned according to their condition.

7.5

Rules for the Therapist

As we are in direct contact with the patient through our hands, it is important that we take good care of ourselves for our own well-being.

> Not all patients require "our best" at all times but rather what is appropriate for them in each situation. This insight gives us more freedom in assigning efficiently our daily ration of vitality.

Even if it appears that we only work with our hands, nonetheless our whole self is participating in the treatment, consciously or subconsciously— and not just at a physical level. The relationships between the part and the whole—the hands and the person—can be experienced as a balanced input of energy if we consider the following three points before starting each treatment.

7.5.1 Correct Posture

A good seating position makes working easier. There are different methods for building up suitable posture. If a method has already proved effective, there is probably no reason to change.

Our proposal. The position of the feet, the legs, and the pelvis is literally of "fundamental" significance because they convey the confidence-building experience that the ground on which we stand and the chair on which we sit are really supporting us. There should be an angle of about 90° between the thigh and lower leg and the feet. In order to be able to experience the natural focus in the **pelvis** more clearly over time, we advise keeping the legs approximately 30 to 40 cm apart, depending on their length, so that the feet are always in connection with the ground without poor posture of the bones and musculature (Lao Tse: "Gravity is the root of grace").

We sit on the chair in such a way that the spine can support itself throughout its full length if the pelvis is well positioned:

- Swaying forward and backward a little, the pelvis is adjusted so that in the initial position it is a little **in front** of the ischial tuberosity.
- The natural lordosis of the lumbar spine is consciously experienced, but is not rigidly fixed. (The term "hollow back" frequently has negative connotations; it simply indicates the physiological swaying of the spine at this point.)
- We ensure that the space between the shoulder blades is and remains free of hypertonus. This can be achieved if the lower end of the sternum is gently moved forward and slightly upward. Thus the posture of the medial thoracic spine, which in many therapists is subject to severe stresses, can be normalized. The arms and hands are connected to the energy flow of the spine quite naturally as a result of this.
- The neck with the cervical vertebrae and head can be positioned normally if the chin is moved slightly in the direction of the sternum and the mandibular joints remain relaxed.

Slightly sloping **seating wedges** can be a useful aid in practicing correct posture, until our body remembers by itself. They should not be used permanently, however.

7.5.2 Observing our Own Breathing

Time and again we subconsciously assume the breathing rhythm of our patients. This is of no benefit to them and can weaken us. If we learn to observe our breathing attentively and patiently, we will discover and maintain our own rhythm more easily.

The best condition for freely flowing respiration is a well-positioned posture which is flexible in itself, for this will allow the breath to find its own way of flowing.

In particular, this should be considered when patients react strongly to the treatment. Almost without exception, we initially associate with the patient's irritation without being aware of it. The disturbance and stagnation of our respiration as soon as an unexpected situation occurs shows very clearly how easily we ourselves can become irritated. Recognizing this as a fact without evaluating it and without judging whether it is right or wrong is a promising step toward the recovery of our own normal breathing rhythm.

> Basically, we should respect our own breathing rhythm and that of the other person, because even in its supposedly "unnatural" form, it is always a spontaneous and honest expression of our current situation in life.

Anyone who would like to find out more about breathing should seek the guidance of a trained therapist to gain practical experience. Breath work is always beneficial in terms of self-development!

7.5.3 A Healthy Distance

The individual length of our forearms suggests a suitable distance between the therapist and the patient's feet. This free space creates a good physical radius of movement which promotes the economical use of our strength and energy.

A healthy internal and external distance between the therapist and the patient helps in obtaining a differentiated overview of the reflex zones while at the same time preventing either person from violating the other's boundaries. Placing the patient's feet on our thigh or in the vicinity of our ribcage is therefore to be avoided.

The more keenly the two sides become involved in the treatment, the more clearly they can determine the necessary and healthy distance between them.

As people in our cultural environment only seldom go barefoot anymore and as some have a disturbed relationship with their feet for esthetic or other reasons, many patients will experience what sensitive and "intimate" parts their feet are, as a result of the treatment.

7.5.4 **Summary**

Apart from the rules regarding sitting posture, breathing, and a healthy distance, it should be remembered that our **mental attitude** to ourselves, our work, and the person on the treatment table play a part in deciding how we feel during and, above all, after treatment. As long as we believe that we alone are primarily responsible for an improvement in the condition of our patient, we delude ourselves and use up unnecessarily large amounts of our own vitality.

> When we accept that our task is solely to evoke, support, and harmonize existing regenerative strength in the other person, we can employ our own physical, emotional, and mental strengths more economically.

This also means recognizing that some patients (and ourselves, too) may subconsciously put us under pressure by giving us to understand that they wish to surrender personal responsibility for their health to us. "Suffering rather than changing something is easier for many!"

Important Note: After each treatment we should wash our hands thoroughly, above all, to neutralize ourselves at an energetic level as well. The more depleted our energy levels, the more the need for **warm** water.

Equally helpful is thorough airing of the room after a treatment and drinking of additional fluids, preferably water, before and after a treatment.

8 Pain—Its Purpose and Significance

8.1

Health, Disease, and Pain

It is rare that a person is completely healthy, and there are many different definitions and views regarding this subject. The French physiologist Du Bois, for example, puts it thus: "People respond to all the factors in their environment, and the manner of their response is the measure of their health." In other words, he regards health as a constantly changing process of adjustment which continues throughout life.

In his book *Dennoch Landarzt,* **Dr. August Heisler** writes analogously that when he meets people who have no experience of pain and disease, he rather avoids them, because he observed that such people often lack compassion and understanding. They are "only" healthy, nothing else. And being healthy alone is not enough for a human being.

Generally speaking, no one welcomes pain or disease and furthermore their occurrence is always inopportune. However, we observe that an increasing number of patients are able to accept that disease and suffering are not simply enemies and troublemakers that have to be fought—they also provide an opportunity for reorientation and encourage a new outlook on life. "Pain creates awareness."

In addition, pain or inflammation is always a **self-preservation response** and plays an important **protective role** in recognizing and accepting limits, such as:

- The child who is cautious where heat is involved as a result of their first, painful experience with the hot stovetop.
- The patient who wisely avoids rotating their injured arm beyond the threshold of pain.
- The woman who learns to avoid some kinds of food as a result of her chronic gastritis.

Naturally, we see our essential task as being to alleviate pain and find ways of making it disappear in part or—according to the regenerative capabilities of our patients—even completely. In traditional reflexotherapy of the feet (RTF), as with other methods, pain presents itself as an **indicator** for the recognition of injuries because usually **healthy organs or tissues do not cause pain**, either in situ or in the equivalent zone on the foot. (Other criteria are paramount in RTF lymphatic treatment in Chapter 29.)

During treatment we work cautiously and alertly **with** the pain felt by patients in certain zones, but never **against** it (Chapters 4.1 and 4.2). As a result of the individually tailored dosage of the therapeutic grips, the patient learns that pain is not an end in itself but that it provides guidance and diminishes sooner when we treat it with respect.

Beginners will sometimes find it difficult to trust the objective testimony of the compiled evidence more than the subjective testimony of the patient. They mistakenly assume that when all is said and done patients "knows best whereabouts something is wrong with them." What is forgotten in the process is that the patient is only aware of the painful symptom but not the background which has led to its development.

Three points requiring clarification:

1. Most people think that the occurrence of pain is synonymous with the **start** of an illness. The reality is different, because every disease process or condition is preceded by a developmental stage or "silent phase" in which the person's powers of self-healing attempt to maintain all the functions in the organism as well as possible. In this so-called preclinical stage, pain **in situ** is still barely perceptible, if at all, but can already be palpated as abnormalities in the **appertaining zones**. It is only when the internal control principle no longer works that the disease becomes subjectively tangible for the patient as a result of pain and/or restricted movement.

2. With **accidents** too, an actual illness seldom begins with spontaneous pain or a fracture because it has individual background causes and internal correlations.

3. Many patients think a troubling **symptom** is an illness. But illness, above all long-term illness, is by no means restricted to the painful site at which the symptom appears. An everyday **example:** In patients with headaches it is not only the head which is affected but the whole person who suffers.

Remember: Patients are usually satisfied when the disorders disappear in the **physical** sphere. However, sometimes the person's powers of self-healing unexpectedly enable responses at **other levels** with the aid of RTF, for example:

- At an **emotional** level, with laughter and/
  or tears providing relief, with the unexpected resurfacing of earlier traumatic events
  (Chapter 17)
- At a **mental** level, through recognition of
  harmful habits (unhealthy eating habits, lack
  of exercise, etc.) and/or
- At a **spiritual** level, with a change of perspective regarding the meaning of illness and the
  concept of fate in life

During a course of treatment it is also observed
that as a result of predominant pain in an organ
or tissue, less intense conditions are **obscured** or
initially overlooked. They only become apparent
when the most noticeable bout of pain has been
overcome by means of repeated treatments. Due to
their lack of awareness of the situation, some patients then think that RTF is making them "worse
than they were before" because they are only
able to feel the previously less noticeable pain as
a result of the more dominant pain diminishing
("Hering's Law," Chapter 14.1).

8.2

Perceptions of Pain in the Zones and Methods of Treatment

When treating the abnormal zones of the foot, the
patient experiences various pain sensations. The
reactions of the autonomic nervous system (perspiring hands, dry mouth, etc., Chapter 4.2) also
point to a subjective sensation of pain in response
to the individual dosage of the grips.

- The most surprising sensation is that of
  intense, almost **stabbing** pain. It occurs most
  frequently on the periostium, for example, on
  the toes, the heel bone and the fibula.
  Method: The small, specific areas are treated
  with the tip of the thumb or index finger while
  keenly observing the patient (**Fig. 10.6**). Slowly
  going deeper into the abnormal zones enables
  the patient to accept the pain, not least because
  he or she finds that it usually subsides rapidly.
- **Well outlined** and clearly defined, often extending into the deeper layers of the foot, pain

is felt at sites with more muscles and connective tissue, usually on the plantar surface.
Method: Basic thumb grips (see **Figs. 3.1–3.4**)
are the most appropriate on the soles of the
feet. Depending on the sensation of pain,
varying the speed and intensity of treatment
is the method of choice.

- The sensation on the webs may be exceptionally **piercing**, triggered by the stretching grip
  customary there.
  Method: The thumb and index finger simultaneously begin stretching the tissue folds
  in the plantar and dorsal space between the
  individual metatarsophalangeal joints and
  continue until the thumb and index finger
  meet (Chapter 3.2.4).
- In the tendons, for instance around the Achilles tendon and malleoli, there is frequently
  venous and/or lymphatic congestion in the
  foot and distal part of the lower leg, above
  all in women. If there is swelling, the pain is
  usually **dull and extensive** in the upper layers
  of tissue close to the skin.
  Method: Treatment here is performed gently
  with the **pads** of the thumbs or fingers and
  specific gripping deep into the tissue with
  the **tip** of the thumb or finger is avoided. The
  alternating strokes of RTF lymphatic treatment are the most appropriate for the area
  around the Achilles tendon (see **Figs. 3.6, 3.7**).
  It is also possible to work around the malleoli
  using gentle thumb and index finger grips.

Exceptions to the sensation of pain are observed
in patients:

- who take **medication** (often a variety at the
  same time) which dampens the perception of
  pain and the responses of the autonomic nervous system and the central nervous system,
  for example, painkillers and sleeping pills,
  beta blockers, psychotropic drugs, drugs for
  rheumatism, and also narcotics.
- who suffer from particular diseases which
  alter sensitivity and the perception of pain
  and may **slow down** reactions such as diabetes
  mellitus, multiple sclerosis, hemi- and paraplegia, fibromyalgia, etc.

- who are in a **coma** or **persistent vegetative state**. Here reactions described by nursing staff and relatives or observed on a monitor can provide information about changes in condition, for example, in the respiratory and cardiac rhythms.

Method: Often in these patients neither local pain in the zones nor the indications of the autonomic nervous system are reliable in assessing the correct dosage for the situation. Therefore in these circumstances initially **gentle** treatment with **neutral** grips is employed. Treatment times are initially limited to 10 to 15 minutes. **Stabilizing/ harmonizing** and/or **eutonic grips** (Chapter 6) are possible at any time and their regulatory effect can be verified spontaneously.

From My Practice

In the early years of my RTF work I took care of a frail, elderly patient suffering from severe pain on the left side of her lower back. On one of my home visits, a footbath had just been prepared for her. As I was pushed for time, I treated her zones in the foot bath. To my surprise, her feet were far less sensitive under water than usual and I was able to increase the intensity of my grips significantly. I later had the same positive experience with other patients who were very sensitive to pain too.

At around the same time, a colleague tried to target the zones with a powerful jet of water during underwater massage. The reactions were more negative, probably because a differentiated dosage of the stimulus was not possible.

9 Limits of Determination of Zones in Writing

Nearly all manual forms of therapy first arose from practical observations and were only later written down. However, the practical observations which we make from findings on our patients' feet are always reliable and more significant than any reference book.

Furthermore, "fixed" treatment processes are a contradiction in terms because therapy as a dynamic process is literally animated and moving. I should therefore like to point out repeatedly the limits of determining certain points in writing and advise training the sensitivity of one's own hands in order to become independent of fixed averages through personal tactile experience.

9.1
Deviations in Related Zones

9.1.1 Physiological Deviations in the Location of Zones

Completely natural differentiations can already be found within the **physiological** range of the organ zones.

Examples

- The zone of the uterus expands in women as a pregnancy progresses.
- The zone of the stomach is smaller after fasting for 10 days than after a lavish meal.
- The zone of the bladder changes in tone and size depending on its content.
- Just as the organs change their position in the body according to whether the patient is lying down or standing, the sites of the zones likewise vary depending on whether the patient is sitting or lying down during treatment, for example, in the case of the stomach and spleen.

9.1.2 Pathological Deviations

Besides natural differentiations when treating patients, we almost always have to deal with pathological changes. Here too the deviations from the norm in situ correlate with the deviations in site or shape of the organs in the body.

Examples

- In patients with floating kidneys both the regular kidney zone and the zone which corresponds to the current pathological site of the kidney indicate abnormalities, both sites being an expression of abnormal conditions.
- In patients with gastroptosis (sagging stomach), a relatively common complaint, the zone of the stomach may often extend into the region of the small intestine, according to the altered site of the stomach as a result of ptosis (sagging).
- In women with a uterine or bladder prolapse, the zones of the pelvis in the medial calcaneus are displaced in a proximal direction.
- Conversely, in people whose **feet** reveal **deformations** which have been inherited or acquired as a result of trauma, the sites of the zones change according to the anatomical and pathological displacement of the foot's bone and tissue structure. I cannot be certain whether anomalies of the feet also bring about deviations in the site of the organs in the body but they may trigger functional disorders in the corresponding organs.

9.1.3 Summary

Beginners will learn to find the zones better if they first gather experience in patients with **precise symptoms**, for example, toothache, acute joint problems, lumbar complaints, or menstrual pain.

The clear pathological condition of such zones can be confirmed easily and objectively.

9.2
Reciprocal Effects of Disorders of the Feet and Organism

9.2.1 Effects of Foot Disorders

There are a number of internal and external causes of strain or pain in the foot region. Whether and when lasting abnormal zones develop as a result depends upon the duration and intensity of the stimulus and the vitality of the person concerned. However, we may assume that there are reciprocal effects between disorders of the foot and their related zones in situ, even if they do not always display perceptible symptoms.

Examples

- Excessive strain caused by extreme hiking or walking, exaggerated practice of a particular sport

- Fatigue experienced in professions involving a lot of standing, especially on concrete floors
- Trauma: injuries, cuts, treading on sharp objects, fractures, sprains
- Hereditary conditions: weak connective tissue, flat feet, fallen arches, spread foot, pes valgus or pes cavus
- Circulatory disorders: paresis, varicose veins, venous ulcers, smoker's leg
- Rheumatism and gout in the whole organism, which can be reflected in the feet as "gouty toes"

Considering all the different ways of observing pathological conditions in the feet, any kind of prolonged disorder in the foot, regardless of the part in which it occurs, may primarily or secondarily also cause pain and discomfort in the related zones and organs in situ.

9.2.2 Effects of Disorders in the Organism

Just as, on the one hand, local discomfort in the feet can have secondary effects on the organism, on the other hand, complaints and pain in the organism are triggers for sensitive zones on the feet.

Examples

- Exhaustion: The zones of the lower spine are usually painful after a long car journey or unaccustomed, strenuous gardening.
- Excessive demands: The zone of the heart shows signs of strain for a short time after exaggerated practice of a competitive sport; the zone of the stomach after a lavish birthday party.
- Prodromal damage: The zone may already be painful in the **"silent phase"** of an illness, during which the patient is not yet aware of it, for example, days before acute sinusitis and weeks before painful restriction of the mobility of the hip joint. **Illness starts before pain occurs!**
- Acute disease process: This affects the zones of the respiratory tract in acute bronchitis, the lumbar spine in acute ischialgia, the bladder in acute cystitis.
- Hyperfunction of organs: The zones of the thyroid gland are affected in hyperthyroidism, those of the colon in ulcerative colitis.
- Hypofunction of organs: The zones of the stomach are painful in the case of hypoacidity or anacidity, the endocrine zones in the case of hypofunction of the endocrine system.

- Flaccidity, atony, atrophy, degeneration: The zones in which the symptoms appear are affected, for example, in patients with uterine prolapse, floating kidney, enteroptosis, rectal prolapse, arthrosis, and the related areas of the organs or joints.
- Hereditary predisposition to disease: With an hereditary predisposition to weakness of the supportive and connective tissue, allergies and diabetes, the zones of the background environment are also painful: frequently those of the intestine, lymphatic system and endocrine organs.
- Accidents: The zones corresponding to the sites of fractures, injuries, contusions and sprains will be painful.

For the practical performance of reflexotherapy of the feet it is irrelevant whether the disorder was in the organ or the feet initially, because the aim of the treatment is always to achieve a balance between all the patient's functions, irrespective of their origin.

9.2.3 Additional Interpretations of Findings in the Feet

In reflexotherapy of the feet (RTF) what is related to disturbed or strained zones on the foot can also be interpreted differently by a specialist.

- Thus, in **orthopaedics** a structural deformity in the longitudinal arch is described as a flat foot; in the topography of RTF, the zone of the spine is located on its medial-plantar edge. Clinically, patients with such a flattening of the longitudinal arch often have diminished lordosis as well, indicating a constitutional weakness of the connective tissue.
- However, in courses in Africa I have observed that the local population usually has a flatter longitudinal arch than in Europe **without** this necessarily being associated with spinal disorders.
- The **phlebologist** speaks of venous congestion around the malleoli; in RTF the described area provides information about possible strain in the abdominal region/pelvis.
- In **surgery** a hallux valgus will give rise to surgical intervention; RTF recognizes zones corresponding to the thyroid gland, neck, and heart in the area surrounding the metatarso-phalangeal joint.
- **Acupuncture** identifies a pressure point on the fourth toe as a disturbance in the energy

flow of the gall bladder meridian; for the RTF therapist it is proves to be a possible disturbance in the region of the molars or the ears.

9.2.4 Summary

Our definition of abnormal zones does not contradict other points of view but supplements them with an interesting range. We have only to decide

which special therapeutic "language" we wish to use and adhere to its individual rules during treatment. Furthermore, all of a person's systems communicate with each other constantly de facto.

Note: Before the seven groups of zones are examined in detail (Chapter 10), the following four diagrams provide a dorsal, plantar, medial, and lateral view of the zones in full (**Figs. 9.1–9.4**). In the following chapters they are discussed in more detail.

Zones of the feet

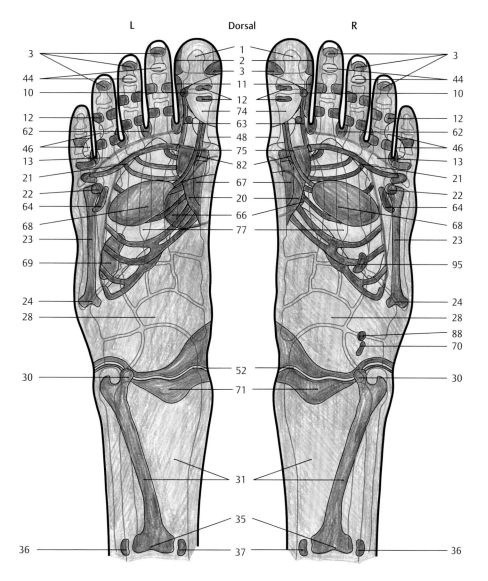

L   Dorsal   R

Bones, muscles, tissues		Sensory organs, endocrine system
1 Forehead	11 Head and neck, lateral	28 Abdominal wall
2 Temporal bone	12 ◼ Teeth	30 Femoral head
3 Frontal sinuses	13 Upper trapezius edge	31 Thigh, ventral
4 Roof of skull	20 Sternum	36 Knee, lateral
5 Lateral skull	21 Clavicle	37 Knee, medial
6 Lower occiput	22 Shoulder joint	40 Tissue, abdomen/
7 Mastoid process	23 Upper arm	pelvis
8 Sternocleidomastoid	24 Elbow	40a Sacrum and
9 Neck muscles	25 Rim of thorax	sacroiliac joint
10 Temporomandibular	26 Scapula	41 Lesser pelvis
joint	27 Diaphragm with	43 Ischial tuberosity
	pars lumbalis	

Sensory organs, endocrine system

44 Eye
45 Visual center
46 Ear
47 Pituitary gland
48 Thyroid
49 Adrenal gland
50 Pancreas
52 Fallopian tube
57 Solar plexus

Fig. 9.1 Zones of the feet (dorsal).

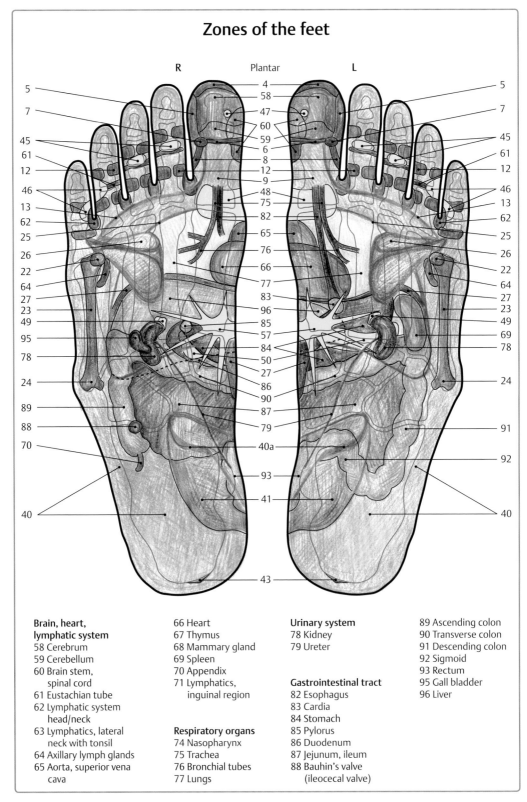

Zones of the feet

R   Plantar   L

Brain, heart, lymphatic system
58 Cerebrum
59 Cerebellum
60 Brain stem, spinal cord
61 Eustachian tube
62 Lymphatic system head/neck
63 Lymphatics, lateral neck with tonsil
64 Axillary lymph glands
65 Aorta, superior vena cava

66 Heart
67 Thymus
68 Mammary gland
69 Spleen
70 Appendix
71 Lymphatics, inguinal region

Respiratory organs
74 Nasopharynx
75 Trachea
76 Bronchial tubes
77 Lungs

Urinary system
78 Kidney
79 Ureter

Gastrointestinal tract
82 Esophagus
83 Cardia
84 Stomach
85 Pylorus
86 Duodenum
87 Jejunum, ileum
88 Bauhin's valve (ileocecal valve)

89 Ascending colon
90 Transverse colon
91 Descending colon
92 Sigmoid
93 Rectum
95 Gall bladder
96 Liver

Fig. 9.2 Zones of the feet (plantar).

Zones of the feet

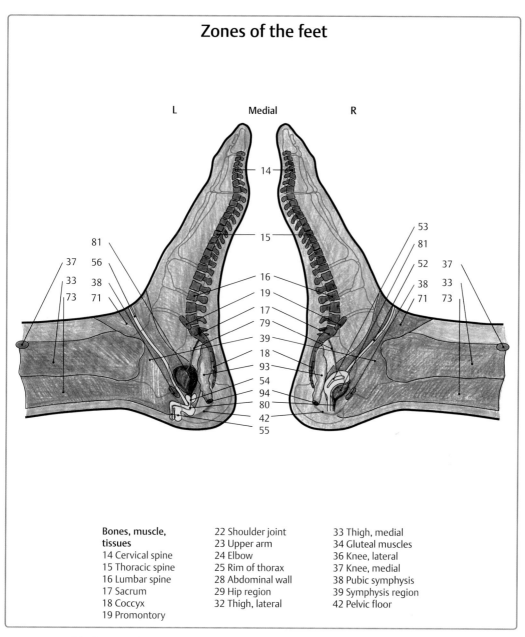

L   Medial   R

Bones, muscle, tissues
14 Cervical spine
15 Thoracic spine
16 Lumbar spine
17 Sacrum
18 Coccyx
19 Promontory

22 Shoulder joint
23 Upper arm
24 Elbow
25 Rim of thorax
28 Abdominal wall
29 Hip region
32 Thigh, lateral

33 Thigh, medial
34 Gluteal muscles
36 Knee, lateral
37 Knee, medial
38 Pubic symphysis
39 Symphysis region
42 Pelvic floor

Fig. 9.3 Zones of the feet (medial).

Zones of the feet

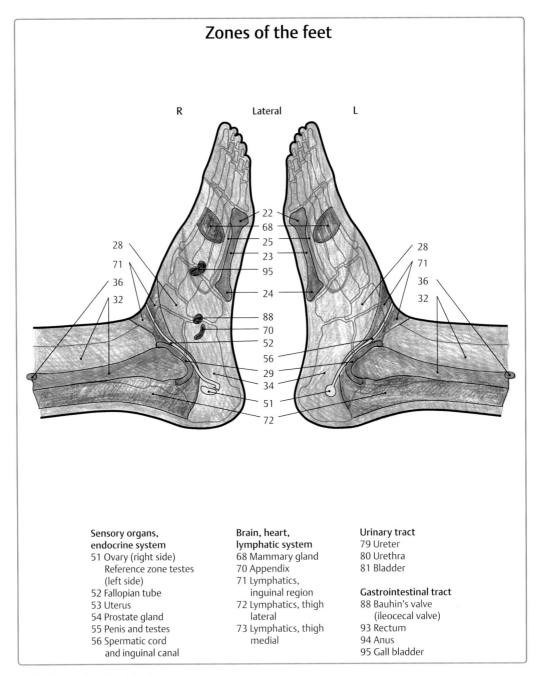

R   Lateral   L

Sensory organs, endocrine system	Brain, heart, lymphatic system	Urinary tract
51 Ovary (right side) Reference zone testes (left side)	68 Mammary gland	79 Ureter
52 Fallopian tube	70 Appendix	80 Urethra
53 Uterus	71 Lymphatics, inguinal region	81 Bladder
54 Prostate gland	72 Lymphatics, thigh lateral	**Gastrointestinal tract**
55 Penis and testes	73 Lymphatics, thigh medial	88 Bauhin's valve (ileocecal valve)
56 Spermatic cord and inguinal canal		93 Rectum
		94 Anus
		95 Gall bladder

Fig. 9.4 Zones of the feet (lateral).

10 The Individual Groups of Zones

10.1

Introduction

A **complete overview** of the reflex zones from plantar, dorsal, medial, and lateral sides can be seen in Chapter 9 (**Figs. 9.1–9.4**). Each of the following descriptions of individual groups of zones is divided as follows:
- General information on the individual zones
- Illustration of the group
- Description of the anatomical position of the zones
- Description of the treatment technique in the individual zones

The illustrations are **color-coded** as follows:
- Green: bones and tissue
- Blue: respiratory organs
- Red: urinary tract
- Yellow: solar plexus, sensory organs, and endocrine glands
- Brown: digestive tract
- Orange: brain, heart, and lymphatic system.

The approved direction of work is shown by arrows marked on the illustrations of the groups. The **basic rule** for localizing the zones is as follows:
- Ventral side of a person = dorsal side of the feet
- Dorsal side of a person = plantar side of the feet.

> While working in the zones it is of great benefit if one is aware of the fact that "feet" mirrror the entire person. Mentally uniting the microsystem and macrosystem of the person thereby increases the quality of the treatment as a whole.

Note: In **Fig. 10.1** I should like to point out the astonishing accuracy and therapeutic significance of the similarity in shape between the person in situ and their feet: 15 important joints and bony transitions on a large scale can also be recognized in proportion as joints and transitions in the feet.

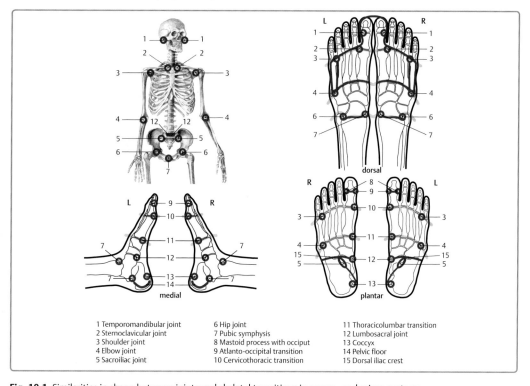

1 Temporomandibular joint	6 Hip joint	11 Thoracicolumbar transition
2 Sternoclavicular joint	7 Pubic symphysis	12 Lumbosacral joint
3 Shoulder joint	8 Mastoid process with occiput	13 Coccyx
4 Elbow joint	9 Atlanto-occipital transition	14 Pelvic floor
5 Sacroiliac joint	10 Cervicothoracic transition	15 Dorsal iliac crest

Fig. 10.1 Similarities in shape between joints and skeletal transitions in macro- and micro-systems.

With this stable "framework" of the joints, the principle of the person, scaled down in the foot, becomes particularly clear and finding all the other zones thus becomes easier.

The pubic symphysis zone on the medial transition from the heel to the ankle bone is also included. Although it is not shown here, it can be seen in **Fig. 9.3**.

In some zone descriptions, there are **overlaps** with groups to be discussed later. Thus, for example, the lymphatic region of the head and neck is not explained with illustrations and text until group 7, the lymphatic system, although it also belongs to the head and neck zones; the pancreas is discussed in group 4, the endocrine glands, but is also part of group 6, which contains the digestive organs.

10.2

Zones of the Head and Neck

10.2.1 General Information

Since projections have been treated on the foot, a phenomenon has been observed for the toes as zones of the head and neck that eludes linear logic but is confirmed in daily practice; namely, on the one hand, the zones of the head and neck can be found concentrated in the two big toes, on the other hand, they are reflected in greater detail in all the toes. Both options are shown in the following illustrations. The zones of the head and neck are supplemented by the zones of the teeth and jaw.

10.2.2 Illustration of the Zones

(Figs. 10.2, 10.3)

10.2.3 Anatomical Location of the Zones

In the Two Big Toes

Unlike the other toes, the big toes contain only two bones on which the zones of the head and neck are located in the same way as in situ.

On the dorsal side we find the zones of ventral (frontal) organs and tissue of the head and neck, for example, the forehead, nasopharynx, and mandibular joint. (This joint is discussed in more detail in Chapter 28.) The zones of the head region are seen from the dorsal side on the plantar side of the big toe, for example, the brain, lower occiput with mastoid process, and neck.

Organs and tissue situated on the median line of the head and neck are represented on the medial sides of both big toes; the outer areas laterally.

From the plantar side of the foot, the similarity in shape between the two big toes and the head and neck is easy to comprehend, thus the rounded shape of the two closely arranged **distal phalanges** of the big toes corresponds to the head, the **end joints** of the toes to the atlanto-occipital joint. The somewhat narrower shape of the two proximal phalanxes resembles the shape of the neck as it narrows from the head.

In the Second to Fifth Toes on the Right and Left

The four toes, consisting of the distal, middle and proximal phalanges, are limited on their medial and lateral sides by interdigital skin folds, while from their plantar and dorsal sides they can each be treated as far as their anatomical beginning in the toe joints. The zones of the eyes, ears, frontal and maxillary sinuses, and teeth are displayed in detail on the toes.

Figs. 10.2 and **10.3** can only show the ventral and dorsal aspects of the toes. However, there are also zones on the medial and lateral sides of the toes, above all those of the tooth–jaw region.

The Tooth–Jaw Region

The zones of the teeth and jaw cover the whole functional unit of the tooth, the tissue of the tooth with its root, the bony structure, the adjacent gingiva (mucosa), and the nerve supply of the maxilla and mandible. They are therefore relatively extensive and cover dorsal, medial, lateral, and plantar areas of the middle and proximal phalanges. The zones of the teeth often extend to the distal and middle phalanx; how far depends on the size of the roots. Usually the places shown in **Fig. 10.2** are the most sensitive, however. We distinguish between

- the maxilla (upper jaw): located in the middle of the middle phalanges of the second to fifth toes;
- the mandible (lower jaw): located around the distal parts of the second to fifth proximal phalanges.

However, on the big toe, the zones of the first incisors (tooth 1) are found more in the dorsal area, directly distal and proximal to the joint between the distal and proximal phalanx.

Medially **and** laterally, each of the toes 2, 3, and 4 has a zone in the distal and proximal areas; the fifth toe corresponds to the wisdom teeth

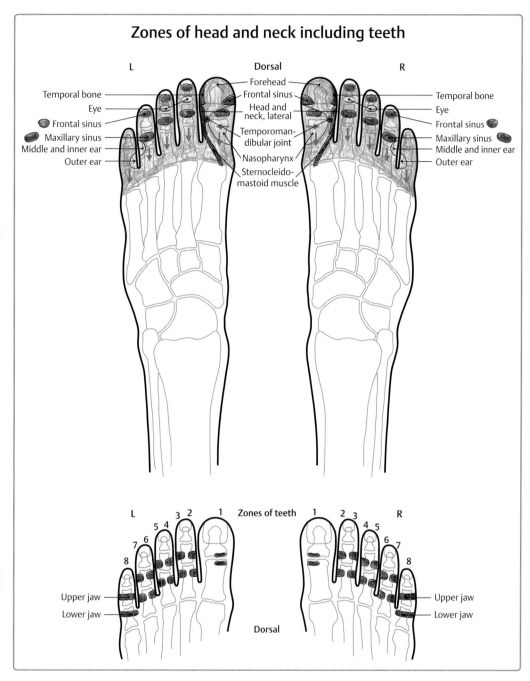

Fig. 10.2 Zones of the head and neck and teeth (dorsal).

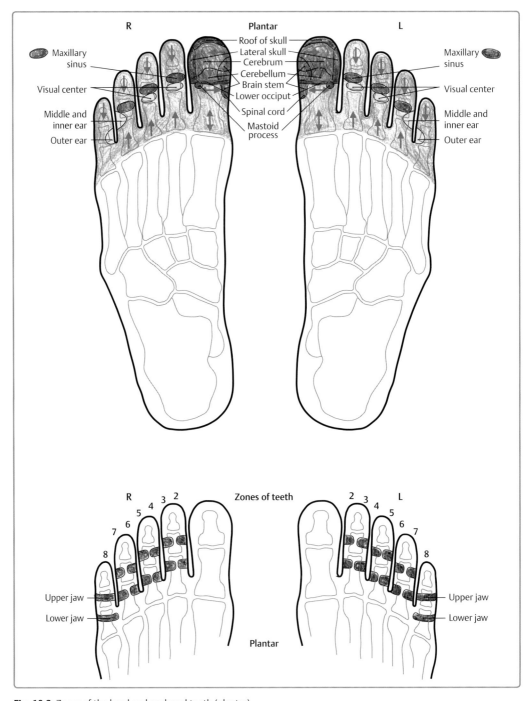

Fig. 10.3 Zones of the head and neck and teeth (plantar).

(tooth 8) distally and proximally from all four sides.

As aforementioned, it is only possible to touch upon the medial and lateral parts in the illustrations of the zones of the teeth (**Figs. 10.2, 10.3**). However, the sides of the toes are often effective in terms of treatment.

10.2.4 Treatment Technique

Treatment of the Big Toes

Unless the therapist has a very long trunk, the treatment should almost always be performed with the index finger on the dorsal surface of the big toe and the thumb on the plantar side.

The nails of the big toes (corresponding to the zones of the forehead) are treated with the thumbnail or index finger nail, the strength of the therapist's own nails permitting (**Fig. 10.4**). They often prove more sensitive than expected.

On the plantar side of the distal phalanx (lower occiput), we work with the vertically positioned thumb in a horizontal direction toward the heel well into the joint between the proximal and distal phalanges (**Fig. 10.5**).

It is rather more difficult to treat the entire length of the lateral side of the big toes as the interdigital tissue covers part of the proximal phalanx and has to be pushed aside by the working finger to a certain extent in order to be able to reach the zones of the transverse processes of the lower cervical spine with the tip of the index finger.

Mobilization of the big toe joints should be performed as follows:

As a saddle joint, the **distal** joint of the big toe is moved into plantar flexion under slight extension.
Important Note about Dosing:
Delicate, cautious, minimal movements should be used initially for patients with skull fractures or brain trauma in order to avoid aggravating the symptoms.

When treating the metatarsophalangeal joint, several variations present themselves, all of which must be performed using cautious extension:
- Gentle up and down movements using good stabilization of the base of the proximal phalanx of the big toe and the head of the first metatarsal bone, or
- Circular movements, both in a medial to lateral direction and vice versa, beginning with small, gradually increasing movements, or
- Semicircular rotation in plantar and dorsal directions.

Beware of overdosing patients suffering from trauma in the neck region and/or from other chronic or acute problems in the region of the thyroid and heart (segmental correspondence with the seventh cervical vertebra).

When mobilizing the big toe, it is advisable to begin slowly and carefully in order to be able to evaluate the patient's current reactions correctly. Usually four to six movements in each direction suffice; now and then, however, more are indicated, above all, to release severe muscular tension in the head and neck.

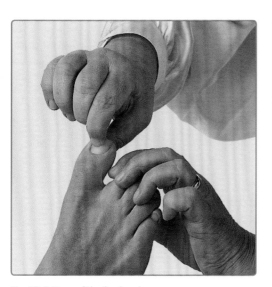

Fig. 10.4 Zone of the forehead.

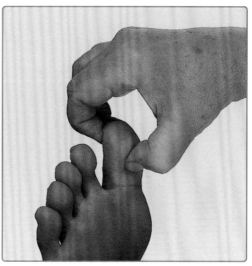

Fig. 10.5 Zone of the lower occiput.

Cautious movements and compressions (instead of extension) from the subtle technique Ortho-Bionomy by **Dr. A. Pauls** are particularly suitable for the structural treatment of the toes. Instead of compression, the term approximation is usually used there (Kain).

Technique for the Second to Fifth Toes, Right and Left

The thumb is used to work on the plantar side of the toes, usually with the index finger on the dorsal side. The lateral borders can also be treated with the index fingers. Like the big toe, the **toenails** are treated specifically with the therapist' own fingernail, emphasizing in particular their proximal parts (zones of the frontal sinuses).

During treatment, toes should remain in their normal position and not be bent too much. The free hand therefore holds and supports the toes being treated at the metatarsophalangeal joints.

The second to fifth toes can also be brought into slight extension. Even with gentle stretching, a surprising "cracking" sound can sometimes be heard, mainly in the metatarsophalangeal joints. This usually provides relief not only in the joint itself, but also in the corresponding zones of the head, neck, and shoulder girdle. Extension should **never** be performed **too vehemently** in order to prevent injuries involving the tissue and joint itself.

Stretching the individual toes not only brings relief to the bones of the feet, but also releases overtension throughout the body, as evidenced by deeper breathing. Recent experience shows that in

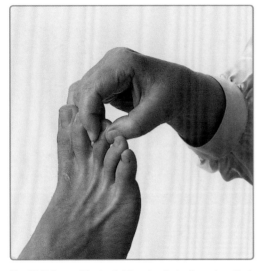

Fig. 10.6 Zone of the teeth (thumb or index finger is active).

addition to the big toe joints, the joints of the four smaller toes can also sometimes be treated more effectively with grips from Ortho-Bionomy.

Technique for the Zones of the Teeth and Jaws

(**Fig. 10.6**)
The zones of the teeth and jaws are always included in a nonspecific manner in the aforementioned treatment of the toes.

For targeted treatment of the zones of the teeth and jaws, we work in half-circles from the plantar surface over the side of the toe to its dorsal aspect, and vice versa. As with all zones, here too the strain within the overall area of the zones of the teeth is often uneven.

The **basis of the proximal phalanges of the toes** is inadvertently presumed to be too distal usually; exact anatomical orientation will help to correct the miscalculation of the position, above all, in a plantar direction.

For treatment indications pertaining to the head and neck group of zones, see Chapter 21.2.

10.3
Zones of the Spine, Thorax, and Shoulder Girdle

10.3.1   General Information

These zones form an "axis of coordinates" in the feet. Placed side by side, the two longitudinal arches touch in the median line, and as the zone of the spine they form the vertical bars, while as the shoulder girdle the two horizontal bars form the horizontal part. Although the spine is usually considered to be part of the skeletal structure, it can also be understood as a central "organ" because of its direct connection with all the tissues and organs within the body through the nervous system, not only in situ but also in the zones of the feet.

10.3.2   Illustration of the Zones
(**Figs. 10.7, 10.8**)

10.3.3   Anatomical Location of the Zones

Zones of the Spine

The appearance of these zones emphasizes particularly clearly the similarity in shape between the bends of the longitudinal arch and the lordosis of the spine. Representing an area in the center of the

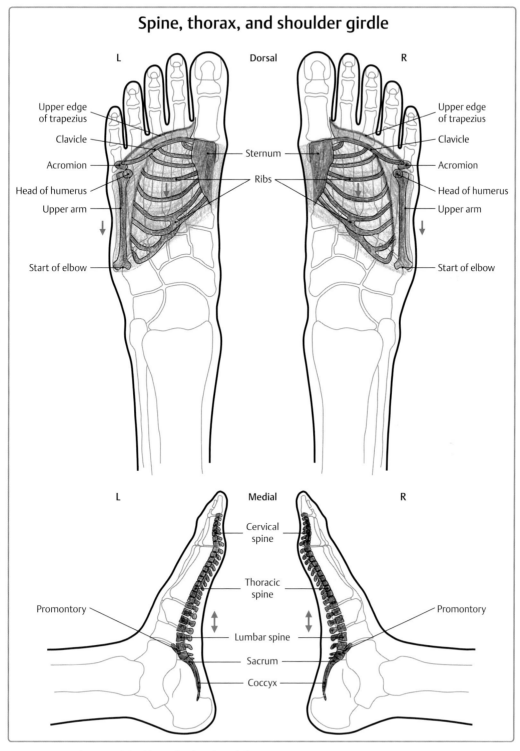

Fig. 10.7 Spine, thorax, and shoulder girdle (dorsal, medial).

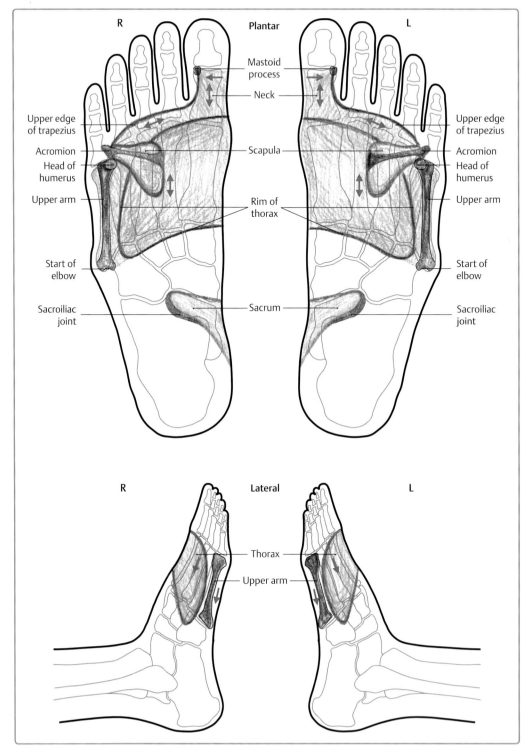

Fig. 10.8 Spine, thorax and shoulder girdle (plantar, lateral).

body, they can be found on the right **and** left foot in longitudinal body zone 1.

Their respective location extends from the medial side of the FitzGerald longitudinal body zone 1 to their lateral side and can therefore comprise the entire width of the vertebrae. The spinous processes, which are particularly suitable for the **neutral** treatment of the vertebrae, are easy to reach in the sinewy muscular area of the medial plantar side.

The more the entire width of the plantar longitudinal body zone 1 is included, the more the vertebrae are included in their entirety, as far as the transverse processes.

The bony part of the longitudinal arch, seen from the medial side, above all, serves to distinguish the individual sections of the vertebrae precisely. It is worth palpating them carefully to be certain in differentiating their various sections (see **Fig. 10.1**).

The Individual Sections of the Spine

- **Cervical vertebrae 1 to 7:** Their spinous processes are arranged on the medial-plantar side of the proximal phalanx of the big toes, the transverse processes on their lateral side. The **distal** phalanx of the big toe corresponds to the lower occiput at the transition to the cervical spine. The **metatarsophalangeal** joint of the big toe characterizes the transition from the neck to the thoracic spine.
- **Thoracic vertebrae 1 to 12:** The spinous processes are located in the medial-plantar tissue along the entire length of the first metatarsal bone. The transverse processes can be detected on the plantar side at the lateral limit of the entire first metatarsal bone.
- The transition from the base of the first metatarsal bone to the first cuneiform bone represents the start of the so-called **Lisfranc's line** which in situ roughly corresponds to the waistline. At the same time, it is also the transition to the lumbar spine. This point requires particularly keen and precise palpation and at the same time is **one of the most important orientation guides** for locating the zones of the central abdominal region.
- **Lumbar vertebrae 1 to 5:** The spinous processes pass from the medial-plantar tissue of the first cuneiform bone to the proximal end of the navicular bone, the transverse processes must be treated on the plantar side at the lateral limit of the first cuneiform bone and the longitudinal half of the navicular bone.

- The medial navicular bone, which protrudes somewhat in many patients, marks the transition to the sacrum with its proximal limit and corresponds to the **promontory**, a well-known weak point not only in the longitudinal arch, but also in situ.
- **Sacrum:** Its upper limit begins on the plantar side at the point of contact of the navicular bone and talus and extends horizontally into the Fitzgerald longitudinal body zone 2 or 3. The diagonal limit runs from the lateral to the medial side. The **sacroiliac joint**, which occupies approximately a third of this section, begins at the point at which its horizontal plane passes into the diagonal plane. As organs and tissue often overlap in situ, here too it is only possible to distinguish from the disease pattern of the patient whether primarily the sacroiliac joint or the small intestine are treated.
- **Coccyx:** The diagonal end of the sacrum, now in the longitudinal body zone 1 again, marks the start of the short section of the coccyx, likewise on both feet.

Zones of the Thorax and Shoulder Girdle

The zones of the **thorax** are located on the plantar and dorsal sides of the metatarsal bones, roughly along the first metatarsal bone to the medial limit of the fifth metatarsal bone. According to the shape of the thorax in situ, the external lower edge extends to the third cuneiform bone and the cuboid bone, while the medial edge leads to the lower third of the first metatarsal bone where it connects with the zone of the sternum.

The metatarsophalangeal joints represent the zones of the **shoulder girdle**, connected segmentally to the liver and gall bladder on the right and to the heart on the left side.

The **shoulder joints** with the head of the humerus as the outer limit of the shoulder girdle can, as in the body, also be recognized as a joint area on the foot: this is the site where the medial part of the head of the fifth metatarsal bone touches the lateral part of the head of the fourth metatarsal bone.

Although the foot essentially resembles the zones of the head, neck, and trunk, starting from the zone of the shoulder joint, the **upper arm** as far as the **elbow** can be treated along the entire surface of the fifth metatarsal bone. The similarity in shape between the upper arm and the fifth metatarsal bone is particularly noticeable.

The **sternum**, located on the median line in the body, is found on both feet on the dorsum of the first metatarsal bone. This zone comprises approximately two thirds of its length; the lateral limit of the first metatarsal bone corresponds to the **sternocostal joints**.

10.3.4   Treatment Technique

Zones of the Spine

(**Fig. 10.9**)
According to the indication, the **spine** can be treated with the thumb in both distal to proximal direction and vice versa. With **neutral** treatment of the spine, we do not work directly on the bony surface of the longitudinal arch, but in the muscle and connective tissue on the medial-plantar side. For **specific** strains, however, we include it.

In order to be able to target treatment of the **promontory** (**Fig. 10.10**) as a zone, we place the thumb on the transition between the navicular bone, talus, and calcaneus and continue on the plantar plane between the navicular bone and talus.

Zones of the Thorax and Shoulder Girdle

These zones can be treated with the thumb on the plantar side from distal to proximal in adjacent lines. As a result of this treatment direction, the slack tissue around the metatarsophalangeal joints (zone of the shoulder girdle) is strengthened, at least passively. If the foot is positioned in outward rotation, the metatarsal area can also be treated from proximal to distal with the same effect.

In the dorsal region of the metatarsal bones only the inter-metatarsal spaces are treated to avoid too strong and direct stimulation of the periosteum. These zones can be treated with ease using the index finger, while the thumb of the free hand holds and supports the plantar side of the forefoot in the center of the metatarsophalangeal joints. The zones of the **upper arm** (**Fig. 10.11**) are treated on the dorsal, lateral, and plantar sides of the fifth metatarsal.

The **shoulder joints** can easily be reached on the dorsal side using the index finger, while the thumb is more appropriate on the plantar side.

The **sternum** (**Fig. 10.12**) can be treated both from distal to proximal or from medial to lateral in several adjacent lines. Usually, the index finger is the most suitable.

For treatment indications pertaining to the group of zones of the spine and shoulder girdle, see Chapter 21.3.

10.4

Zones of the Urinary Tract, Bones and Tissue of the Pelvis to the Knee

10.4.1   General Information

To provide an overview, this extensive area is divided into two main groups. The zones of the

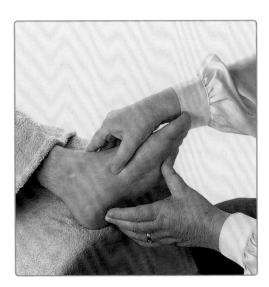

Fig. 10.9 Zones of the spine from cranial to caudal.

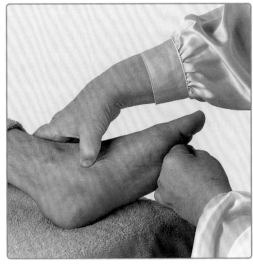

Fig. 10.10 Skeletal orientation for the zone of the promontory.

General Principles

urinary tract comprise both of the kidneys, the ureter, bladder, and urethra.

In detail, the zones of the iliac bones with the gluteus muscles, pubic symphysis, and symphyseal area and the hip joints from ventral, lateral, and dorsal sides are found within the zones of the **pelvic girdle**. The medial, ventral, lateral, and dorsal sides of the thighs and knees are arranged in the distal part of the lower leg.

10.4.2 Illustration of the Zones
(**Figs. 10.13, 10.14**)

10.4.3 Anatomical Location of the Zones

Zones of the Kidneys, Ureter, and Bladder

As the size and/or location of all the zones, in particular that of the **kidneys**, may vary physiologically, the average location of the zones is plotted around the base of the third metatarsal bone as far as the third cuneiform bone. From there the sensitive thumb will, by causing pain, be able to detect where the kidney zones are individually located in the event of illness or ptosis.

The zones of the **ureter** lead toward the sacrum and their lower third is medial to the flexor tendon of the hallucis longus muscle. They continue from their plantar surface to the medial insides of the heels and onward into the zone of the bladder.

The zone of the **bladder** is located equally on both feet as a projection of an organ in the center of the body. It is located on the medial-proximal part of the calcaneus and its upper limit partly touches the talus. In the bladder zone in particular, variations in the location and tone can often be noticed in situ depending on the content and strain on the bladder, for example, during pregnancy or with postoperative urine retention.

In males the zone of the **urethra** is surrounded by the prostate gland and passes through the penis near the beginning of the Achilles tendon immediately after the bladder, slightly proximal to the upper inner edge of the calcaneus. In females the zone of the urethra directly leads into the perineum. The illustration (**Fig.10.13**) shows the female and the male urinary systems on the medial heel view of one foot each, although both female and male systems are treated on the respective zones of both feet. In practical work they can hardly be differentiated.

The zones of the **perineum** run across the proximal part of the calcaneus on both feet and are of major physiological as well as possibly therapeutic significance for women during and after delivery (Chapter 22).

Zones of the Pelvis and the Thigh to the Knees

The plantar part of the calcaneus is related to the tissue of the lower **abdomen** and **pelvis** from

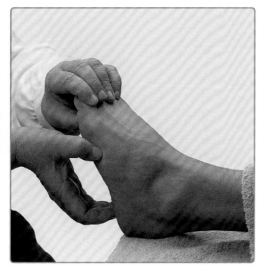

Fig. 10.11 Zone of the upper arm.

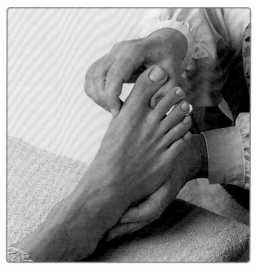

Fig. 10.12 Metatarsophalangeal joint. Somewhat dorsal: medial part of the zone of the sternum.

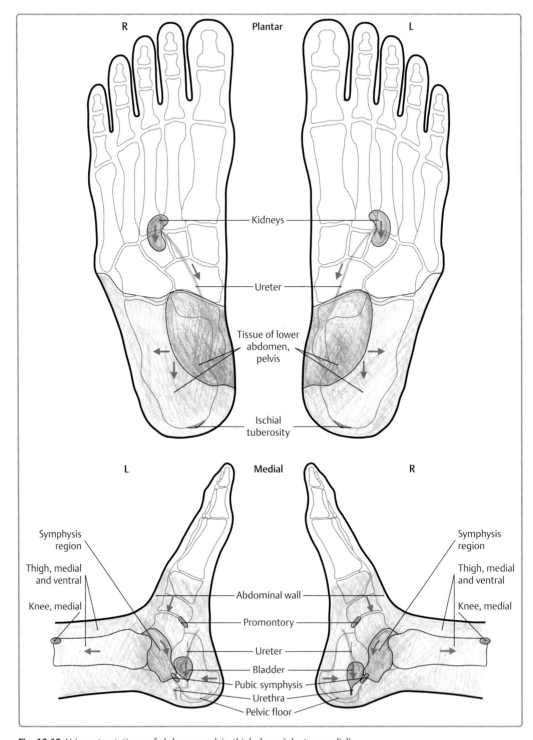

Fig. 10.13 Urinary tract, tissue of abdomen–pelvis, thigh–knee (plantar, medial).

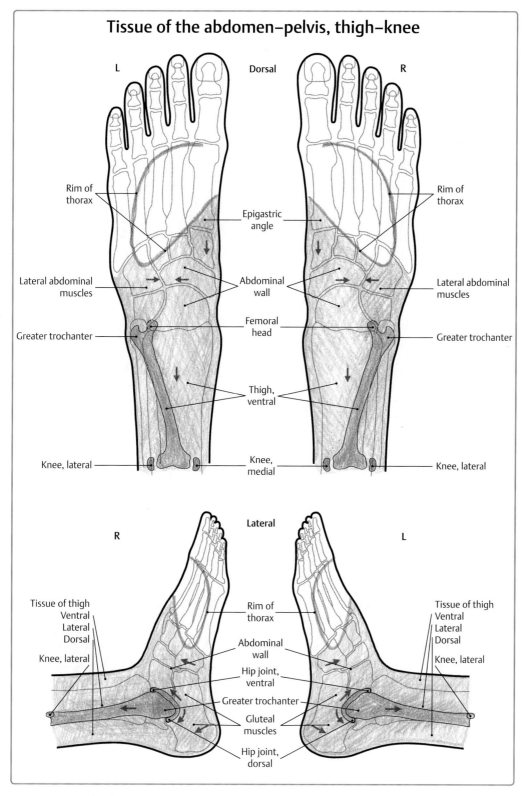

Tissue of the abdomen–pelvis, thigh–knee

L

Dorsal

R

Rim of thorax

Epigastric angle

Lateral abdominal muscles

Abdominal wall

Lateral abdominal muscles

Greater trochanter

Femoral head

Greater trochanter

Thigh, ventral

Knee, lateral

Knee, medial

Knee, lateral

Lateral

R

L

Tissue of thigh
Ventral
Lateral
Dorsal

Rim of thorax

Tissue of thigh
Ventral
Lateral
Dorsal

Knee, lateral

Abdominal wall

Knee, lateral

Hip joint, ventral

Greater trochanter

Gluteal muscles

Hip joint, dorsal

Fig. 10.14 Tissue of abdomen–pelvis, thigh–knee (dorsal, lateral).

behind. However, the tissue here is often tough. These zones on the medial areas of the tarsal bones as far as the inner malleoli can be reached with less effort.

The zone of the **pubic symphysis** can be palpated most clearly on a small medial groove where the calcaneus meets the rear part of the talus on both feet.

The tissue underneath the medial malleolus along the talus is called the symphyseal **area**. This requires a brief explanation. There is a **similarity** between the shape of the foot and a seated person, but the **similarity** in shape is not true to scale at all points. Thus, for example, the thorax is larger in situ than the pelvis; however, as a reflex zone the pelvis appears larger than the thorax as the entire tarsal area is related to it. This comparison makes it easier to understand why the entire length and width of the medial part of the talus is described as the zone of the symphyseal **area**. In addition, it has been observed for decades that this point is very effective in the treatment of disturbances in the pelvic organs.

The ventral, lateral, medial, and dorsal **muscles of the thigh** can be found from the mortise to approximately a hand's width above the (patient's!) knuckles and finish in the zones of the knee. The section along the periosteum of the distal fibula corresponds to the zone of the iliotibial tract.

The zones of the **knee** can be subdivided as follows: the medial area is to be treated on the ventral side of the tibia, while the lateral part should be treated on the ventral side of the fibula. The **patella** lies between the two. The **popliteal fossa** can be found on the dorsal side of the lower leg opposite the patella.

The tissue on the proximal two thirds of the lateral calcaneus is related to the **gluteus muscles**; the **lateral abdominal muscles** can be treated somewhat more distally as far as the cuboid bone, third cuneiform bone, and the lateral part of the navicular bone.

The entire zone of the **hip joint** can be reached by working around the lateral malleolus; the head of the femur can best be found at the bony connection between fibula and talus from the dorsal side of the foot; the laterally most protruding point of the lateral ankle corresponds to the **greater trochanter**.

10.4.4 Treatment Technique

Zones of the Kidneys, Ureter, and Bladder

As the zones of the **kidneys** are usually smaller than the distal phalanx of the therapist's thumb,

we should take care to palpate them precisely, passing into the zone of the ureter in a linear fashion (**Fig. 10.15**).

The zone of the **ureter** is usually treated following the direction of the flow of urine. Only in the event of a **kidney stone** in the ureter do we first work in the opposite direction from the bladder to the kidney.

At the transition from the plantar to the medial side, the zone of the ureter passes very close to the zone of the sacrum. In 1930s the zone of the bladder was treated there by E. Ingham, in the direction of the medial malleolus. Today we assign this point to the **innervation** of the pelvic organs, in other words, **indirectly** to the bladder as well. The bladder as an organ behind the pubic symphysis arose as a result of multiple practical examinations. **Both** the zone of innervation and that of the organ are treated if there is a corresponding indication.

Zones of the Pelvic Girdle and Lower Extremities to the Knee

In the **zone of the pubic symphysis** it is advisable to apply the therapeutic grip cautiously, as overreactions may occur surprisingly quickly here, probably due to the fact, among other things, that pertaining to the pelvic organs as this area does, it may also be functionally disrupted by emotional strains on the endocrine system (difficulties in partner relationships, hormonal disorders, sexual abuse, etc.). It can be treated selectively as a small, elongated area using the tip of the index finger.

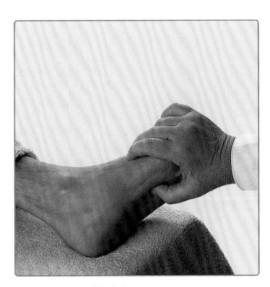

Fig. 10.15 Zone of the kidney.

I have treated several pregnant women with a loosened pubic symphysis—from approximately the seventh and eighth month of gestation onward—using reflexotherapy of the feet. This resulted in improvement of the major difficulties they complained of while sitting, standing, or walking.

For treatment of the symphyseal **area**, we clearly place the foot in the center of the treatment table and hold it in external rotation with the free hand. The therapist bends keeping the spine straight until the thumb can be gently drawn in a semicircle along the talus from distal to proximal.

While it is possible to work very firmly with the thumb on the plantar side of the heel as a zone of the **abdomen–pelvis area**, on the medial side of the heel gentle fingertips or thumb grips should be employed.

On the lateral edge of the foot the lateral **abdominal and gluteus muscles** (**Fig. 10.16**) are treated with one or two fingertips from the cuboid bone to the proximal end of the calcaneus. If the hand can perform good supination, the thumb can also be used there.

The front quarter of the zone of the **hip joint** (**Fig. 10.17**) around the lateral malleolus is almost always easy to reach with the thumb; for the rear quarter in the direction of the Achilles tendon the index finger is usually used.

The medial and ventral sides of the **thighs** (**Fig. 10.18**) are treated with the thumb and the lateral and dorsal sides with the fingertips. If the iliotibial tract requires special treatment (e.g., if there is a scar on the outer thigh in situ), it makes

more sense to use the thumb for this section. For this, good supination of the hand under the heel and slight inner rotation of the foot are necessary. Care should be taken not to apply too much pressure to the foot during inner rotation.

The zones of the **knee** are treated selectively with the thumb or index finger. In the event of disorders of the knee, they may be painful within a radius of approximately 1 to 2 cm.

For treatment indications for the group of zones pertaining to the urinary tract, pelvis to the knee, see Chapters 21.3 and 21.4.2.

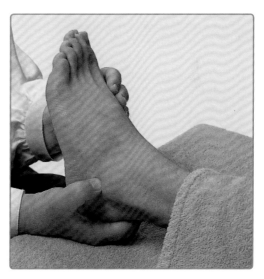

Fig. 10.17 Zone of the hip joint.

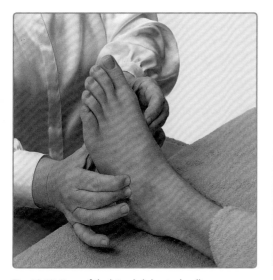

Fig. 10.16 Zone of the lateral abdominal wall.

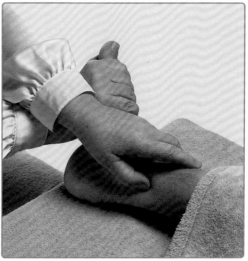

Fig. 10.18 Zone of the medial thigh.

10.5

Zones of the Endocrine System

10.5.1 General Information

A minimum of treatment experience has been available hitherto for the **pituitary gland** in this system. In the course of practice, I have had only a few opportunities to examine it (pre- and post-operatively) in patients with **tumors** of the pituitary gland. The evident pain and responses confirm that the zone of the pituitary gland can be treated at the specified point. This zone is also treated in other hormonal disorders (e.g., menstrual cycle complaints).

With the other endocrine glands, it is significantly easier to find and treat the zones.

> **Important:** If **one** endocrine gland is dysfunctional, all the others should be treated at the same time because their functions are coordinated.

10.5.2 Illustration of the Zones

(Figs. 10.19, 10.20)

10.5.3 Topography

The **pituitary gland** can be accessed from the plantar side on the medial edge of the periosteum of the distal phalanges of both big toes where the bone widens into its base.

The **thyroid gland** can be treated on both the dorsal and plantar sides. The dorsal zone is on the proximal third of the proximal phalanx of the big toes, over approximately two thirds of their width. The plantar site surrounds the two metatarsophalangeal joints and is more extensive than the dorsal site. Strictly speaking, it is the zone around the seventh cervical vertebra, in other words, a **reference zone** for the thyroid gland, because the seventh cervical vertebra is located in situ opposite the thyroid gland. If this tissue is congested and thickened by additional connective tissue, the site is known as a "widow's hump."

The **thymus** will be discussed in connection with the lymphatic system, though it could also have been included in the endocrine system (Chapter 10.8).

The **adrenal glands** are located at the distal end of the kidneys and partially protrude somewhat into the space between the bases of the second and third metatarsal bones.

The **pancreas** can be divided into different zonal areas: the **head** is located on the right foot between the base of the first metatarsal bone and the first cuneiform bone; the center and caudal end are located on the left foot between the bases of the first, second, and third metatarsal bones, laterally adjoined by the zone of the spleen.

The zones of the **genital organs** are arranged medially on both feet between the center and proximal third of the calcaneus. In women the uterus is located here. It leads directly into the vagina which connects with the pelvic floor, known as the perineum.

As the tarsal bones, as zones of the lower abdominal region and pelvis, are significantly wider and larger in proportion than the abdomen–pelvis area in situ, the **ovaries** and **fallopian tubes** can be treated laterally as well as medially on the calcaneus.

The medial points of the fallopian tubes and ovaries are not shown in the figures; they are partly identical to the uterus and continue to approximately the beginning of the talus. From a **lateral** direction, the ovary can be found in the center of an imaginary diagonal line between the lower edge of the outer malleolus and the rounded rectangular tip of the heel and continues from there in a somewhat distal direction.

The **fallopian tubes** connect the ovaries to the uterus on the right and left foot, starting from beneath the lateral malleolus. In the male the **testes** and the **penis** are connected to the **prostate**, the location of which approximately corresponds to the location of the uterus in the female pelvis, on the upper inner edge of the calcaneus.

It is true for both the male and female genital zones that the **inguinal canal** largely corresponds to the zone of the fallopian tubes. However, similar to the lateral position of the ovary and the fallopian tube, the testes, the inguinal canal, and the spermatic cord can also be treated in a lateral to medial direction.

10.5.4 Treatment Technique

The zone of the **pituitary gland** is treated selectively in a medial to plantar direction with the tip of the thumb pointing toward the heel (similar position to that for the zones of the occiput and eustachian tubes). We include it as an essential part of treatment of the endocrine system for hormonal disorders and insufficiencies.

In patients with head and skull trauma, tumors, or operations in the head area, however, only the sedating grip is used here consistently, or it is omitted completely.

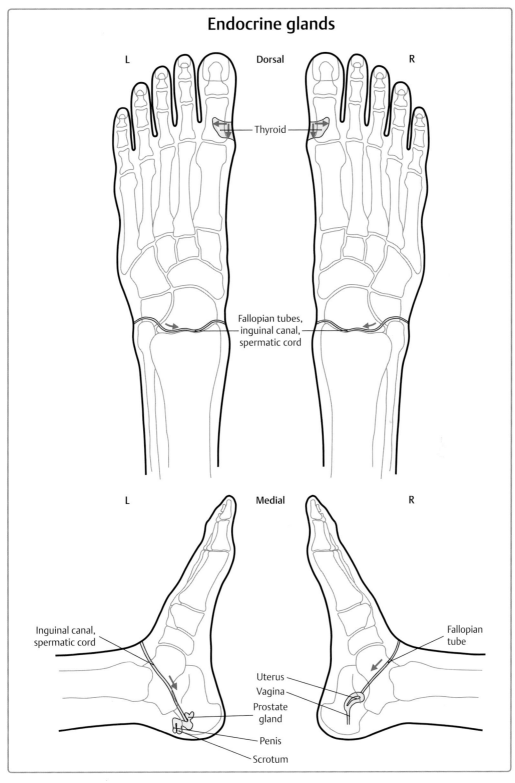

Fig. 10. 19 Endocrine glands (dorsal, medial).

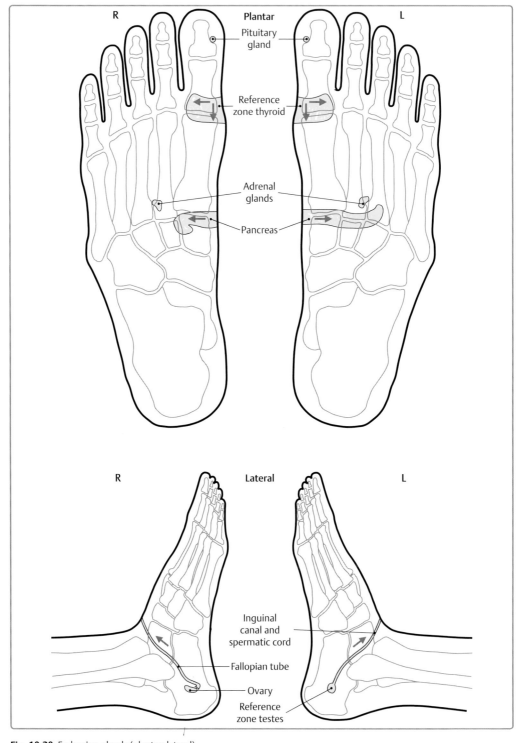

Fig. 10.20 Endocrine glands (plantar, lateral).

The dorsal part of the **thyroid gland** can be treated in a medial to lateral direction with the index finger while the thumb is used for the plantar side. An overly strong lateral flection of the metatarsophalangeal joint of the big toe and a change in the position of the first metatarsal bone is frequently observed as **hallux valgus** in patients with disorders of the thyroid gland. As a consequence, treatment of disorders in this area should be cautious, and mobilization of the first metatarsophalangeal joints of the big toe must also be gentle, for example, employing Ortho-Bionomy treatment techniques.

The **adrenal glands** can scarcely be differentiated from the kidneys; their distal part is selectively treated for disorders (e.g., in patients suffering from asthma, rheumatic conditions, or allergies) in a gently tonifying manner.

The **pancreas** is treated from medial to lateral on the right foot (pancreas head), on the left (central and caudal part) likewise from medial to lateral along the Lisfranc's joint line as far as the base of the fourth metatarsal bone. It goes without saying that in **diabetic** patients the blood-sugar level must be monitored particularly carefully during treatment. (For more detailed treatment indications, see Chapter. 21.5.2, section "Diabetes mellitus.")

The **genital organs** are selectively treated from medial and lateral directions, either with the index finger or gently with the thumb. Similar to the treatment technique in the lymphatic zones of the groin (Chapter 10.8.4, section "lymphatic system"), the connection from the external to the internal genitals—in the woman corresponding to the **fallopian tubes**, in the man the **inguinal canal** and **spermatic cord** (Fig. 10.22)—is treated with the thumb. In both men and women, the medial zones usually prove to be more painful.

The zones of the **prostate**, **scrotum**, and **testes** are located as close to each other as they are in situ. The zones are treated with the index finger or thumb: prostate on the proximal edge of the zone of the bladder, testes in the vicinity of the upper inner calcaneus edge.

In both men and women the genital zones are relatively sensitive to touch, even in the absence of chronic or acute diseases. As the endocrine system has a close functional connection with the autonomous nervous system and both are related to our moods, pain in these zones may also indicate problems and difficulties relating to partnerships or traumatic experiences in childhood or adolescence. Toxins and waste materials from the pelvic and digestive organs often accumulate in the **pouch of Douglas** (peritoneal fold between rectum and genital organs). As the digestive and genital organs partly overlap here, these zones should in general be treated with caution initially.

For treatment indications pertaining to the group of zones of the endocrine system, see Chapter 21.5.

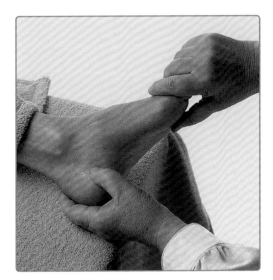

Fig. 10.21 Zones of the pelvis (start).

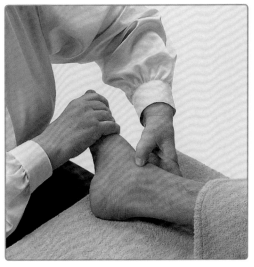

Fig. 10.22 Treatment of the zones of the fallopian tubes/ inguinal canal.

10.6

Zones of the Respiratory Organs and Heart

10.6.1 General Information

The zones of the respiratory organs start in the dorsal area of the two big toes as the **nasopharynx** and together with the zones of the heart and upper abdominal organs, they cover the whole midfoot area as far as the fifth metatarsal bone.

The **heart** and **lungs** provide the two most clearly perceptible rhythms—the heartbeat and respiratory rate—and are connected to each other. The **diaphragm** joins them as a third "organ" and

establishes a highly dynamic connection between the thoracic and abdominal organs.

The mobility of the diaphragm always tells us a lot about a person's vegetative and emotional state.

10.6.2 Illustration of the Zones

(Figs. 10.23, 10.24)

10.6.3 Topography

Zones of the Respiratory Organs

The **nasopharynx** covers the largest area of the dorsal side of the big toes. Starting on the medial part next to the two big toenails as the frontal sinuses, it contains not only the nose but also the posterior

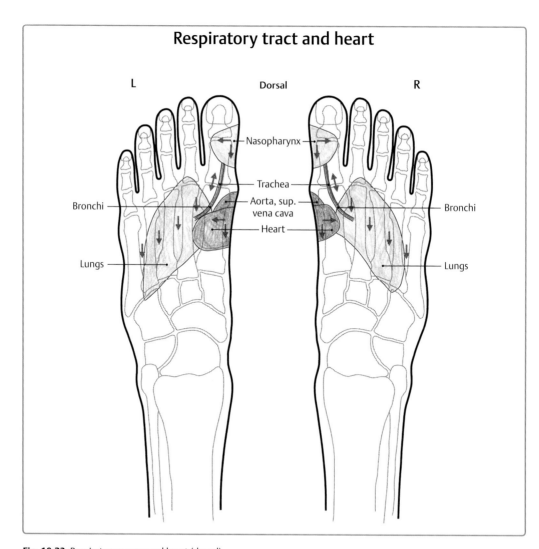

Fig. 10.23 Respiratory organs and heart (dorsal).

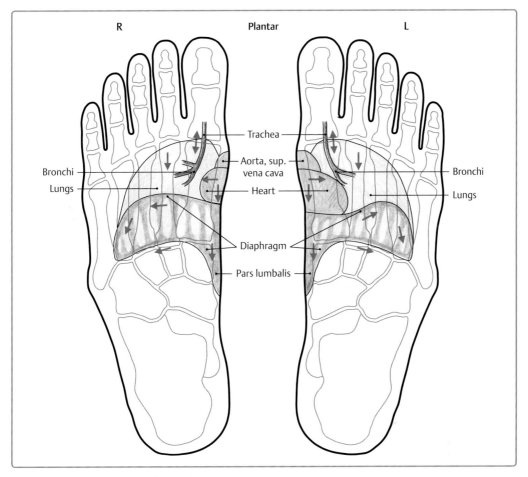

R   Plantar   L

Trachea

Aorta, sup.
vena cava

Bronchi

Lungs

Heart

Bronchi

Lungs

Diaphragm

Pars lumbalis

Fig. 10.24 Respiratory organs and heart (plantar).

apertures of the nose and the maxillary sinuses. It partially overlaps the oral cavity.

The **trachea** passes near the tendon of the extensor hallucis longus muscle and leads to the **bronchial tubes** in a linear connection. The trachea, bronchial tubes, and lungs are accessible on the dorsal and plantar sides. The ventral lung section of the ribs is demarcated in the dorsal area of the foot; on the plantar side the lung extends in a medial direction as far as the tip of the sternum, in a lateral direction as far as the base of the third and fourth metatarsal bones.

The large muscle of the **diaphragm** is found on the lower edge of the metatarsophalangeal joints leading in a proximal direction to Lisfranc's line.

As overlapping organs in the body also appear as overlapping zones, some of the areas of the metatarsal bones are also related to other organs at the same

time, for example, the liver, spleen, and stomach, as discussed in detail in the following chapters.

Zone of the Heart

The **heart** can be reached from both the dorsal and plantar sides in the distal part of the two first metatarsal bones. The zone extends to the left as far as the edge of the second metatarsal bone, in accordance with the left-sided emphasis of the heart. The distal part of this area, connecting directly to the metatarsophalangeal joint gap of the big toe, is related to the large supply vessels from the trunk, the **aorta**, and the **superior vena cava**.

The zone of the heart ends lengthwise both on the plantar and dorsal sides, on the right and left, halfway along the first metatarsal bone and is located, easily discernible on the plantar side, distally of the zone of the diaphragm.

10.6.4 Treatment Technique

Zones of the Respiratory Organs

The index finger is usually employed in vertical or horizontal lines on the dorsal side of the big toe, which corresponds to the nasopharynx.

Usually, the preferred direction of work is from distal to proximal in the area of the trachea and bronchial tubes. If the expectoration of phlegm from the respiratory tract is to be promoted, treatment can take place in the opposite direction, toward the nasopharynx. As longitudinal body zone 1 is particularly wide as a result of the anatomical structure of the foot (the big toe and the first metatarsal bone occupy the largest area in comparison with the other four toes), it is advisable to extend the examination of the trachea and bronchial tubes to the lateral margin of longitudinal body zone 1 in the event of diseases of these organs in order to find the individual focus of treatment.

The same considerations should be borne in mind when treating the zone of the esophagus, the anatomical location of which partially coincides with that of the trachea and bronchial tubes.

The **lungs** are treated like the thorax: on the dorsal side with the index finger (**Fig. 10.25**), and on the plantar side with the thumb.

If the foot is brought into outward rotation in a relaxed state, the **diaphragm** can easily be treated from the medial to lateral side in lines one below the other from the lower margin of the transverse arch to Lisfranc's line. In patients suffering from severe respiratory malfunction, it has proved effective to work deep into the tissue on the proximal parts of the metatarsophalangeal joints, which correspond to the upper edge of the diaphragm, using a technique with the thumb showing in the direction of the heel. Usually the respiration becomes calmer and deeper spontaneously. The **pars lumbalis of the diaphragm**, being the partial origin of the diaphragm, is situated in front of the lumbar spine at approximately the level of the third and fourth lumbar vertebrae and may be treated somewhat plantar of the lumbar vertebrae. This point plays a major role in patients with diseases of the respiratory tract; it cannot be differentiated from the zone of the intestine. As the cause of this group of patients' complaints frequently lies in a disturbed intestinal environment, it requires particularly attentive treatment.

Zone of the Heart

The same treatment technique can be used for the **heart** as for the sternum: on the dorsal side with the index finger in vertical or horizontal lines, and on the plantar side with the thumb. When treating the heart zone from its plantar side, particular care must be taken not to start from the proximal phalanx of the big toe, as this corresponds to the neck, but anatomically precisely from the head of the first metatarsal bone (**Fig. 10.26**).

For treatment indications pertaining to the group of zones of the respiratory organs and heart, see Chapter 21.6.

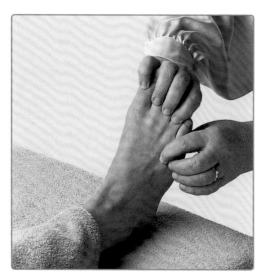

Fig. 10.25 Zone of the lateral thorax and lungs, dorsal view.

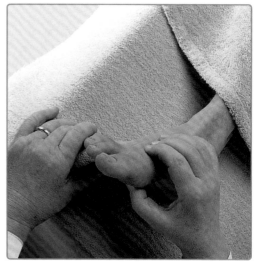

Fig. 10.26 Plantar heart zone, right side.

10.7

Zones of the Digestive Tract

10.7.1 General Information

This system represents the most extensive group of zones and its physiological sequence of food intake, processing, and excretion is explained. The liver and gall bladder can be treated subsequently or in direct connection with the stomach. When treating the digestive organs, we should bear in mind that the process of digestion is not only restricted to its physiological aspects, but also includes the ability to "digest" disturbances at an **emotional** level. The similarity between the shape of the intestine and the brain also indicates therapeutically useful connections.

10.7.2 Illustration of the Zones

(Figs. 10.27, 10.28)

10.7.3 Topography

For the third time the dorsal side of the big toe signals the starting point of a group of zones in the center because the nasopharynx and the **oral cavity** partially overlap.

The **esophagus** is in the same place as the trachea on the right and left foot as far as the start of the bronchial tubes and then continues on the plantar side of the left foot as far as the lower third of the first metatarsal. There the first section of the zones of the digestive tract ends with the sphincter muscle of the **cardia** at approximately the level of the superior edge of the diaphragm below the first and second metatarsophalangeal joints.

The **stomach** extends on the left foot in the lower third of the first, second, and third metatarsal bones as far as the cuneiform bones, and on the right foot around the base of the first metatarsal bone as far as the first cuneiform bone. According to size, location, and volume in situ, however, the zone of the stomach on the left side ends laterally with the second metatarsal bone and second cuneiform bone. The transition into the small intestine as the zone of the **pyloric sphincter** is around the base of the first and second metatarsal bones on the right foot.

From there the large area of the small intestine extends along the cuneiform and partly the cuboid bones on both feet. It reaches as far as the proximal parts of the calcaneus. Its three sections of duodenum, jejunum, and ileum cannot be distinguished from each other during treatment, however.

Only the transition from the ileum (last part of the small intestine) to the cecum (first part of the colon) can be clearly found on the right foot as the **ileocecal valve**. It forms a small pointed area between the cuboid bone and calcaneus, at approximately the transition to the outer third of the foot. This zone can also be accessed easily on the back of the foot, opposite the plantar side.

We can find a circumscribed small area marking the zones of **Oddi's sphincter** and the **papilla of Vater** at the site where the duodenum surrounds the head of the pancreas in a semicircle, approximately between the first and second cuneiform bones and near the Lisfranc's line; it is particularly noticeable in patients suffering from liver, pancreas, and gall bladder disorders.

The zone of the **ascending colon** begins on the plantar side in the lateral third of the right foot in the calcaneus. It leads to the **hepatic flexure** at the base of the fourth metatarsal bone and further to the **transverse colon**. Curved somewhat proximally, this occupies the space of the three cuneiform bones on the right and left foot as far as the **splenic** flexure in the proximal third of the fourth metatarsal bone. From there the descending colon leads into the outer third of the left foot as far as the calcaneus, where the S-shaped loop, the **sigmoid**, is connected. As an organ situated in the middle of the body, the **rectum** is positioned in front of the sacrum on both feet and followed by the final sphincter of the digestive tract, the **anus**, in the proximal part of the medial calcaneus.

By far the largest part of the proximal metatarsal bones and the distal parts of the cuneiform bones on the right foot are covered by the zone of the **liver**. The **gall bladder** is situated on the lower edge of the liver, usually around the base of the third metatarsal bone, sometimes somewhat further laterally. As with the zone of the ileocecal valve, the gall bladder can be treated on the back of the foot, opposite its plantar zone. The left lobe of the liver is identical in parts to the stomach on the left foot.

Although the **pancreas** is partly connected to the digestive tract, it has already been described in more detail in Chapter 10.5 on zones of the endocrine system.

10.7.4 Treatment Technique

The zone of the **oral cavity** is treated with the index finger in the distal half of the proximal phalanx of the big toe including the distal phalanx of

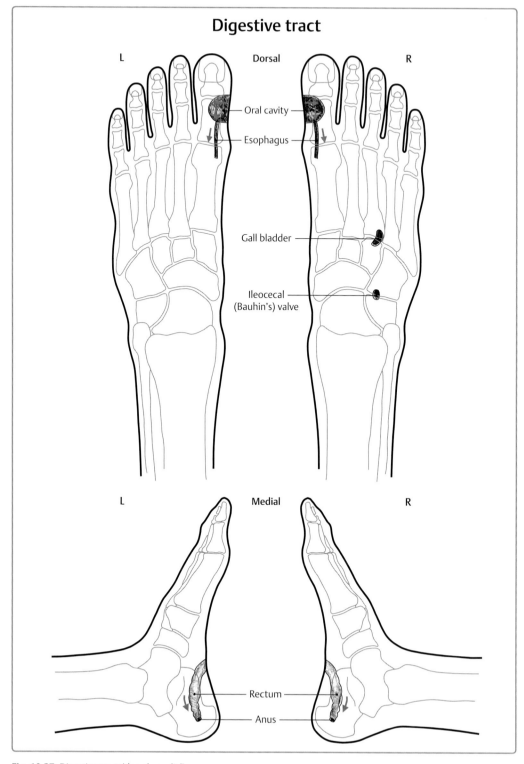

Digestive tract

L Dorsal R

Oral cavity

Esophagus

Gall bladder

Ileocecal
(Bauhin's) valve

L Medial R

Rectum

Anus

Fig. 10.27 Digestive tract (dorsal, medial)

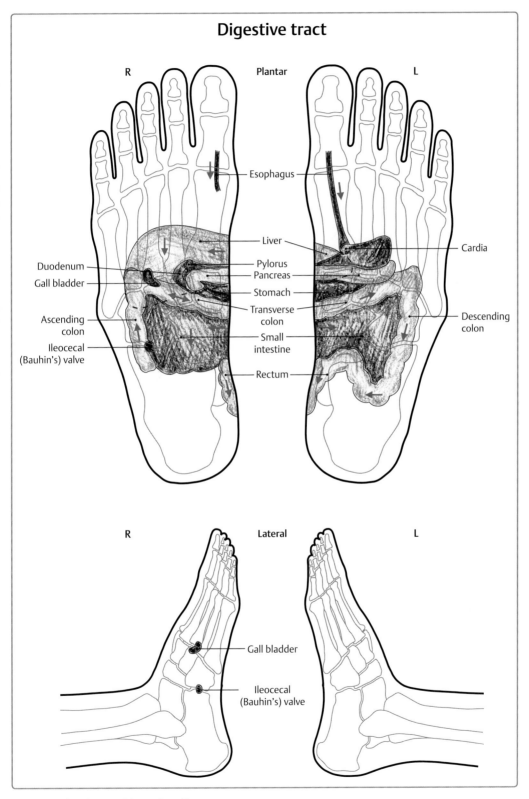

Fig. 10.28 Digestive tract (plantar, lateral).

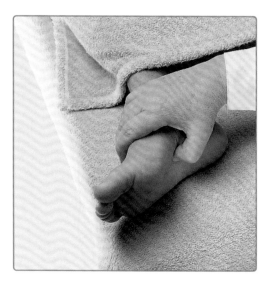

Fig. 10.29 Zones of the intestine.

the big toe from the dorsal side, as well as the dorsal beginning of the **esophagus**. The continuation on the plantar side of the esophagus is performed with the thumb.

Both the **stomach** and the **small intestine** (**Fig. 10.29**) can be treated most easily on the outwardly rotated right and left foot in consecutive horizontal lines in a medial to lateral direction.

The ascending, transverse and descending **colon** to the **sigmoid** is treated in the direction in which peristalsis moves the content of the colon. Only the right side of the transverse colon can also be treated in the opposite direction, that is to say, from medial to lateral, because peristaltic movements in this part of the colon are still in both directions.

If the tonus of the last part of the colon, the **rectum**, is sluggish and defecation is impaired as a result, this zone can also be treated in the opposite direction to excretion in order to stimulate better bowel movements.

The zones of the **cardia, pylorus, ileocecal valve,** and **gall bladder** are treated selectively with the thumb on the plantar side and with the index finger on the dorsal side. The zone of the anus on the rear edge of the right and left medial calcaneus can be treated with the thumb or the index finger.

The zone of the **liver** can be treated on both feet in distal to proximal or medial to lateral direction. Experience shows that the lower and outer edge of the liver is most frequently afflicted on the plantar and dorsal side (identical to the hepatic flexure of the colon).

For treatment indications pertaining to group of zones of the digestive tract, see Chapter 21.7.

10.8

Zones of the Lymphatic System and Solar Plexus

10.8.1 General Information

As an independent, comprehensive treatment within RTF, a separate chapter (Chapter 29) is devoted to the lymphatic system in this new edition of the book. However, the individual description of the lymph zones has been retained here so that beginners, who have not yet learned about RTF lymph treatment (Course III), can orient themselves.

Within the scope of the zones of the lymphatic system, the most important nodules, vessels and organs are mentioned. However, it should be remembered that the lymphatic system is just as widespread as the circulatory system and that no matter which area we treat, we are indirectly connected to both the bloodstream and the lymphatic system.

Unlike the venous and arterial system, however, the lymphatic system is not a closed system but begins in the intercellular spaces of the peripheral tissue layers.

The zone of the plexus celiacus, better known as the **solar plexus**, could also be discussed in the context of other systems. That it is related to the lymph zones is, on the one hand, a matter of presenting it as clearly as possible and, on the other hand, the autonomic nervous system and lymphatic system forming a functional unit.

10.8.2 Illustration of the Zones
(**Figs. 10.30, 10.31**)

10.8.3 Topography

Lymphatic System

The area of the nasopharyngeal cavity, shown at the dorsal center of the big toes, is particularly well supplied with lymphatic tissue and organs and includes **Waldeyer's lymphatic ring**.

In situ, as in the corresponding zone on the foot, the **lateral lymph nodes** of the neck extend from both the mastoid process and the temporomandibular

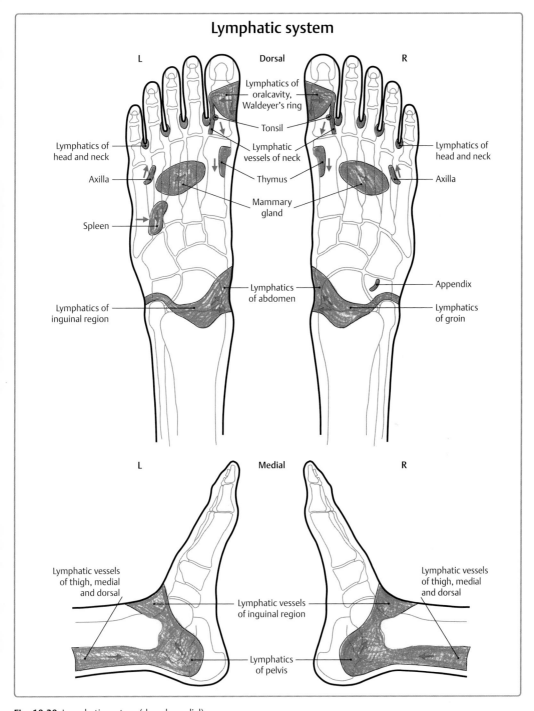

Fig. 10.30 Lymphatic system (dorsal, medial).

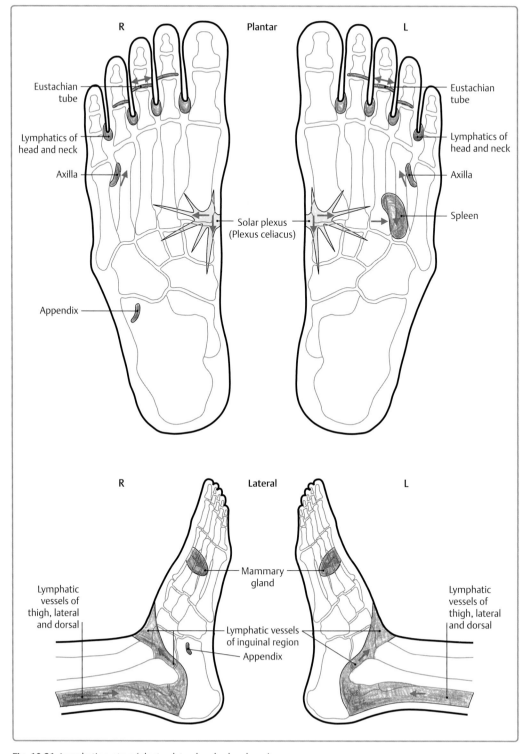

Fig. 10.31 Lymphatic system (plantar, lateral and solar plexus).

joint to the clavicle. The zones of the **tonsils** are centrally located and can clearly be touched when the dorsal proximal phalanx of the big toes is horizontally bisected in a lateral direction.

The lymphatic system of the head and neck can also be reached in the interdigital spaces as was customary in the past, before the zones of the lateral lymph nodes were defined to the precision with which they are known today.

The **eustachian tube** (Fig. 10.31) can easily be reached on the right and left foot from the plantar side in the joint space between the middle and proximal phalanx of the second, third, and fourth toes.

The zone of the **thymus** cannot be differentiated from the sternum, especially as its size and position may vary greatly.

The **axillary lymph nodes** are near the shoulder joints, somewhat proximal of the medial head of the fifth metatarsal bone, on the dorsal and plantar sides of both feet.

The **mammary gland** on the medial part of the dorsal metatarsal bones leads from the lateral edge of the sternum to the vicinity of the axilla.

The zone of the **spleen** is located on both the plantar and dorsal sides of the left foot on the lower third of the fourth metatarsal bone. The dorsal zone has been added to the illustration (Fig. 10.30) to emphasize the importance of the spleen (Chapter 21.8).

The zone of the **appendix** can be palpated on the plantar side of the right foot. It is usually located somewhat proximal of the zone of the ileocecal valve. However, it must be remembered that it may vary considerably in size, shape, and position.

Like the ileocecal valve, the appendix is also easy to find on the lateral/dorsal side of the foot; it is likewise located opposite the plantar point on the distal part of the calcaneus in longitudinal body zone 4.

The lymphatic system of the **pelvis** covers almost the entire proximal part of the calcaneus medially and laterally. The connecting line between the lateral and medial malleoli on the dorsum of the foot represents the zones of the **lymphatic nodules and vessels of the inguinal area**; they extend in a broad strip along the ankle joint and expand medially into the lymphatic areas of the lower abdomen and thighs.

The entire distal area of the lower legs contains the lymphatic areas of the **thighs**, therapeutically most useful medially and laterally along the Achilles tendon as far as the bony structure of the tibia and fibula.

The lymph area around the **knees** can be treated in the extended radius around the knees, and that of the **popliteal fossa** at the same level as the knees, opposite the patella on the dorsal side of the lower leg.

Solar Plexus

The zone of the **solar plexus** extends on the right and left foot from the base of the first metatarsal bone to the first cuneiform bone and is identical to the zone of the stomach in its central parts.

10.8.4 Treatment Technique

Lymphatic System

Waldeyer's lymphatic ring, insofar as it affects the nasopharynx, is treated with the fingertip and the lateral lymph nodes on the neck with gentle grips or with alternating strokes using the tips of both index fingers (see Chapter 3.2.3), especially in patients with lymph disorders in the head and neck. With care and some practice, it is easy to distinguish whether these strokes can be performed smoothly or the flow falters. The strokes are longer if there is good permeability in the tissue; for congestion they are shorter and repeated often.

The **interdigital skin folds** (Figs. 10.30–10.32) between the toes can be stretched distally using the thumb and tips of the index fingers (Chap. 3.2.4). This is useful if there is no special and acute indication for the lymph area of the head and neck. As the interdigital space between the big toe and the

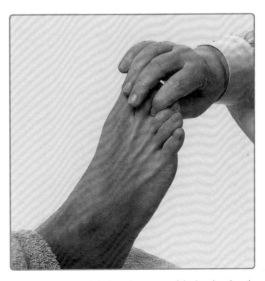

Fig. 10.32 Zones of the lymphatic area of the head and neck.

second toe is particularly wide, the skin fold there is stretched both from the lateral side of the big toe and the second toe.

If there are **acute** lymphatic symptoms in the head and neck (e.g., with toothache, otitis media, or sinusitis) it is advisable also to perform the strokes in the interdigital spaces in a distal to proximal direction. The simplest way is to put the tips of the index fingers in the tissue folds between the toes and to stroke them in alternating fashion in the direction of the metatarsophalangeal joints. When the tissue tone at these points has improved, the stretching grip can be also be used again for further treatment.

The **lymph nodes of the axilla** are treated gently with the index finger or thumb on the medial head of the fifth metatarsal bone, both on the dorsal and plantar sides. In the absence of specific medical problems, the zones of the **mammary glands** can be treated dorsally with the index finger in the inter-metatarsal spaces. This treatment is similar to that of the lungs and thorax (see Chapter 10.6.4).

If congestion, pain, or postoperative care necessitates more extensive treatment, the grip known as **velvet paws** is employed whereby two fingertips from each hand are positioned opposite each other and the two thumbs support the metatarsophalangeal joints from the plantar side. While the hands gently move out of the extension into a normal position in alternating fashion, the fingers move onto their tips and provide a gentle but distinct stimulus in the central third of the dorsal metatarsal bones. The relaxed wrists likewise resume slight

dorsal flexion in an alternating fashion. While the two fingertips of one hand move forward in small steps, those of the other hand move backward. The direction of work leads from near the sternum into the axilla.

The plantar zone of the **spleen** (**Fig. 10.33**) in the proximal third of the fourth metatarsal bone can be treated effectively with the thumb, the dorsal zone with the index finger. The same rule can be applied to the **appendix:** the plantar zone is treated selectively by the thumb, the dorsal zone by the index finger.

The **medial lymphatic area of the pelvis** is gently treated in several lines in the direction of the inguinal region using the thumb; the lateral area around the calcaneus is usually easier to reach with the index and middle fingers. If good supination of the hand is possible, the thumb can also be used.

The thumb also treats the **lymphatic area** of the **inguinal region** from the lateral to the medial side. The lymph nodes and vessels flow in front of the medial malleolus into the lymph nodes of the inguinal area.

The **medial lymphatic areas of the thigh** can be treated with gentle alternating strokes using the two thumb tips flat against each other from proximal to distal as far as the medial malleolus and the medial edge of the calcaneus (**Fig. 3.6**). **Laterally**, the third and fourth fingertips likewise provide alternating strokes from proximal to distal along the Achilles tendon (**Fig. 3.7**).

Solar Plexus

The solar plexus is treated on the plantar side of the right and left foot using the thumb, usually bimanually. As the initial condition of the autonomic nervous system is not always spontaneously evident (depending on the individual background to the disease, and the activity of the sympathetic or parasympathetic nervous system), when treating this zone we can let the patient choose: for a few seconds we offer the option of both the sedating grip and gentle tonifying of this zone and decide in favor of the version which has proved appropriate for the patient.

For treatment indications pertaining to the group of zones of the lymphatic system and solar plexus, see Chapter 21.8.

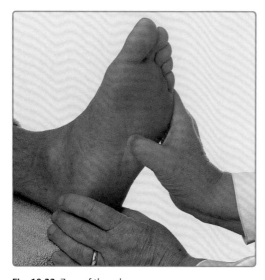

Fig. 10.33 Zone of the spleen.

Part II
Practical Part

11 The First Treatment as an Assessment

11.1

The Initial Perception of the Feet

To a certain extent the quality of our work literally lies "in our own hands." "Touch" conveys, besides the mere physical connection, additional information on a subtle level. Our own awareness of what we do, and our attitude when working has an effect on the whole treatment. Further, our hands should be warm or warmed up first. Rubbing the palms together vigorously, for example, not only actively generates warmth, but also increases their tactile qualities.

First we attune ourselves to the patient by placing our hands gently on their feet for a few seconds. The attentiveness of our hands allows us to perceive subtle initial information about the patient in general, as well as about his or her particular condition at that moment.

If the patient is embarrassed, shy, or very ticklish, the feet should remain covered during this first contact. If established gently, it can promote trust and must not feel oppressive or distressing under any circumstances.

During the first assessment we differentiate between **visual inspection** of the feet and **palpation** of the zones.

11.2

Visual Inspection

It is advisable to examine the patient's feet without initially drawing any therapeutic or diagnostic conclusions. Only after acquiring some practical knowledge can correlations with possible disorders be derived from visual inspection. In principle, however, only **subsequent palpation** can determine whether a zone really has an abnormal reaction or not.

As visual inspections alone fail to provide an adequate objective basis for treatment, we should not relay **any concrete observations** to patients concerning these findings since it may unsettle them and undermine our credibility unnecessarily.

For example, some disorders can already be construed in the zones at a time when no abnormalities of any kind are discernible (**prodromal stage**); some only indicate **general** weakness without their manifesting as an illness. Some tissue findings simply have external causes too, such as extreme sports, ill-fitting shoes, etc.

Sometimes visible symptoms persist after a disorder or illness has abated, perhaps because their causes are still latent and the abnormality of the zone is to be interpreted as a secondary symptom.

The normal tissue tone of the muscles of sportsmen should be examined in order to avoid interpreting well-trained, well-developed muscle groups as afflicted zones.

When inspecting the feet visually the following sequence has proved helpful:
- **Structural analysis of the foot:** longitudinal arches, shape and position of the toes
- **Tissue characteristics:** venous and lymphatic congestion and swelling in the tissue, changes in the subcutaneous tissue, and slackening or shortening of the tendons and muscles
- **Conspicuous features of skin and nails:** calluses, rhagades, verrucas, blisters, injuries, mycosis of nails or in the interdigital tissue, moles, scars, etc.

11.2.1 Structural Analysis of the Foot

The significance of the foot as a weight-bearing arched base for the whole person is recognized in orthopaedics, physiotherapy, and numerous other manual treatments in which the foot is principally seen from the perspective of structural interrelationships. Such viewpoints are not contradictory to RTF as there is often an **interactive correlation** between malposition of the skeletal structure of the feet and malfunction of organs, joints, and bones that manifests itself in painful zones.

Examples
- As the zones of the spine are related to the longitudinal arch, distinct **fallen arches and flat feet** will influence these zones and with them the spine in situ.
- Weakness in the metatarsophalangeal joints can have a disturbing effect on the zones of the shoulder girdle, respiratory organs, and heart.
- Patients with obvious problems of the neck, cervical spine, and thyroid have the typical **hallux valgus** position of the first metatarsophalangeal joint more frequently than

others. Sometimes pathological processes in these zones may arise both as a result of the orthopedic deformity and as a result of scar following a hallux valgus operation.

- Retraction and weak tone at the level of the first **cuneiform** bone in the direction of the **navicular bone**, corresponding to the zone of the lumbar spine, can often be observed as a consequence of the pathologically stressed longitudinal arch.
- **Hammer toes** and other malformations of the toes can influence the zones of the head. Sometimes visual inspection of the toes leads to the presumption that there might be disorders in the dental region and sinuses. I have observed more than once that after holistic treatment of teeth (e.g., removal of silver amalgam, decayed, or devitalized teeth) it became easier to mobilize the toes and they became less congested.
- **Footwear fashion** should also be considered in this respect; ultimately, however, the interaction between the toes and the head area exists regardless of whether the abnormality was triggered by the wrong kind of shoes or due to complaints in the head region (e.g., chronic sinusitis, severe dental strain, migraine, etc.).
- **Collapsed cuneiform bones can** affect the zones of the colon and the lower spine. These connections became obvious to me when a doctor was sending his patients to me for treatment after they had undergone chiro-practic and manual repositioning of the tarsal bones. Many reported that after the reposi-tioning of the cuneiform bones (which partly represent the zones of the digestive tract) not only had their whole posture up to the neck improved, but even chronic digestive prob-lems had noticeably improved.
- Injuries to the **malleoli** and the **calcaneus** are related to the pelvic organs and hip joints via the zones and can cause problems and diseases there.

11.2.2 Tissue of the Foot

Lymphatic and venous **congestion** and **edema** are found especially in the region of the ankles, the Achilles tendon, and on the dorsal part of the feet near the five metatarsophalangeal joints, particularly in women. Retraction or sluggishness of the tissue can be observed both on the plantar and medial sides of the feet, often clearly circumscribed.

From My Practice

In my experience, sportsmen and women with poorly healed injuries or fractures of the ankle joints or with scars on the medial or lateral malleoli later tended to suffer from pelvic or hip problems, partly of a structural–muscular nature and partly of a functional nature, which they had not had before.

Every now and then I noticed that the nailing through the calcaneus that was necessary for extension treatment where fracture of the lower leg occurred, was directly related to the subsequent development of malfunctions, and even acute inflammatory processes in the pelvic organs of such patients who had been involved in accidents. After treatment of these small scars with neural therapy on the medial and lateral sides of the calcaneus (precisely the zones of the pelvic organs) and a few treatments of the zones of the foot, the problems usually vanished as quickly as they had appeared.

Note:

Neural therapy according to Dr. Ferdinand Huneke (1891–1966): "Therapeutic local anesthesia with the aim of healing sites of chronic irritation (e.g., scars, chronically inflamed tonsils, devitalized teeth). A solution containing procaine is frequently injected (subcutaneously)" (Pschyrembel Naturheilkunde).

Examples

- Many patients with **digestive problems** have cushionlike raised tissue on both feet, located in the zones of the intestinal tract (cuboid bones, navicular bone, and parts of the calcaneus in both feet). During a series of treatments and/or through a change in eating habits and improvement of the intestinal flora, we observe that these "swellings" often decrease, at least partially, in line with the patient's improved bowel function.
- Women with serious complaints in the **urogenital organs** (e.g., prolapse of uterus and bladder) often undergo changes in the tissue quality and color of the region around and beneath the inner ankle toward the heel.
- In children suffering from **pseudocroup** and **asthma**, as well as **cystic fibrosis**, swollen, congested areas in the dorsal area of the metatarsal bones, as zones related to the thorax, are not uncommon.

- Some patients have significantly more congested tissue around the lateral malleolus, corresponding to the zone of the hip, directly after an **endoprosthesis operation** of the hip. This resolves itself without any special treatment in the following weeks, as the patient's condition improves.
- Tissue congestion around the **Achilles tendon** as far as the medial and lateral parts of the calcaneus often occurs in women with impaired **fluid excretion** and/or lymphatic flow. The intensive, but not necessarily vigorous, treatment of these areas alone can initiate good diuresis.
- Often women who are familiar with the relationships of the zones report in the final stage of their **pregnancy** that the tissue tone, shape, and color of the medial sides of their heels, which are related to the pelvic organs, change from day to day.

11.2.3 Skin and Nails

Skin of the Feet

On the one hand, unsuitable footwear and restrictive, synthetic socks or stockings are hard on the feet and, on the other hand, the feet are often neglected. Therefore, observations of the skin can be very informative.

When noticing changes in the skin, the **type** of change is not of primary importance, but rather the **site** at which the change is apparent. Thus, a corn near the fifth metatarsophalangeal joint could be related to shoulder problems; a corn between the second and third toes could be indicative of eye disorders.

It is of secondary importance whether there is a corn, mycosis, or rhagade in the zones of the shoulder or eyes. The visible abnormalities only draw attention to the fact that there may be a disturbance in that particular zone.

The following **changes in the skin** on the foot as far as the lower leg are important in a visual inspection:

- Verrucas (warts), cracked skin in the interdigital spaces, Athlete's foot sore spots, corns, blisters, unusual pigmentation, reddening, pallor, scabby skin, rhagades, perspiration, ulcers (e.g., ulcus cruris), calluses, changes in color, scars.
- Particular attention should be paid to any changes in size, color, and tissue composition in moles and nevi (birthmarks) (possibility of malignancy).

Examples

- In women who have experienced a difficult delivery (a very large baby or other complications) changes are often observed in their skin around the zones of the pelvic organs on the **medial sides of the calcanei**, such as venous or lymphatic congestion and/or telangiectasis (bluish-colored superficial veins with a broomlike appearance).
- Calluses around the medial part of the **first metatarsophalangeal joint** can be observed in patients suffering from neck, thyroid, and/or heart problems.
- Tourists who have eaten food and drink with which their digestive organs are unfamiliar while abroad may suffer from small blisters filled with lymphatic fluid in **the center of the plantar part of the feet** (the zones of the **gastrointestinal tract**) weeks later. The blisters empty themselves after some time, causing irritating itching while healing. As long as there is a toxic load on the digestive tract—although often without recognizable symptoms—new blisters may develop and consequently heal during the course of improvement.
- **Athlete's foot**, usually occurring as interdigital mycosis, is a special phenomenon because although both feet are exposed to the source of the infection (swimming pool, sauna), the mycosis hardly ever spreads across the whole foot, not even across all interdigital spaces. It can be observed on typical areas that are often connected with a disorder or weakness in the related area of the head/neck. The interdigital space between the **fourth and fifth toes** is exposed to fungal infections remarkably often. In this area we find the lateral areas of the head and neck, zones of the tonsils, lymphatics of the sides of the neck, middle and inner ear, maxillary sinus, molars, and wisdom teeth. Diseases or weaknesses of these groups of organs and tissues create a correspondingly weakened environment on the skin in the related areas of the foot, which is particularly susceptible to Athlete's foot infection.

Athlete's foot as a parasitic condition always requires a predisposed—that is, weakened—skin environment in order to establish itself and can therefore persist in certain sites of the feet for weeks, months, or even years. As soon as the application of antimycotic tinctures or ointments is stopped, the infection breaks out again because the symptoms were merely suppressed.

Against this background it may be understood that external influences (tight shoes, source of infection in swimming pools, saunas, and bathrooms, unsuitable footwear, insufficient skin care, careless drying between the toes) are only **superficial** reasons for the existence of interdigital mycosis and that relationships with the zones (and meridians) are to be seen as an important aspect.

For the above reasons, **externally natural substances** should be used for Athlete's foot, for example, tea tree oil, coffee charcoal (prescription: Carbo Königsfeld, Müller/Göppingen), oak bark footbaths, one's own urine. However, what is more important is the **internal** improvement of the acid to alkaline-base balance in the digestive tract through a change in diet and herbal or homeopathic remedies because Athlete's foot is only a **symptom** of overall metabolic stress.

From My Practice

Decades ago I had a highly compelling experience regarding the interaction between zones and organ disorders when one of my patients had a flare-up of severe facial neuralgia after the fourth treatment. From the outset, I was only able to partially treat the patient's toes and interdigital spaces because for many years she had had pronounced Athlete's foot between the fourth and fifth toes that was resistant to treatment.

Her dentist extracted the seventh tooth on the top left, which had been devitalized for a long time owing to root treatment. Her acute facial pain soon subsided. What surprised me and the patient the most was that the Athlete's foot infection immediately started to heal and within three weeks a healthy, well perfused new layer of skin had formed.

From My Practice

The medical history of patients with chronic diseases (e.g., renal and hepatic insufficiency, rheumatic complaints) has often revealed that foot perspiration had been previously suppressed by synthetic means for an extended period of time. If the regenerative power of the sick person was so strong that the "detoxification valve" of foot perspiration (often smelling penetratingly sour) re-emerged during a course of treatment, there was also the possibility of improving the chronic symptoms. "Treatment homework": a change of diet, increased fluid intake, saltwater footbaths in the evening, washing with diluted fruit vinegar, footwear made of natural materials.

Toe Nails

Inspection of the feet includes checking the shape, consistency, and color of the individual toe nails.

On the one hand, an obvious deviation from the norm (e.g., deformed and mycotic nails) may indicate a general tendency toward malfunction or the onset of an illness in the head area; on the other hand, it is just as important to consider that various **acupuncture meridians** begin and end near the toe nails.

To avoid causing unnecessary concern, we should therefore deal with the information in a particularly responsible and restrained manner and adhere to the principle that we **do not share** with the patient our findings from the inspection.

11.2.4 Temperature of the Feet

In the **transitional phase between inspection and palpation** we apply gentle and attentive strokes with both hands—perhaps even with our eyes closed—to all sides of the feet in order to obtain information about their temperature.

Examples

- A **hypotonic** person tends to have cool or cold feet even in summer and in warm rooms. Often we find the toes, corresponding to the zones of the head, to be the coldest parts.
- If there is **inflammation** in the pelvic organs (mostly observed in females), the heels, representing the zones of the pelvic organs, are more congested and sometimes unnaturally warm compared to the temperature of the rest of the foot.
- In patients suffering from acute **inflammation of the joints**, the correlating zones may be significantly warmer than the surrounding tissue, for example the fifth metatarsophalangeal joint in "frozen shoulder"; the lateral malleolus in acute or chronic hip problems.
- With chronic **degenerative** processes, on the other hand, the local tissue tone is often slack and the skin in the outlined area too cool.

We can both **see** and **feel** skin changes which indicate pathological changes in the temperature of the feet: too much redness or pallor, coldness or heat, perspiration of the whole foot or of certain parts such as, for example, on the medial areas of the heels and the dorsal areas of the big toes.

Through observant examination of the temperature of the feet during gentle stroking, we can also differentiate whether both feet are of the same temperature or whether there is a difference between right and left, plantar, and dorsal parts and further develop our sensitivity.

The temperature of the feet may change very quickly during a treatment. Obvious initial differences between the toes and heels, the soles and backs of the feet, and the right and left foot often even out after only a few minutes.

The **time required** to compile the visual findings of the structure of the foot, tissue composition, conspicuous features of the skin and nails and temperature of the foot is approximately three minutes initially but with some practice, 20 to 30 seconds should suffice.

The **results of the visual findings** are recorded in pencil or ballpoint pen on the **treatment card** (**Fig. 11.1**).

11.3

Palpation

It has proved useful to carry out palpation immediately after the visual inspection and stroking movements. It is carried out on the plantar side with the basic thumb grip; the index finger is better suited on the dorsal side.

The patient's **spontaneous response** to the therapeutic stimulus—facial movements, utterances, or signs from the autonomic nervous system such as moistened hands, show if and where abnormal zones exist.

11.3.1   Establishment of a Reliable Measure

To find a reliable measure for detecting the zones that need treatment, we usually choose a zone on the foot which is painful in most patients, for example, the lumbar spine or small intestine. Here we work with the examining basic grip 6 to 8 times in millimeter steps in order to enable better the assessment of the patient's spontaneous reactions.

If the patient feels hardly any pain or discomfort, we may increase the intensity of the grip. If the patient shows signs of pain by wincing, with sudden exclamations, or with hands suddenly moistening after the first touch, we must adapt ourselves to the patient's momentary condition by reducing the force of our grip somewhat. In this way, we ascertain a useful **basic and reliable measure** on the basis of which we can largely orient ourselves throughout the entire initial findings in all the zones.

As the same intensity of grip triggers different sensations and responses at different points on the foot, we have good opportunities for comparison between a healthy and a diseased zone.

As the tissue can vary to quite an extent throughout the feet, there may be some **variations** necessary regarding the intensity of the examining grip:
- Near the periosteum (toes, medial sides of the calcaneus) we reduce the intensity.
- We can increase the intensity of the grip in places where the layers of tissue are thicker (calcaneus from the plantar side, tissue around the plantar toe joints, etc.).
- We usually work with gentle, alternating strokes on sites where the tissue is normally more sensitive (lateral and medial sides of the Achilles tendon).

11.3.2   Practical Application of Palpation

The first assessment shows tangibly the patient's current condition and is performed in the following way:

Both feet are palpated systematically and evenly **once** in millimeter steps using the rhythmical basic grip and checked for abnormal zones.

Abnormal zones are recognized:
- by the pain experienced in a zone, and/or
- by overreactions of the autonomic nervous system, and
- by palpation (with some experience and sensitivity).

Only in the **follow-up treatments**, which unlike the initial findings represent the **actual therapy**, are the painful areas treated repeatedly (Chapter 12.2.1).

Throughout the entire treatment, wherever possible, both hands are on the foot, alternately working or supporting it. Alternating the treatment from left to right and vice versa, clearly shows that we also record the person's "microsystem" as an organic whole and do not divide him or her into two halves by first treating one foot completely and then the other.

Two ways of carrying out the initial findings have proved effective in practice.
1. Classification according to **affiliation with zone groups**, as described in detail in Chapter 10.

We check the seven groups in turn for painful areas:

- Head and neck
- Spine, thorax
- Urinary tract and tissue of the pelvis, thigh to knee
- Endocrine system
- Respiratory organs and heart
- Digestive tract
- Lymphatic system.

2. Classification according to the **anatomical structure** of the feet:
We check for painful zones:
- Toes (zones of head and throat)
- Metatarsal bones (zones of the thorax, shoulder girdle, and upper abdomen)
- Tarsal bones with the calcaneus and malleoli (zones of the abdomen and pelvis)
- Distal parts of the lower legs (zones of the thighs and knees).

As the zones of the **spine** run through all the aforementioned areas of the foot, they are examined as a whole in order to obtain a better overview.

The first assessment takes longer, above all for beginners, than the subsequent treatments. To work economically one can, as a general overview, check the condition of the zones of the head at first in its smaller scale on the two big toes (**Fig. 28.1**). However, for follow-up treatments the larger scale of the head zones on all toes (Chapter 10.2) should be chosen as they can be treated more efffectively there.

11.3.3 Differentiation between Symptomatic and Background Zones

During the first assessment we usually find numerous abnormal zones. We differentiate between symptomatic and background zones and we keep to this system throughout all follow-up treatments.

It should be noted that patients are only aware of their symptoms **subjectively**. Through the first assessment we can form a therapeutically holistic picture **objectively** by recording all symptomatic **and** background zones.

Symptomatic zones are the zones of those organs that the patient complains about, for example, the zone of the stomach with gastritis, the zone of the shoulder joint with frozen shoulder (periarthritis humeroscapularis), and the zone of the lower spine with lumbar pain.

Background zones are all areas on the feet that are painful or need treatment **in addition to the symptomatic zones**. Often they refer to connections within the musculoskeletal system, germ layer similarities, or to functional organic connections. For example, patients with low back pain often have to be treated in the cervical spine, with chronic sinusitis in the zones of the pelvic organs, and with disorders of the colon in the zones of the brain (similarity in shape).

We also come across background zones for which we as yet have no plausible explanation. Here we might touch on connections between the **physical** and **psychological** level, or even concealed aspects which may reveal themselves only during a course of treatment. Even if we do not "understand" the meaning of all background zones, we should accept them as existing and include them in the treatment, knowing that they are an important part of the patient and their disease. Sometimes we are just too emphatically body-oriented and forget that a person consists of more than just the sum of his or her physical organs. Thus, we may get in touch with the emotional level or components connected with the build-up of the patient's personality and destiny. For example:

- Painful zones in the digestive tract may occur when difficult life situations cannot be "digested" easily.
- Abnormal pancreatic zones may appear because of a lack of "sweetness" in life.
- Zones of the inner ears (equilibrium) are tender when the balance of one's life is disturbed.

All processes of life, even disturbed ones, are specifically or latently connected to the whole person and appear as a differentiated network in constant interaction with one's whole being. The existence of this network should be taken into account during each treatment to avoid a one-sided approach.

Due to these complex relationships, the background zones cannot be established or "learned" schematically in advance.

Practically speaking, this means that patients with similar or even the same symptoms can have different background zones, according to the individual context that has led to the illness.

> As the symptomatically oriented approach to patients and their disease is prevalent while the strained environment and deeper relationships of an illness are often neglected, I feel urged to emphasize the **significance of the background zones** as a necessary supplement to the symptomatic zones. A symptom can only arise on an existing strained background.

Symptomatic and background zones should be understood as complementing each other. Only a well-balanced application of both can guarantee **truly holistic treatment** with good results. I consider the relationship between symptomatic and background zones comparable with the tip of an iceberg and its large underwater part, which usually requires more attention because of its hidden dangers.

11.3.4 Examples of the Same Symptomatic Zones with Different Background Zones

The symptomatic zones of three patients with **hip problems on the right side** were always around the right lateral malleolus, corresponding to the zone of the hip joint and its surrounding tissue. During the first assessment, the **background zones** can, and often do, differ widely from patient to patient according to the different background of the symptoms.

Example 1: This patient showed structural–muscular relationships as the background: lower spine with sacroiliac joint, promontory, temporomandibular joint (form analogy), symphysis, gluteal and lateral abdominal musculature, thigh and knee. The right **shoulder** (in situ and as a zone) must be treated collaterally (on the same side), the **left** hip joint contralaterally (on the opposite side), likewise in situ and as a zone (Chapter 21.4).

Example 2: Here **metabolic disorders** emerged as the background. This usually involves zones of the small intestine and colon with the ileocecal valve, the stomach with the cardia and pylorus, liver/gall bladder and urinary tract, and solar plexus to compensate for the autonomic nervous system.

Example 3: In this patient chronic **inflammatory sites** and **scars** came into consideration as background zones: abnormalities of teeth 13, 23, 33 and 43 (energetically related to the hip joint [see Chapter 26]), right lower abdomen (chronic enteritis?), pelvic organs, appendix, inguinal hernia or thigh scar, spleen, kidneys, and lymph for the removal of noxious substances (toxins).

11.3.5 Summary

The practical consequence of these lines of thought regarding palpation is simple. Freed from theoretical reflections on if and how we ought to name and classify the zones, we can simply sit at the patient's feet and investigate all the zones as to whether they need treatment according to the order of the seven working groups (or according to the anatomical structure of the foot) using the basic grip.

Thereby, we consequently come across the abnormal symptomatic and background zones, because both are recognized in the same way: by **pain** and/or **irritations of the autonomic nervous system.**

> The differentiation between symptomatic and background zones is, strictly speaking, an aid with the aim of leading therapists to acknowledge that, although only the symptom causes discomfort and pain, even a **sick** person is a **whole person** and therefore there must be central connections for each peripheral symptom.

11.4

How to Work with the Treatment Card

Fig. 11.1 shows an example of a completed treatment card.

> We choose different colors to denote the abnormal zones:
> - **Black** for the results of visual inspection
> - **Red** for the symptomatic zones
> - **Green** for the background zones

This choice is independent of the different colors we use to depict the groups of zones, where the color red is related to the urinary system and green to the musculoskeletal system.

First Possibility, recording the palpation findings:

Each of the seven groups of zones is individually palpated:
- Head and neck,
- Spine, thorax and shoulder girdle,
- Urinary tract, bones and tissue of the pelvis, thighs, and knees,
- Endocrine system,
- Respiratory organs and heart,

Treatment card for reflexotherapy of the feet

Name: **Mary Smith**   Date of birth: **7.8.50**

Address: **Maywood, NJ**   Tel no.: **98765**

Prescribed by: *Dr. Newman*

Symtoms and/or diagnosis: *Lumbar syndrome*

Important medicines: **Analgesics 2–3 /week for approx. 7 weeks**

Previous illnesses: **Sinusitis, bronchitis as a child**

Mental state, sleep, dreams: **Easily irritable, only falls asleep after midnight, wakes up frequently.**

Accidents, operations, other scars: **Appendectomy in 1962, fracture of right upper arm in 1985, scar on left knee**

Blood pressure: **76 / 132**

Births, perineal sutures, complications, the "pill"? **1 birth in 1978, long painful perineal suture, on**

the "pill" until start of menopause

Previous therapies: **Back exercises, fangotherapy and movement therapy, 5 injections on account of pain.**

Dental status: SiAg = silver amalgam   Dev. = devitalized   Infl. = Inflammation

18 SiAg	17 SiAg	16 SiAg	15	14	13	12	11	21	22	23	24	25 dev	26	27 SiAg	28
48	47 SiAg	46 Infl	45	44	43	42	41	31	32	33	34	35	36 SiAg	37	38

Initial findings: visual inspection – **black**, symptomatic zone – **red**, background zones – **green**
Intensity of the zones: very badly affected – **strong**, badly affected – **moderate**, little affedted – **slight**
Final results/altered zones: zones clearly affected – **circle in blue** – zones no longer affected – **delete in blue**, new zones – **blue**

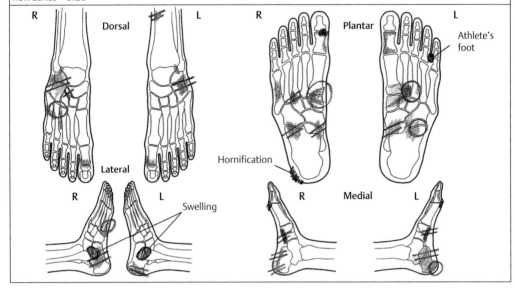

Fig. 11.1 Treatment card Reflexotherapy of the feet (continued on next page).

Date:	Reactions in the treatment intervals:	Treated or noticeable zones Reactions during treatment:
8.4		First treatment
11.4	Lumbar spine unchanged, increased flatulence, good diuresis at night as well.	Lumbar spine, intestine, right kidney. Autonomic nervous system low resistance to stress. Reacts very well to Yin-Yang grip and sedation via solar plexus zone.
14.4	Less pain when lying down and standing up, malodorous bowel movement.	Spine, above all cervical spine, abdominal wall, intestine. Respiration deeper, "rumbling" in stomach during treatment.
18.4	Slept restlessly for 2 nights, dreamt more. 1 day diarrhea. (Discussion of diet, emphasis should be placed on basic food).	Lumbar spine, lesser pelvis, lateral abdominal muscles highly sensitive. A lot of sedentary grips, longer resting time after treatment.
21.4	Spine more mobile, flatulence less, left knee painful for 1 day. Mentions skiing accident many years ago.	Spine, upper abdomen, nasopharynx, kidneys. Abdominal wall on right and left tonified as significantly less painful.
26.4	Slight pressure in head, onset of a cold. Lumbar spine and right buttock hurts more again. Increased "rumbling" in intestine.	Lumbar spine and sacroiliac joint, buttocks, intestine, hip. Scar zone appendectomy right abdominal wall. Strong emotional reaction with crying at the end of scar RTF.
29.4	Good diuresis, lumbar spine, buttock complaints better. Sleep more refreshing, can usually sleep through the night now. Cold has developed into a runny nose, head feels less congested.	Right kidney, head, spine. Can only process gentle stimuli. Talks about family problems. Hand perspiration resolves spontaneously as a result of grip for regulating respiration.
7.5	Improvement continues in lower back, neck slightly tense. Excretion via intestine good.	Lateral abdominal wall, spine, sacroiliac joint, buttocks, hip, intestine. Normal tolerance of strain.
12.5	Spine almost pain-free in spite of light gardening, also feels better mentally.	Final results

Patient's own exercises, accompanying measures: *Regular swimming. Drink more! Should not eat any raw vegetables or fruit in the evening.*

Result: After how many treatments did the condition change significantly? *Fewer complaints from 5th RTF onward*
Which complaints have changed a) from *a therapeutic perspective: Mobility of the spine in all directions good, excretion from intestine and kidneys more intense*
b) from **the patient's perspective:** *Significantly fewer complaints, except with long car journeys (some tensions). Improved mood.*
Additional observations (e.g. weight change, reduction of medicines): *Has lost 2 kg (excretion of retained water). Does not need analgesics any more.*

Treatments performed by: (write name clearly) *O. Summer*

- Digestive system,
- Lymphatic system

Immediately afterward, the abnormal zones are recorded on the treatment card before the next group of zones is examined (Chapter 11.3.2).

Second Possibility: When we decide to examine the zones for the **anatomical classification** of the foot, we record each of the abnormal zones according to the individually palpated sections:
- Toes—zones of the head and neck
- Metatarsal bones—zones of the thorax and upper abdomen
- Tarsal bones—zones of the abdomen and pelvis
- Distal parts of the lower legs—zones of the thighs and knees
- The longitudinal arch as a zone of the spine can be checked over its entire length at the start of palpation and recorded in its entirety (Chapter 11.3.2).

> To differentiate the respective **intensity** of the irritated zones clearly, we apply three different degrees of pressure when using the colored pencils:
> - Highly irritated zones: **intense**
> - Irritated zones: **moderate**
> - Less irritated zones: **light**

Some areas on the feet correspond to several zones. They need not be palpated several times because they correlate to overlapping organs as they are located in the body.

The **message** an irritated part of the foot wants to convey to the therapist is more important than attempting to name it: spontaneous pain and/or symptoms of severe vegetative irritation indicate an area requiring treatment.

11.5

Exceptions with Regard to Performing the First Assessment

Usually, the first treatment serves as an assessment, but sometimes there are reasons for postponing the assessment or omitting it completely:
- If **acute treatment** (Chapter 16) is indicated, the initial assessment may be performed after the subsidence of acute complaints where necessary.
- If the patient shows **signs** of **strain** (cold, moist hands and feet, oversensitivity to pain,

extreme exhaustion, or obvious nervousness) it is advisable to start with a few unspecified treatments to improve his or her general condition. These treatments will mostly consist of stabilizing grips combined, if appropriate, with gentle and rhythmic tonifying of the zones of the digestive tract, lymphatic system, spine, and endocrine system.
- **Severely sick or terminally ill patients** do not require an extensive first assessment, but rather a light touch and, perhaps, gentle mobilization of the feet. Stabilizing grips may be performed in combination with light strokes. Holding both feet attentively with warm hands can bring some relief. If the patient is suffering from great pain, brief first-aid treatment may be chosen.
- No first assessment is necessary with patients suffering from **chronic neurological diseases** such as Parkinson's disease, multiple sclerosis, hemiplegia, or tetraplegia, where the nerve supply is partially or completely destroyed. To a certain extent we can use the signs of the autonomic nervous system (Chapter 4.2) to find the correct level of treatment, but our attention is mainly focused on the symptomatic zones and a few obviously connected background zones. Both feet are also given a gentle general massage to increase the blood circulation and thereby warm them.
- A first assessment is not suitable for patients taking strong **painkillers** (psychopharmaceuticals, allopathic sleeping pills, cortisone, or narcotics) over a long period because these medications veil the symptoms and their backgrounds.
- With **long-term drug addicts** (abuse of medicines, alcohol dependence, etc.) a first assessment is usually not suitable because their perception in general is often disturbed, so we are handicapped by a lack of information about the sensations experienced. However, these patients experience treatment of their feet as highly beneficial and stabilizing.
- Treating **babies** and **small children** usually involves treating the entire surface of the feet due to their small size. According to the illness, the symptomatic zones can be emphasized during the general treatment.
- Patients with **multiple physical or mental handicaps** are treated as described for babies or small children. They particularly enjoy this kind of attention and respond well with im-

proved function of the excretory and respiratory organs, regenerative powers permitting. Their tactile awareness can also be increased significantly. Children with multiple physical or mental handicaps also "treat" each other's feet with great enthusiasm and interest when instructed to do so and thus "hone" their fine motor skills. In addition, they cultivate interpersonal contact in this way and should be supported and affirmed in doing so.

11.6

Finishing a Treatment

11.6.1 Rest after Treatment

Those patients who still have cool or cold feet at the end of the treatment should be given additional warmth in the form of a hot water bottle, a warm footbath, or other means of passive warmth. Frequently, however, putting on their warmed-up socks or stockings again is sufficient.

The more irritated and weak a patient feels, the more emphasis should be placed on the **resting period** to give the treatment a good chance of being well "digested." Patients should be covered comfortably and be allowed to lie in a quiet room for about 20 minutes. However, many of our patients, like ourselves, have a disturbed relationship to leisure and rest time and thus should be patiently taught how important relaxation and recuperation are for a good treatment result. "How long **must** I rest?" is a typical question.

Correctly understood, this little "oasis" of undisturbed rest could be a first step toward experiencing the blessing of releasing any tensions, whether physical or mental.

Some patients feel encouraged by this experience to include short phases of rest more naturally in their daily routine, and they will surely benefit from it.

In order to neutralize the energy after the treatment, we should wash our hands thoroughly, air the room well, and have a drink so that **we** also feel good (Chapter 7.5.4).

11.6.2 Suggestions for Active Involvement of the Patient

Before patients return to their familiar surroundings, they should be informed about observing changes in their condition during the treatment intervals. These must be assessed as **reactions in the treatment intervals** (Chapter 14) and signify

individual responses to the therapeutic stimulus of RTF.

Reactions may already begin in the resting phase and can extend over hours or days until the next treatment. Such observations are understood to be a kind of therapeutic "homework" for patients and educate and activate them to observe their health and disease, as well as the effects RTF can have, with greater interest.

Systems in which Reactions Can Be Observed

Obtaining reliable answers from the patients requires sound information on the part of the therapist. The following examples represent only a selection from a wide range of possible reactions in the treatment intervals (for more details see Chapter 14).

Examples

- Concerning the **symptoms:**
  "I can raise my arm a bit higher."
  "My sore throat is not as painful."
- Concerning the **head and neck region**:
  "Yesterday evening I felt strong pressure in my forehead; today my nose has been running and this has reduced the pressure."
- Concerning the **spine** and **joints**:
  "I don't have low-back pain when I get up in the morning."
  "The movement of the right knee was restricted for a few hours, but this has now resolved itself."
- Concerning the **kidneys and bladder**:
  "Last night I had to get up twice to urinate, the urine was quite clear/opaque, and now, as on frequent occasions previously, I have an increased urge to urinate again."
- Concerning the **endocrine glands and autonomic nervous system**:
  "On the same evening as the treatment I had more vaginal discharge, but my period started almost painlessly."
  "I feel calmer and my hands are much less damp than they were."
- Concerning **respiration and the cardiovascular system**:
  "Sometimes I notice that my breathing extends deep into my pelvis of its own accord—that does me good."
  "Last night I woke up with strong palpitations. After half an hour they subsided and I fell asleep again."
- Concerning the **digestive tract:**
  "My stools smell more offensive than before.

However, after defecating again, my abdomen feels better."

- Concerning the **lymphatic system:**
"My ankles are less swollen in the evening since the treatment."
"The scar on the right side of my chest is less painful now and I can move my arm backwards more freely."
- Concerning the **skin:**
"The itching was more intense on the first day after treatment. Now it has subsided again and my skin looks better."
- Concerning **sleeping habits:**
"Although I slept less, I still woke feeling greatly refreshed."
"Waking up this morning I remembered a very strange dream; I am still thinking about it."
- Concerning **mood:**
"In the evening after your treatment I had to cry seemingly for no reason. Since then I have felt relieved."

Other changes which occur regardless of the effect of RTF are often important too, for example, changes

- in eating habits,
- as a result of travel,
- in the family and professional sphere,
- of a climatic nature.

The beginning of menstruation or unforeseen events such as accidents or news of pleasing or depressing incidents may also bring about changes in health.

Significance of the Patient's Feedback

For the **therapist**, the mentioned changes undergone by the patient during or since the last treatment are the first indicators that some zones might have changed or that old zones have disappeared. This must be taken into account in the current treatment.

Patients learn to observe and report on processes and to take greater responsibility for themselves.

Reactions in treatment intervals not only relate to disturbing changes and disagreeable symptoms becoming more acute, but very often to the **subsidence of pain and disappearance of the symptoms**.

11.7
Summary

In my experience, the **result of a treatment** depends on a number of factors which may vary from person to person:
1. The quality of the chosen **method**. RTF is a regulatory therapy, that is, it works with personal regenerative force and avoids unilateral overrating or suppression of symptoms.
2. The **professional** qualities of the therapist. As diseases become increasingly complex, the demand for sound professional knowledge and the necessity for good training grow.
3. The **personal** qualities of the therapist, which play a role in any manual work in the sense of per-sonare (the Latin word "person" emphasizes the meaning: "personare" means to "sound through"). Sensitive patients notice whether we are attentive to them or are distracted by external and internal disturbances.
4. The patient's existing **vitality** and **will to recover their health**. There are very subtle, constantly changing connections between disease, regenerative force, and health. Du Bois, a French physiologist of the last century, came up with the following definition: "Each person reacts to all the factors of their environment, and the nature of their response is the measure of their health!"
5. The **background to a person's disease** and the acquired and inherited disturbances and experiences associated with it.
6. The patient's insight and endeavor to actively support the healing process by taking up recommendations which can alter and improve their lifestyle.
7. The individual's **mission and destiny in life**. Disease provides a person with highly personal constellations as an opportunity for inner maturation and development.

Regeneration as a response to RTF usually takes place in three phases:
1. In the **rest period** after the treatment
2. In the **treatment intervals**, in the form of various reactions
3. After completing a **course of treatment**, above all, if the patient is prepared to make some changes in their way of life or, if necessary, alter it completely.

12 Performing the Follow-up and Final Treatments

12.1

Overview

Only the first treatment, which is the assessment, is always performed in the same manner because, regardless of the patient's symptoms, **all** the zones are checked systematically to detect abnormal areas.

All **follow-up treatments** include consideration of various factors that may have changed from one treatment to the next. Any subsequent treatment will focus on those zones which

- emerge from a description of the patient's responses,
- were marked as abnormal in the initial findings, and
- may have arisen in addition during the course of treatment.

We learn precisely which zones these are when we take into account and inquire about particular aspects as per the following points **before** the follow-up treatment:

1. **Checking the visual and palpatory findings.** As no further detailed records are kept until the final findings and there are only brief written notes about the reactions experienced on the reverse side of the treatment card, the **initial findings** in red, green, and black help to provide a quick overview of the initial situation each time.
2. **Inquiring about changes in the symptoms.** The question about changes in their complaints is the most important one for patients and is therefore asked first, for example: "How is your neck?", "Is there any change in your stomach irritation?", or "How is your right knee today when walking?"
   As many people have forgotten to observe the changes in their condition, sometimes they do not know how to reply. To obtain a reliable answer, we can ask a more specific question: "Is your condition better, worse, or the same since the last treatment?"
3. **Referring to previously recorded reactions.** By briefly reading which reactions we recorded in the previous treatment intervals on the reverse of the treatment card, we can recall which of the patient's organs and/or systems have reacted to the treatment up to now.
4. **Inquiring about reactions since the last treatment.** Experience shows that reactions occur most often in the **excretory organs:**
   - Digestive tract
   - Urinary tract
   - Skin and mucous membranes

   Changes in **mood** and **quality of sleep** are also relatively common. Additional factors may trigger changes in health without needing to be classified as reactions to the RTF treatment:
   - Family and professional changes
   - Changes in the weather
   - Different eating habits, fasting, travel, invitations

   Changes of this nature are also taken into account in subsequent treatment.
5. **Palpation of the zones noted during the first assessment.** As the patient's description of their present state and reactions is always personal and subjective, we objectify it by means of brief palpation of the zones which were recorded during the first assessment. This enables us to discover which zones need more treatment. Some of the recorded zones are **less sensitive**, others completely **pain-free**, while some are momentarily **worse**, perhaps because of a temporary and significant reaction phase if, for example, the excretory organs are activated and stimulated more intensely as a spontaneous response to the treatment stimulus applied.

12.1.1 Summary

From the results of information gathered from attending to the five points listed above we obtain useful indications as to which zones should be at the forefront in the respective follow-up treatment. Whether we treat the symptomatic zone first or do not include it until later in the course of treatment has no major bearing on the result of a treatment.

The outcome of a treatment depends less upon rigid adherence to the sequence of the groups of treatment zones than upon skilled, person-centered handling of the painful areas on the foot and upon finding the appropriate treatment dosage.

12.2

Approach in the Follow-up Treatments

12.2.1 Treatment of Abnormal Zones

During the follow-up treatments, the zones in question are treated repeatedly—usually twice, thrice, or four times—for a few seconds at short intervals. The short treatment intervals produced in this way for the individual zones mean that the effect of the grip can develop and the tissue has an improved blood supply before the next stimulus is applied. The zone will consequently be less sensitive to pain.

We consider a zone to be normalized when
- it is less painful, and/or
- it no longer triggers overreaction by the autonomic nervous system,
- it feels warm and soft when palpated, and when
- the tissue has a pink sheen.

Variations in Treatment

If individual zones still appear exceptionally painful even after repeated application of stimuli for several seconds, deliberately slow "**creeping**" into the depth of the tissue may be employed. Taking into account the patient's pain threshold, the intensity of the grip is gently increased. We wait for the pain to subside before the next grip is performed in the same attentive manner. This variation is similar to the **sedating grip** (see Chapter 3.2.5).

If a zone is already very painful when first touched, the varied sedating grip can likewise be employed in this way. If, in addition to the pain, strong autonomic overreactions are triggered in a zone, it usually suffices to place the tip of the thumb or finger gently and calmly on the zone until the patient's condition has stabilized.

12.2.2 Points of Emphasis

It is not necessary to treat all irritated zones with equal attention. However, over time we should recognize **points of emphasis** as a result of practice and observation from questions asked **before** the treatment. As a rule, six to eight zones per treatment, sometimes a few more, should be deliberately and selectively treated.

Similar to the ripple effect caused by a stone when thrown into water, treatment is a dynamic process, communicating with additional, functionally related zones and **reorganizing the whole organism.**

From My Practice
In my first year of teaching reflexotherapy of the feet (RTF) I recognized the dynamic process of treatment acting on remote organs very clearly as a result of the response I received from one of the female course participants. On the second day of the course she mentioned that her menstruation had started a week earlier than expected "although we only treated the zones of the head and neck yesterday."
When informed that the zones of the pituitary gland and the thyroid were already included in the practical exercises in the head and neck region, she was able to understand that there was a connection between the preceding treatment and her menstruation beginning early, particularly as she also reacted similarly to a change of location or work.

12.3

Final Treatment

As a rule, a final check-up is performed after a series of treatments in order to inspect all the zones objectively. This gives patients and therapists the opportunity to obtain an overview of the results of the treatment.

12.3.1 Performing the Final Treatment

As at the beginning of the course of treatment, we perform a **visual inspection** to note which changes have taken place in the
- anatomical structure of the feet,
- tissue of the feet, and
- skin and nails.

Then all the zones are **palpated** again briefly in seven working groups or according to the anatomical structure of the foot in order to objectify the patient's descriptions of changes in their complaints.

Recording the Final Findings

For practical reasons we use the same treatment card as for the initial findings and record the results in **blue**:

- Circle in blue, zones which are still clearly painful or irritated.
- Cross out in blue, zones which are no longer abnormal.
- Add in blue, new abnormal zones.

With the same gradual differentiation as for the initial findings, highly irritated zones are marked **boldly** in blue, less irritated zones are marked **less boldly** in blue, and zones that are hardly painful at all are marked **very lightly** in blue.

12.3.2 **Summary**

The primary aim of a course of treatment is for the patient to experience the maximum subjective improvement possible, not to eliminate all painful or tender zones by the end of the course.

A distinct improvement culminating in the complete healing of the patient's ailments is to be expected in patients with **acute** diseases which have developed in a short period, above all, if they have a fair amount of physical and inner regenerative strength. Even if some painful zones can still be found after six to eight treatments, the course can be finished because **some things just need more time to heal**.

Time and again, **chronically ill patients** demonstrate such a strong will to recover that many of their aggravating symptoms can be **alleviated** or severe pain borne more easily because their overall vitality has been mobilized by RTF.

In chronically ill patients many zones may undergo qualitative changes and even demonstrate significant improvement over a specified period of time. However, these patients continually require a fresh array of treatments and, in addition to other regenerative applications, should undergo one or two shorter courses of RTF treatment every year.

13 Duration of and Intervals between Treatments

13.1

Duration of the First Assessment and Follow-up Treatments

We should leave ourselves sufficient time for the **first assessment**, above all as beginners, because new experiences require calm and practice. When I first began in private practice, I often gave my new patients appointments at the end of the day or doubled the treatment time.

At the beginning each patient should be allotted a full hour; this also provides the opportunity to become better acquainted with each other. Having gained more experience, approximately 45 minutes will be sufficient.

The **follow-up treatments** are much shorter, approximately 20 to 30 minutes. In the follow-up treatments, however, a **different choice** of zones for treatment is almost always made as a result of the reactions which have taken place. This leads to the need for flexibility in terms of time because

- in an acute reaction phase 15 minutes might be sufficient,
- during the next treatment, time may also be needed for a brief conversation,
- on another occasion it may be necessary to include new zones, for example, because of the onset of a cold.

13.2

Treatment Intervals

Usually reflexotherapy of the feet is provided like other methods of physical therapy, two to three times a week.

Sometimes it is more beneficial if treatment is provided for three to four days in succession, above all, if the patient's response is stable and they take enough time for the resting phase after each treatment.

With **acute** pain, treatment is daily or even several times a day (Chapter 16).

In the situation of long-term patients and the **chronically** sick, if their symptoms permit, after the initial regular series of treatments the frequency can be slowly reduced to once a week, once every 14 days, or once a month.

One or two intense **series of treatments** a year at long intervals, during which other treatments may be provided, are usually more effective for the **chronically** sick than continuous treatment with the same method.

13.3

Duration of a Treatment Series

A series should last for as long as the therapeutic measures bring about a **change** and/or **improvement** in the patient's condition—usually 6 to 12 treatments.

If patients possess good regenerative forces, their health will improve after only a few treatments; in patients whose reactions are slower, as many as 15, 20, or even more treatments may be necessary.

In deference to their independence and autonomy, I let patients decide for themselves when they deem the time to be right for a further series of treatments and only make therapeutic recommendations based on their present symptoms.

Experience shows that a **good basis** is already laid by the first series of treatments for further series and that these usually require fewer sessions as a result.

14 Reactions during Treatment Intervals

14.1

General Information

Reactions in the periods between two treatment sessions are a response to the therapeutic stimulus and present themselves as changes in the patient's condition. They often occur between the **second** and **sixth** treatment, usually lasting several hours, sometimes even days and are characterized by their great variety. The principle that a chain is only as strong as its weakest link is confirmed by the way in which the organs or systems that are most affected or weakened often react first.

Reactions are an important transitional phase between disease and health and can affect all the physical organs and systems as well as the whole person at an emotional, psychological, or mental level.

The first most clearly perceptible reactions are at a physical level. Here it is often the **excretory organs** which constitute the appropriate vehicle for the removal of existing toxins, harmful substances, metabolic residues, and end products from inside the body.

Hering's Law (named after the homeopathic physician C. Hering, 1800–1880) also frequently applies to the response and healing phases of reflexotherapy of the feet (RTF), above all, in those with chronic disease:

- The symptoms disappear from the inside to the outside, and/or
- from top to bottom, and/or
- in the reverse order to that in which they arose.

From a **therapeutic** perspective, reactions are useful and necessary on principle for without reactions no changes can be achieved in the present condition.

From the **patient's perspective,** reactions may be pleasant or disturbing. However, they must in any case be assessed positively, even if they are sometimes subjectively described as "deterioration" due to ignorance of their internal correlations.

The analogy with a good spring clean helps some patients to accept the acute phase of reactions and enhances their understanding of the fact that it is precisely the unpleasant attendant symptoms that provide a major opportunity for improvement during the regeneration process.

The **special nature of the patient's reactions**
- is linked to the internal and external background of the patient's illness,
- provides an overview of previous and current ailments, and
- points to the available opportunities and resources that can be activated in order to change and improve the current phase of their condition.

14.2

The Most Common Reactions

With the following list it should be remembered that biological processes cannot be defined by schematic, linear thinking but always present themselves in the following manner:
- interconnected,
- overlapping with other systems, and
- in a rhythmic and dynamic form.

The result of any treatment, including with regard to responses and their effects, primarily depends on the **overall regenerative capacity** of the patient and **not** on the name of a disease. Often an **improvement** in the ailments is the first encouraging reaction.

For the sake of clarity, the reactions are classified as described in detail in Chapter 10:
- Head and neck
- Spine, thorax
- Urinary tract, tissue from the pelvis, thigh and knee
- Endocrine system
- Respiration, heart and circulation
- Digestive tract
- Lymphatic system

Three further groups are added to this list, which must likewise be addressed with respect to reactions to treatment:
- Skin and mucous membranes
- Sleep, regeneration, dreams
- Mood, mental state

When reactions within groups of organs are discussed below, this does not mean that they arise solely as a result of treatment of these groups of organs.

The types of reaction and the choice of transport route via which they take place can be supported but not fundamentally influenced from outside.

Head and Neck

Headaches of various kinds and origin sometimes cease after a short phase of reactivation.

Sinuses discharge secretions which are watery or viscous in consistency.

Blood pressure readings and their amplitude may change in both hypertonic and hypotonic conditions.

The conjunctiva of the eyes often reacts in allergic patients with a decrease in exudate and reduced reddening and swelling.

Chronic inflammatory tendencies in the nasopharyngeal cavity and neck abate.

Spine, Thorax, Joints, and Muscle Groups

Functional complaints in the spine (e.g., pain after accidents, ischialgia) and restriction of movement in the large and small joints improve, sometimes accompanied by a short, acute period of pain. The quality of the posture improves.

Myogelosis, especially in the shoulder girdle and back, become less painful as the muscle tone normalizes.

Urinary Tract

Often the kidneys and bladder discharge more urine. This may become cloudier or clearer, the smell may change and become more or less intense, and laboratory examinations may reveal more urinary waste substances.

Patients suffering from an **irritated bladder** throughout the day or night usually experience an improvement after a few treatments if their regenerative qualities are well developed.

Practical Advice

If a patient's bladder irritation develops into an **inflammation with fever**, we must respect our professional limits and those of RTF and, where necessary, refer the patient to a doctor. With such decisions, it is important for further progress that the symptom is not suppressed but rather supported by natural remedies promoting self-healing so that deeper reorganization can take place in the ailing background systems.

Endocrine and Nervous Systems

In many patients suffering from an endocrine deficiency, RTF may constitute a supportive concomitant treatment. If the patient is taking hormones, we can and must reckon with additional reactions as a result of the treatment (Chapter 16.3).

As **menstruation** represents a hormonally determined response of the mucous membranes, excretions may change. Bleeding may become heavier or lighter, severe pain before or during menstruation diminishes significantly. Vaginal discharge may be heavier or disappear. **Gynecological complaints are one of the most promising indications for RTF.**

Time and again the cycle also changes in terms of length and frequency in women with weakened endocrine and nervous systems, usually resulting in the next period starting earlier. **In very rare cases** it has also been observed that intrauterine devices (the "coil") alter their position or the menstrual cycle changes even when taking contraceptives. Furthermore, not all women are adequately aware that oral contraceptives may be **ineffective** in the event of severe diarrhea rendering the organism unable to absorb them. There is a duty of care to provide this information!

In **diabetics** it is particularly important that the blood sugar level be checked more frequently as it may already change significantly as a result of the first treatment.

Patients with **hyperthyroidism** respond to the correct dosage of treatment with greater tranquility and calm. If possible, they should be treated in the morning because their sleep may be disturbed if they receive too strong a dose.

Respiration, Heart, and Circulation

One of the most common observations is that respiration becomes more regulated, that is, deeper and calmer. Expectoration is easier in patients with asthma, bronchitis, or bronchiectasis; the color, consistency, and odor of the phlegm may change.

The disturbing effects of functional cardiac complaints such as tachycardia and minor angina pectoris disorders diminish. Many patients report after only a few treatments that their **chronically cold feet** and blood circulation in general have improved and that venous congestion has decreased.

Practical Advice

In patients suffering from severe heart disease, the zone of the heart should not be at the center of the therapy to avoid aggravating the complaints (Chapter 16.3).

Digestive Tract

Bowel excretions usually become more voluminous and frequent as well as temporarily malodorous, mucilaginous, and discolored. Flatulence either increases or decreases.

Rarely, spontaneous vomiting or diarrhea occurs for one or two days. In the event of more persistent diarrhea, a more precise diagnostic examination is indicated.

Aphthae and thrush in the oral area may subside and hemorrhoid pain decrease.

Practical Advice

In patients who suffer from **chronic** intestinal disease (ulcerative colitis, mucous colitis, Crohn's disease), the zone of the intestine should never be vigorously tonified because the patient may become increasingly dehydrated and further disruption of the electrolyte level may occur as a result of excessive irritation (see Chapters 16.3 and 21.7).

Lymphatic System

Patients with primary or secondary disorders or diseases of the lymphatic system often react to RTF with a significant increase in urinary output. A measurable **reduction in the volume** of the congested arm may often be observed in women after a mastectomy. The effect may be intensified by means of special treatment of the zones of the lymphatic system within RTF (Chapter 23).

There is a decrease of congestion in the feet and legs that occurs during the day. A tendency to chronic infections of the upper respiratory tract declines, particularly in children, who nowadays often suffer from lymphatic disorders starting at a young age (Chapter 22).

Skin

The skin becomes more active in terms of excretion and receptiveness and takes on a healthier appearance as a result. Perspiration may increase or decrease at first depending on the patient's initial condition. Now and then pustules or urticaria (nettle rash) appear briefly.

Frequently a disturbing and unpleasant body odor develops for a while and this should not be suppressed by artificial deodorants under any circumstances. (Examine and change eating habits, if necessary!)

The symptoms of existing acute or chronic skin irritations and conditions (e.g., eczema) abate; sometimes the symptoms are aggravated for a short time. Areas of open skin between the toes often clear up of their own accord after a few treatments.

Practical Advice

If acute skin reactions persist or become significantly worse, interim consultation of a doctor is advised in order to curtail this process using corresponding remedies, preferably those that do not simply suppress superficial symptoms. **Classical homeopathy** offers a wide range of opportunities for far-reaching treatment. It is essential that prescribed dietary rules should be consistently followed.

Mucous Membranes

The mucous membranes of the nasopharynx and bronchial tubes can cleanse and stabilize themselves by increasing or decreasing the discharge of secretions.

In men and women there may be a discharge from the vagina or urethra, sometimes so concentrated that it irritates the tissue of the mucous membranes and skin. More often, however, above all in women, an existing **discharge** eases significantly, changes in odor and color and disappears completely.

In women more often than in men, the lining of the genital organs is plagued by chronic recurring fungal infections. Treatment with RTF should be accompanied by a specific change in diet to improve the entire environment of the mucous membranes, including those of the intestine.

Raised Temperature and Fever

A short febrile attack or raised temperature in response to RTF is usually an obvious attempt to deal with toxins and waste material internally.

This being so, the fever is a sign of a **healthy immune system** and should not be tackled with antibiotics because this obscures the course of the illness, as only the symptoms are suppressed. Whether and when the administration of antibiotics is regarded as essential for the course of a particular disease should be decided by the doctor in consultation with the patient.

Practical Advice

Apart from the well-known remedy of wet compresses applied to the lower legs, an **enema** is a household remedy for naturally providing relief and regulating a high temperature.

Activation of Earlier Diseases

Diseases which have not been completely cured, or which have been suppressed instead of being healed, may briefly reappear in a milder form. This reaction should not be understood as an aggravation of the patient's condition, but rather indicates that the therapy can lead to the healing of chronic, hidden processes via an acute phase.

Practical Advice

If the patient possesses a good amount of vitality, a whole series of earlier diseases may be reactivated at short notice and encourage healing, in the sense of a "progressive vicaration to diminish the toxins accumulated in the deposition phases". This is certainly not a cause for concern but promotes good cooperation between the patient and doctor and clear psychological guidance for the patient.

Sleep and Dreams

With regard to the quality and quantity of sleep, some patients react to RTF with an increased need for sleep that should be heeded; others are particularly unsettled or require less sleep than usual and yet feel more refreshed and ready for action the next day.

Dreams, both pleasant and worrying, are significant signals from the subconscious and perform important spiritual "tidying up." Sometimes it would also be advisable to suggest getting support from a good psychotherapist or responsibly led self-awareness group in order to enable old, hitherto subconscious or suppressed problems to be processed more easily.

When patients entrust their private lives to a professional in order to process upcoming life-themes, the latter's absolute integrity and credibility is of vital importance.

Mood and Mental State

Restlessness or anxiety may now and then increase for a few hours as an initial reaction but often the experience of having their feet touched gives patients a feeling of being grounded and less nervous, indecisive, and fearful.

Growing inner awareness and poise may be revealed in
- more open encounters with other people,
- freer expression of feelings in the form of laughter, tears, attentiveness, joy, rage,
- increased readiness to undertake ventures and make changes, and
- active endeavor by the patient to find their own place within the family or among friends.

> In general, there is insufficient awareness of the clarifying, cleansing, and strengthening powers of **Classical Homeopathy** (Samuel Hahnemann) in dealing with both inherited diseases and deep-seated emotional problems.

14.3

Dealing with Strong Reactions

14.3.1 General Information

In the event of unexpectedly strong reactions (rarely happens), we can choose different forms of care and support for the patient. However, at times like these patients should always feel reassured that they can depend on us and that, if necessary, we will notify their specialist or physician that their reactions are to the treatment stimulus and not indicative of a new disease. Under the right conditions, we thus avoid the administration of medication that merely conceals and suppresses the symptoms again.

14.3.2 Care during Strong Reactions

There are a number of possibilities open to us:
- We offer **interim treatment** which focuses on the acute symptoms (Chapter 16).
- A treatment session may be **omitted** to enable the intensity of the reactions to subside gently.
- If patients are extremely anxious, they may be treated daily, now and then even **briefly several times a day**. Preferably, stabilizing grips are chosen to allow the nervous system to recuperate. Treatment time is usually restricted to 10 to 15 minutes.
- The next treatment does not focus on the symptoms but rather the related groups of organs or systems. By treating these, intense reactions in the symptomatic region are eased. The **background zones** are often of great value as they represent the basis on which the symptoms were able to arise.

Examples

Severe headache. The zones of the intestine, upper abdomen, or genitals may be tonified because for many people, the causes of headaches lie in the digestive tract and in women, in the lower abdominal area as well.

Heavy colds in the head and throat region. We apply the tonifying stimulus to the pelvic organs, lymphatic system, and intestine (development of mucous membranes from the same germ layer).

Acute asthmatic attack. As a rule, patients react well to tonification of the zones of the adrenal glands, small intestine (severe hyperacidity), liver and gall bladder, pelvic floor with anus, and to sedating grips. (Sphincter muscles usually react to stress stimuli with spasticity.)

14.3.3   Examples of Severe Reactions

On occasion, the following occur:
- a latent headache develops into a **migraine**,
- severe **urticaria** appears over the entire body, usually disappearing again without special treatment after a few days,
- we trigger **renal** or **biliary colic**,
- a heavy **phase of diarrhea** signifies intensive cleansing of the intestine,
- patients develop acute **toothache**,
- women in the menopause have unexpected **vaginal bleeding**.

We also support patients during periods like those suggested in Chapter 14.3.2. If and when soothing medication is administered in addition is usually decided on the basis of a given situation often not occurring for the first time and in the event of which those concerned can then fall back on earlier behavioral strategies.

However, duty of care requires that, without delay, the attending physician be notified of suspicious reactions suggestive of more serious, previously undetected diseases.

From My Practice
On three occasions over the years—on two occasions in children and one in a young woman—I have witnessed how RTF has caused a chronic lymphatic deficiency to develop into **acute appendicitis** by way of fever, nausea, and pain, necessitating an operation. After appendectomy, these three patients underwent further RTF treatment and as a result became much stronger and more stable than before.

However, it is much more often the case that—sometimes after a slight, short-term more acute period—chronic recurring complaints in the right lower abdomen are completely healed with one or more series of RTF, especially in children.

14.4

Negative Reactions, New Diseases

Genuinely negative reactions which clearly aggravate the existing situation in the long term may arise if
- the therapist has worked for too long and with too much force during treatment,
- treatment overemphasized symptoms in an unbalanced manner, and/or
- contraindications were not taken into account.

Nowadays people are more sophisticated and consequently often also more rapidly afflicted than before. There has been a significant increase in sensory overload and the use of medications.

We should therefore observe particularly carefully the reactions of those who are noticeably weakened and overloaded through taking many different forms of medication during treatment intervals, in order to detect when a reaction phase **lasts too long** or **takes on a life of its own** and under unfavorable conditions a new or different disease develops as a result (**very rare!**).

14.5

Summary

Usually, reactions as a direct response to RTF cease after a few hours but sometimes only after 3 to 6 days. If they last longer, the therapist should thoroughly investigate the background to the delayed reaction.

With a multitude of treatments on offer today and in view of the fact that not all of these are motivated by a desire to improve people's health, **all** those involved (those prescribing, those performing the treatment, and those receiving it) should exert their influence to avoid **too many different** treatments being administered in too close succession.

Above all, the effects of stimulation-specific treatments should be allowed to develop over a period of at least a few hours, if not even a whole day, uninterrupted by other forms of therapy.

This presupposes good professional insight and an overview of the different forms of treatment offers prevalent today and their modes of action.

15 Right–Left Interchangeability of Zones of the Feet

15.1

General Information

For decades William FitzGerald's assignment of body zones to the **same** side in the feet had for the most part proved its worth in my practice. Contrary to his findings, however, I repeatedly observed that in disorders and complaints in bilateral organs, joints, and groups of muscles the point on the foot which corresponded to the symptom-**free** side of the body reacted just as strongly to the treatment stimulus as the affected point, or even more strongly.

Initially I assigned this to the principle of contralateral effects known to me from physical therapy (Chapter 18.4). Later, however, my observations of a right–left relationship of the areas affected by symptoms were confirmed by experienced doctors using **acupuncture** and **neural therapy**.

In some patients I then gradually began to specifically treat only the side corresponding to the complaint-**free** side of the body in accordance with the previous assignment of zones; that is, I only treated the zone of the shoulder on the **left** foot, although there was a shoulder injury on the **right**. Sensitivity to pain at the newly selected points did not prove uniform but the results were striking enough to continue devoting much of my time to this.

In the course of my observations over the years, I also began to examine the zones of the **unilateral** organs. For example, I observed that in some patients the point that corresponded to the gall bladder zone on the right foot reacted just as strongly or even more so on the left. Strangely, more than once acute biliary colic was triggered exclusively and spontaneously only as a result of treatment of the **left** foot. It was clear that the right–left reversal was present so often that I could not simply dismiss it as accidental.

Wholly unexpectedly at first, course participants supported me for years by coming to further courses with their own, similar observations of the right–left reciprocal effect and for their part found their observations confirmed by my practical experiences.

This background led me to extend the hitherto familiar and exclusive view held by FitzGerald of

same-sided assignment to include the spectrum of right–left interchangeability of the zones.

FitzGerald's arrangement is retained in the detailed illustrations of the zones in this book, in other words: right half of the body, **right** foot. In addition to the illustrations of **all** the zones (**Figs. 9.1–9.4**), this chapter includes a slightly smaller drawing of the right–left reversal as important information, repeatedly confirmed in practice, in other words: right half of the body, **left** foot (**Fig. 15.1**) and vice versa.

I should like to pass on these experiences and observations to stimulate the **expansion of therapeutic approaches** within reflexotherapy of the feet and do not regard them as a restrictive either/or principle.

15.2

Practical Aids for Differentiation

The right–left relationship should be considered as a possible variation in the treatment process in the very first assessment; above all, with regard to the **symptomatic** zones (Chapter 11).

If we want to clarify the side on which the relevant zone can be found, at the start of each new treatment session we briefly examine the symptomatic zones on their anatomically corresponding side on **both** feet simultaneously. As a rule, we will obtain a response which accords with one of the following three statements, and the patient's reaction will indicate unmistakably the right path to the area requiring treatment:

- The zone on the **same** side is more sensitive to pain (FitzGerald's rule).
- The zone on the **opposite** side is more sensitive to pain (right–left interchangeability).
- **Both sides** react equally or with only a slight difference in terms of the quality and quantity of pain experienced.

It is important to examine both feet **simultaneously** because if examined in succession, the treatment of one side might have already influenced the as yet untouched side, thus falsifying the results.

Right–left interchangeability of the reflex zones

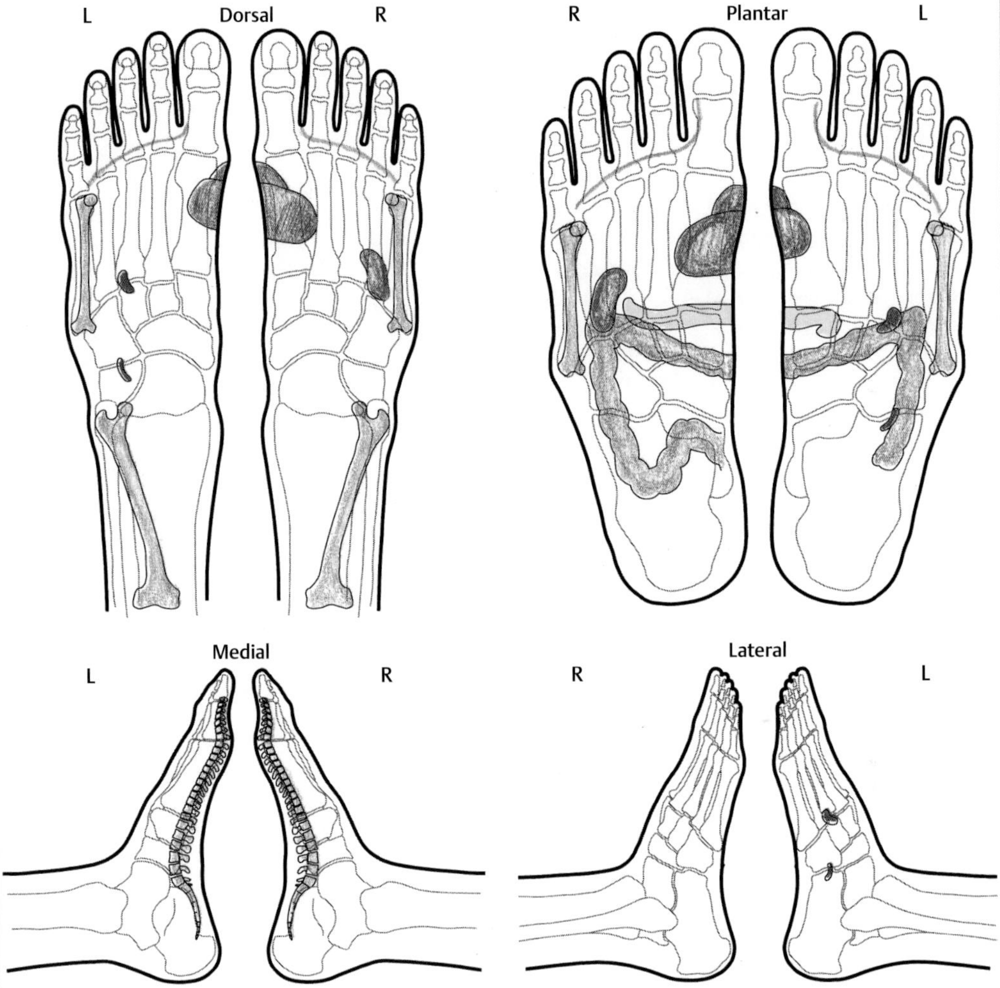

L   Dorsal   R   R   Plantar   L

L   Medial   R   R   Lateral   L

This illustration represents those zones in which right–left interchangeability is particularly easy to recognize: the heart, spleen, gallbladder, pancreas, large intestine, and appendix.

In **therapy**, depending on the patient's illness, this interchangeability can naturally relate to **all** the zones, including the bilateral organs and joints.

Palpation will always indicate which zones currently require treatment.

Aid to understanding: in both top views of the feet we imagine seeing a scaled down person standing opposite us from the **front** (dorsal side of the foot) and from the **rear** (plantar side of the foot) and are thus able to classify the sites of the organs in their mirror image more easily.

Fig. 15.1 A selection of some zones of the feet in right–left interchangeability.

The different variants do not alter the practical performance of a treatment because **all** the points on the foot in need of therapy are always included, regardless of whether they are on the right or left side or of their zone designation (Chapter 11.3.2).

15.3

Summary

Anyone who would like to familiarize themselves with the possibility of right–left interchangeability of the zones in a simple manner should look at their own feet, placed next to each other, as if they were sitting opposite a scaled-down figure of themselves.

It is thus easy to "see" the left half of the body in the right foot and the right half in the left foot.

It has long been obvious to me that a rigid separation between right and left does not have the significance usually conceded to it in customary one-sided thinking.

In all holistically oriented branches of therapy, the balancing and linking of opposites lies at the center of treatment, not only of the right and left sides, but also of above and below, behind and in front, inside and out. By widening the field of vision in this way therapy can become genuinely "whole" again, in the sense of holistic and complete.

16 Management and Treatment of Pain in Acute Situations

16.1

General Information

Situations arise in which patients require urgent treatment for acute pain or illness, for example:

- Acute hay fever
- Ischialgia
- Cystitis (without fever)
- Asthma attacks
- Biliary or renal colic
- Hemorrhoid pain
- Migraine
- Earache, especially in children
- Pylorus spasm
- Premenstrual or menstrual pain
- Painful restriction of movement of joints
- Torticollis, especially in early childhood
- Unexpectedly heavy bleeding
- Accidents such as whiplash injuries, sprains, bruises
- Toothache
- Cervical or intercostal neuralgia

With **intense pain** or other acute complaints, we apply the **sedating grip** (Chapter 3.2.5) to the symptomatic zone immediately rather than making a detailed initial assessment. This grip soothes the painful related point in the body.

In addition, we **tonify** the zones that are functionally related to the painful area. These are background zones directly relevant to the current acute situation. If some of these prove very painful, the sedating grip may also be applied first.

After the pain and complaints have **subsided**, the symptomatic zones may also be tonified—gently at first, and then later with greater intensity.

Important note: The symptomatic zones are always examined on **both** feet in the sense of right–left interchangeability (Chapter 15). The sedating grip is applied to the clearly affected point (sometimes both right **and** left).

16.2

Performance

16.2.1 Treatment of the Symptomatic Zone with the Sedating Grip

Performing this grip in its active phase is similar to performing the basic grip:

- Touch the symptomatic zone gently.
- Bring the distal phalanx of the thumb from a horizontal into a vertical position by swinging the arm.
- Apply the therapeutic stimulus deep into the tissue. Unlike the customary basic grip, this position is calmly maintained until the strong pain in this zone has eased significantly. In general, this takes 5 to 10 seconds, sometimes more, sometimes less.
- Only now is the tension of the grip released, and the relaxed thumb swings gently back into its initial position.

The entire symptomatic zone is treated point by point in millimeter steps using the sedating grip, coordinating the release of pressure with the easing of the pain in the zone.

As soon as the patient appears strained and the autonomous nervous system severely irritated, we perform a **stabilizing grip** and pause for a moment.

If the intensity of the pain persists for longer than 15 seconds or if it eases only slightly, the **solar plexus** zone is treated (sedating grip!) and the painful zone then carefully re-examined again.

With all First Aid treatments, the equivalent symptomatic site on the other foot is also examined to see how painful it is and, if necessary, it is treated likewise with the sedating grip (Chapter 18.4). Apart from the thumb, the index finger may also be used for this.

16.2.2 Simultaneous Treatment of Functionally Related Background Zones

Sometimes simply treating the symptomatic zones with the sedating grip is sufficient. Usually, however, acute pain eases faster and the results are longer lasting if we tonify additional zones which are functionally related to the existing complaint.

Exception: If the background zones are very close to the symptomatic zone, they are not tonified. For example, in the event of acute pain in a wisdom tooth the zones of the ear are not tonified.

The **choice of background zones** can be made in accordance with the following criteria:

- Musculoskeletal functional range (e.g., in patients with epicondylitis): lower cervical spine and neck, upper thoracic spine, scapula, shoulder joint and muscles including the trapezius and arm
- Ontogenetic connection to the same germ layer (e.g., mucous membrane disorders): interrelationship between the digestive tract, nasopharynx and bladder – genital system
- Systemic connections (e.g., tonsils–appendix; thyroid gland–ovary; liver–spleen; eyes–kidneys, pancreas)
- Segmental connections (e.g., sacrum – organs of the lower pelvis; middle of the thoracic spine – stomach)
- Areas with similar shapes in which the joints or organs can be treated alternately, (e.g., humerus–femur; temporomandibular joint – hip joint; brain–intestine, Eustachian tubes – fallopian tubes)

With all **inflammatory processes** the zones of the intestine and spleen are treated at the same time, both usually with tonification.

Examples

- **First Aid** for a patient with acute **toothache:**
  Sedating grip in the zone of the affected tooth. It often proves necessary to treat the zones of the adjacent teeth with the sedating grip as well. Now and then, however, the sedating grip may aggravate the toothache. In this kind of situation, **first** the lymphatic zones of the head and neck are stroked, both laterally on the metatarsophalangeal joint and on the interdigital spaces between the individual toes, in order to promote drainage. The background zones may also be treated. Then the sedating grip should be repeated carefully and slowly in the symptomatic zone.
  Tonifying of the zones of the intestine (relationship between teeth and the digestive tract).

- Women with severe **menstrual pain:**
  Sedating grip in the zones of the uterus, ovaries, lower spine with sacroiliac joint and solar plexus.
  Tonifying of the zones of the intestine, gluteal muscles, pelvic floor, pituitary gland, nasopharyngeal cavity (development from the same germ layer). When the acute phase of pain has eased, the symptomatic zones of the uterus and ovaries may first be tonified gently and then later possibly more vigorously. Alternating strokes in the zones of the lymphatic system of the thigh and inguinal areas (assignment to the genital area).

- Patient with **biliary colic:**
  Sedating grip in the zone of the gall bladder (plantar and/or dorsal).
  Tonifying of zones of the small intestine, right side of the neck, shoulder girdle and joint (segmental relationships).

- **Renal colic:** (Chapter 21.4.2)

- Child with **earache:**
  Careful and slow performance of the **sedating grip** on the zones of the ear and mastoid process.
  Tonifying of the zones of the cervical spine, intestine and/or pelvis and kidneys (correlation via mucosal structure from the same germ layer and via meridian energy). Gentle treatment of the lymphatic chains of the neck to relieve the symptoms.

- Patient with **whiplash** of the neck:
  Sedating grip (always performed carefully and slowly) on the zones of the neck, back of the head with mastoid process, thoracic spine, inner ear (sense of balance).
  Tonifying of the sacrococcygeal region (craniosacral connections) and the adrenal glands (experience involving shock).

- If the symptoms **worsen:** sedating grip also on the lower spine and omit symptomatic zone completely for one or two treatment sessions. Gentle treatment of the lymphatic chains of the neck. Pay careful attention to the dosage limit.
  Treatment for about 10 minutes daily or even several times a day for around 3 to 4 days proves effective at the start of therapy. The performance of many stabilizing grips in the interim is particularly important here.

- Patient with acute **hay fever:**
  Sedating grip in the zones of the nasopharyngeal cavity. Tonifying to encourage

discharge via the nasopharyngeal cavity can also take place after the acute phase with the intensity dependent on the sensitivity of the patient. Gentle treatment of the zones of the lymphatic chains of the neck and/or treatment of the interdigital tissue for relief of the symptoms.

Tonifying of the zones of the kidneys, pituitary gland, thymus, small intestine, pelvic organs (development of mucous membranes from the same germ layer), spleen, pancreas, stomach.

- **First Aid** for patients with **acute circulatory weakness:**
Position the legs higher than the head. Balanced tonifying treatment (not too vigorous), several times in succession and lasting for only a few seconds in each zone, performed in the following sequence:
  - Pituitary gland
  - Occiput with neck
  - Heart, thyroid gland
  - Adrenal glands (identical to kidney)
  - Spleen
  - Genitals
  - Solar plexus

Tonifying the abdominal and pelvic organs in addition supports basic metabolic processes and enables the patient to regain their general equilibrium so that they are less agitated. Medication to stabilize the circulation and Bach flower essences number 39 - **Rescue Remedy** can also be used for this purpose, although these measures are not always necessary.

16.2.3 Summary

Practical Information

- Often, acute care helps to overcome the most aggressive phase of pain. Sometimes it helps to bridge the time until other measures are possible, for example, with acute toothache. After the acute phase has passed we must decide, through careful observation of the patient's present condition, if and when it is necessary to ask for further medical advice.
- The stronger the pain and the more sensitive the symptomatic zones, the more we advise:
  - either starting treatment with the background zones (functional connections with the symptom), or

- slowly and carefully increasing the intensity of the sedating grip in the symptomatic zone—that is, slowly increasing the intensity of the grip in the tissue until we reach the maximum possible.
- If the pain in the symptomatic zone remains constant for longer than 15 to 20 seconds, we first choose the same anatomical site on the other foot and return to the former later on.
- If the pain in the symptomatic zone does not subside at all, **only** the background zones are tonified. During the next treatment session, however, the symptomatic zone should be checked again. It then often proves to be less painful.
- If the pain in the symptomatic zone fluctuates during the sedating grip, in our experience there may be a **disturbing focus** in the organ, tissue, or meridian—for example, scars, chronically inflamed organs, or tooth decay. In this situation, neural therapy or holistic treatment of the teeth will be the methods of choice. Reflexotherapy of the feet (RTF) should be continued as an additional measure.
- Sometimes, contrary to all our expectations, the symptomatic zone is not painful in patients suffering from acute ailments. An examination of the same anatomical site on the other foot (Chapter 15) or the detection of background zones in such situations usually leads to a good treatment outcome.
- Practice has shown that the desired treatment outcome can also be achieved with some acute treatment if the symptomatic zone is completely **disregarded** and only the affected background zones are treated.
- After the acute phase has subsided, it is often wise to perform a thorough initial assessment to ascertain as far as possible the disturbed environment in which the painful symptom was able to develop and to treat it in follow-up sessions.

People tend to forget that the symptoms are only the visible "tip of the iceberg." Only if the background (of the "iceberg") is changed can the symptoms also change because they have arisen as a result of the background zones.

> **From My Practice**
> During the first months of my attempts with RTF, I had an astonishing experience that helped me to understand connections of this nature more deeply. A patient came to me with severe pain and obvious restriction of movement of her **left shoulder** (periarthritis humeroscapularis). Neither the left nor the right shoulder zones responded to the therapeutic grip. Puzzled, I palpated both feet and encountered an extremely painful zone of the descending colon and the sigmoid, which I tonified intensely. The patient then had a voluminous and offensive-smelling bowel movement and was able to spontaneously move her shoulder with less pain and in a larger radius.
> Shortly thereafter, when examining the field of acupuncture, I learned that the **meridian of the large intestine** also supplies energy to the shoulder on its way from the index finger to the nostril. As a result of this powerful experience, I coined the term "causal zones," later renamed "background zones."

16.3

Careful Treatment of Symptomatic Zones in Special Diseases

As patients today often have more complex, multi-layered diseases than before, we advise **not** focusing on the symptomatic zones in the groups of patients listed below during initial treatment.

> If the stimuli in the symptomatic zone are too strong and one-sided and the background zones are not taken into consideration, the patient's complaints may worsen rather than abate.

Subsequently, in particular when the patient's condition has stabilized, the treatment can also be intensified somewhat in the symptomatic zones.

16.3.1   Examples

- Symptomatic region of the **head and neck:** patients with
  - Hypertension
  - Craniocerebral trauma and head surgery
  - Tumors in the head, whether benign or malignant, operated on or not
  - Apoplexy
  - Glaucoma
  - Epilepsy
  - Alzheimer's disease

- Whiplash in the head–neck region
- Avoid excessive treatment in the (symptomatic) **head and neck zones**. (For further information, see Chapter 21.2.)
- Symptomatic region of the **spine** and **joints:** patients with
  - Paraplegia as a result of accidents or other serious diseases (e.g., tumors)
  - Joint endoprosthesis (e.g., hip)
  - Avoid excessive treatment of the symptomatic zones of the corresponding sections of the **spine** or replaced **joints.** (For further information, see Chapter 21.3.)
- Symptomatic region of the **urinary tract:** patients with
  - Serious chronic, degenerative kidney disease (e.g., glomerulonephritis, patients on dialysis)
  - Kidney stones which cannot be excreted in the normal way due to their size
  - Avoid excessive treatment in the (symptomatic) **kidney zones**! (For further information, see Chapter 21.4.)
- Symptomatic region of the **endocrine glands:** patients with **hormone** deficiencies or who are taking hormones such as preparations for the pituitaries, thyroxine, cortisone, insulin, contraceptives or hormone patches in the menopause.

The **symptomatic zones** here are the organ zones directly affected by the hormonal preparation, for example, the pancreas in diabetics, the uterus and ovaries in women who are taking contraceptives, etc. Here too excessive treatment stimuli must be avoided.
N.B. In diabetic patients excessive, over-vigorous treatment of the pancreatic zone can result in an unexpectedly rapid and significant fall in blood sugar levels. The critical period is approximately 12 to 16 hours after treatment (patients should be advised to check their blood sugar more frequently). (For further information, see Chapter 21.5).
In women who take contraceptives, the increased risk of deep vein thrombosis and other diseases is well known and should also be heeded accordingly in RTF (Chapter 5.2.1).

- Symptomatic region of the **cardiovascular system**: patients with
  - Angina pectoris or after myocardial infarction
  - Heart surgery, pacemakers, or bypass operations
  - Other serious heart disease

- Avoid excessive treatment in the (symptomatic) **heart zones**. Direct energetic connections between the heart and **spleen** are well-known in acupuncture. It therefore makes sense to treat the spleen zone before the heart zone. (For further information, see Chapter 21.6.)
- Symptomatic region of the **respiratory organs**: patients with asthma (including in the intervals **free** of attacks) are also treated carefully in the **zones of the bronchi and lungs** (symptomatic zones) because with overemphasis on one side, there is a risk of triggering an acute attack. (For further therapy advice, see Chapter 21.6.)
- Symptomatic region of the **digestive system**:
  - Patients with acute or chronic inflammatory bowel diseases: diarrhea, ulcerative colitis, mucous colitis, Crohn's disease. Avoid excessive treatment in the (symptomatic) **zones of the intestine,** both the small and large intestine. (For further information, see Chapter 21.7.)
  - Patients with **large gallstones**: If the treatment in the symptomatic zone of the gall bladder is too intense and protracted, it may trigger hepatic colic. (For further information, see Chapter 16.2.2.) This relates to large kidney stones.
- **Postoperative treatment**:
  The symptomatic zone relates to the organ operated on; for example, the zone of the stomach after a gastrectomy, the zone of the appendix after an appendectomy, including the respective areas of the abdominal wall concerned (scars).
  We regard patients as **newly operated on** until the wound has healed well, usually in 8 to 12 days, more major operations may take longer. The symptomatic zone is only touched gently for about 1 to 2 minutes initially. Then, possibly as early as a few days after the operation, brief, soothing treatment on a daily basis has a highly regenerating effect. Together with other measures, it helps to overcome the stress of the anesthesia and operation. Treatment of the zones of respiration, heart, digestive tract, and lymphatic system (spleen) is particularly important. Stabilizing grips must be included in every treatment session. Initial treatment sessions should not last longer than 10 to 15 minutes each.
- Patients taking **anticoagulants**:
  Patients who take phenprocoumon (Marcumar),

for example: Avoid excessive stimuli in the **liver zone** because the Quick values may change as a result.
- With chronic neurological diseases, the zone of the **brain** and the **spine** is regarded as a symptomatic zone. In patients with multiple sclerosis, Parkinson's disease, especially in the **acute stage:** Avoid excessive stimuli in the symptomatic zone. The same applies to apoplexy, paraplegia, and tetraplegia. (For further information, see Chapter 24.1.)
- **Implants:** In patients with **implants** the symptomatic zone is the zone related to the joint or organ. Avoid excessive treatment in these zones. (Transplants count as contraindications.)
- **Cancer:** In patients with **cancer** the symptomatic zone is the point at which the primary tumor is located in the body. Treat this point slowly and carefully with the sedating grip and avoid strong stimuli overall. (For further information, see Chapter 24.1.)

Instructions for careful treatment also apply to all other **critically ill patients.**

For **pregnant women** too, we advise a cautious approach in the zones of the **uterus, fallopian tubes**, and **ovaries**. As pregnancy is not an illness, however, these zones need not be omitted. The series of treatments starts in approximately the fourth month of pregnancy and may be continued once or twice a week until the birth (and beyond). (For further information, see Chapter 5.2.2, penultimate paragraph.)

16.3.2 Summary

The instructions to work with special care and attention in the symptomatic zone in the aforementioned groups of patient do not under any circumstances mean that RTF treatment should be omitted. It is only intended as a **precautionary measure to avoid unpleasant overreactions** because, above all in the case of beginners, there is a constant tendency to attach more importance to the symptom than the person as a whole.

However, if therapists feel **particularly uncertain,** they can omit the symptomatic zone completely in the aforementioned groups of patients during initial treatment sessions. Careful observation of the patient's reactions and a description of the reactions which have occurred provide indications for further treatments and creates trust in RTF.

17 Therapeutic Support for Intensely Emotional Reactions

17.1

General Information

Therapists who attend our courses rarely have special training to deal with the emotional reactions of patients. In addition, these patients usually come to us with seemingly physical diseases and complaints.

However, it appears increasingly—sometimes to the surprise of both sides—that a disease which is initially presumed to be "only" physical has a significant emotional basis.

The following considerations and practical information have proved their worth when supporting a patient during intense phases of emotional reaction. They concern reactions familiar to us from reflexotherapy of the feet but which may also be observed in other forms of treatment.

- In order to avoid one-sided fixation at certain levels—"It is all just psychological" or "My illness is definitely only something to do with my stomach"—we should view any kind of pathological process from an understanding of **correlations** and less on the basis of intellectually fixated causal links. Given the complexity of some illnesses, we can rarely establish unequivocally whether "the chicken or the egg" came first. From a therapeutic perspective, this decision is not necessary either, because it does not alter the course of treatment.
- It is more important to recognize spontaneously when more support is needed at a physical level and when at an emotional level, and to be alert to this aspect during treatment.
- In order to avoid being caught off our guard by patients' strong emotional reactions and being better prepared to deal with these where necessary, we advise asking the following specific questions in the **first treatment session** as part of the case history:
  - Do you have memories of serious life events which placed or continue to place a heavy psychological strain on you?
  - Do you have a family history of emotional stress?
  - Do you take medication or drugs to stabilize your mental state?

We can thus react more appropriately to situations if deeper emotional connections emerge. Naturally, such "intimate" questions should be asked sensitively.

Patients **decide for themselves** what and how much they would like to tell us about their psychological condition. However, we bear no responsibility for reactions caused by a patient's background about which we have not been informed.

The more alert we are ourselves in dealing with our **own** traumatic experiences, the sooner those being treated will be able to open up to us psychologically. This includes our learning to distinguish,

- what the patient's actual condition comprises,
- what constitutes our wishful thinking and our expectations,
- what such reactions trigger in us ourselves.

In addition, we can be sure of developing greater certainty in dealing with such reactions as a result of experience and careful observation.

- We should be aware of our **own limits** in this regard and make these clear if necessary, for example, by providing instructions for further special care if we feel overstretched. In our experience, treatments such as breathing therapy, biodynamic, and other psychotherapeutic methods which incorporate both psychological and physical aspects, lead clearly and comprehensively to the next steps involved in processing central issues in a person's life.

17.2

Practical Information

With strong emotional reactions, we can choose from the following options:

- Apply one or two of our proven stabilizing or Eutonic grips
- Offer something to drink
- Place our caring hand somewhere on the patient that both parties may discern is an appropriate place
- Suggest a different position or stance or sit the patient upright

- Bring up the topic in conversation or remain silent and alertly attentive
- Add more covers or offer a hot water bottle.

Bach Flowers Remedy No. 39, known as Rescue Remedy, has also proven its worth (Dr. E. Bach: English physician, who at the start of the last century developed a special branch of homeopathy). One or two drops on the tongue, in the center of the palm or on the sternum, if necessary, repeated a few times, support stabilization.

- In the process of dealing with a topic, patients can always **determine for themselves** if and when they would like to stop. If we receive a sign that the patient has had enough for the time being, we should try to understand why by asking a suitable question. The answer may, for example, be: "I am frightened that it is bringing up too much" or "This has already happened to me a number of times and until now I have never gone any further". In addition to respecting this decision, however, we should ensure that the current experience is not suppressed again. We therefore encourage the patient: "Give yourself time and allow yourself to breathe calmly again." With regard to ourselves, we should make sure that our breathing does not falter either. We can also gently encourage further processing of this experience at a later time.
- The (re-)experiencing of stressful feelings is **one** way of really processing deep-seated problems. In addition to the emotional reaction, there should be a **discussion** so that the emotional change initiated does not get "stuck" and is felt consciously. Just the simple question: "How does it feel now?" points in this direction. We assume the role of listener and avoid being distracted by accounts of individual experiences. A discussion, which should, however, be limited in time, also produces a healthy distance from the preceding, usually unanticipated emotional experience.
- If we ourselves feel overstretched or uneasy in the situation which has arisen, it helps both parties if the patient sits up. (Experience from bioenergetics suggests that being in a horizontal position invites the unconscious to go deeper.)
- With severe reactions, it can help to provide a healthy distance by ceasing any direct touching as this may be too indicative of proximity. However, it is worth asking whether continued touching is felt to be helpful. People usually know what is good for them in such situations.
- We should bear in mind that any kind of touch makes **interpersonal proximity** far more clearly perceptible than eye or linguistic contact because it includes the body–skin threshold.
- For every treatment in which strong emotional reactions occur, a period of **subsequent rest** is particularly important to enable the emotions to abate. During the subsequent rest period, patients should feel that they are also being cared for in this phase. Some sleep for half an hour or even a whole hour and wake up refreshed and relaxed. A brief concluding conversation can usually provide a sound way of returning to everyday reality.
- **Very rarely:** If a patient "drifts" within a strong emotional reaction, that is, if contact is lost, we should ask them to open their eyes and keep looking at us and talking to us. Very simple questions are appropriate for this: "Did you have a jacket with you?" Or: "What did you have for breakfast?" Again and again it has proven useful to have one's own first name repeated clearly audibly several times in succession. The treatment that was started prior to this situation is not continued.
- It will be helpful for us if we maintain our own breathing rhythm and adjust our posture. After coping with such shared experiences, usually unanticipated, we should request professional advice with regard to further treatment.

17.3

Additional Experiences

If a person reacts intensely at a psychological level, it is not because we have done something "wrong." What appears spontaneously in the other person was already present in them beforehand; we have not caused it but rather provided the stimulus for its expression and potential resolution.

> Reactions always depend on the individual experience of the person concerned and their personal opportunities for processing that experience.

Beware of subjective, well-intentioned interpretations and attempts at explanations! It is enough if we support what is happening with empathy and gentleness of touch or a few words, for example,

"I know that feeling too" or "Other people have had similar experiences."

Dreams can also help to clarify a difficult situation. We should therefore advise the patient to make a mental note of them, and to describe them during the next treatment session. In our experience, dreams should never be interpreted in a one-sided intellectual way but the message of their images viewed holistically.

It is much appreciated by patients if we say they can contact us in the intervening period before the next treatment if the experiences during treatment have upset them.

17.4

Summary

It is always important to note that in phases of strong emotional reaction patients indicates the direction of further treatment based on the needs shown. Under no circumstances should we urge them to develop in a way which seems meaningful to **us**.

When supporting such processes, it is important that we make it clear (even though we ourselves are aware of this) that everything that happens is covered by our duty of **professional confidentiality**.

18 Treatment Combinations

18.1

General Information

Combination of treatments should be set against a background of practical experience and sound expertise. If several methods are combined in **one** treatment too early and because of uncertainty, this usually results in an indiscriminate mixture which satisfies no one.

Reflexotherapy of the feet (RTF) should therefore be given a chance to prove its effectiveness by being the only treatment offered to some patients in addition to their existing therapy program.

Naturally, a course of treatment would make most sense for those patients, as well as their friends and relatives perhaps, who are not currently taking any medication or undergoing any other kind of therapy.

The more certain we become in observing changes and reactions during treatment, the more naturally we are able to combine a number of particular aspects of different methods to provide optimum treatment.

18.2

Approved Combinations

18.2.1   In Physical Therapy

RTF can be combined with the following methods to good effect:

- Physical therapy
- Traditional massage
- Manual lymph drainage
- Balneotherapy
- Inhalations, respiratory therapy
- Feldenkrais work, Alexander technique
- Chirotherapy
- Ortho-Bionomy
- Osteopathy, craniosacral therapy

Once some experience has been gained, the aforementioned methods may be combined in a single RTF treatment or offered at intervals on the same day.

18.2.2   In Clinics, Rehabilitation Centers, and Sanatoriums

Several of the aforementioned therapies can be combined within the framework of focused care for patients in hospitals and sanatoriums, where it is customary for inpatients to receive a series of daily treatments and a variety of medications.

Whenever possible, a **neutral period** of approximately 60 to 90 minutes should be ensured between two different kinds of treatment, thus allowing the applied therapeutic stimulus to be processed.

Given the variety of treatment options, decisions about the number of daily treatments should not be taken on a primarily commercial basis.

> Treatment carried out to excess, too often, too quickly, or without the patient's active participation, rather than being beneficial puts more of a strain on the patient's health over time as it cannot be adequately "digested."

18.2.3   In Medical Practices

RTF has proven useful in combination with the following methods:

- **Manual therapy** and **ortho-bionomy** or similar measures in preparation and follow-up treatment to support and facilitate functional chains of movement
- **Neural therapy** for follow-up treatment of scars, muscle groups, joints, and organs
- **Classical homeopathy** to support acute and chronic treatment processes
- **Bach Flower** remedies and/or **anthroposophical** and other natural remedies to alleviate strong reactions
- **Dietary measures** and fasting cures to promote the function of the excretory organs
- **Gynecological** treatments for many pathological processes, for example, the prolapse of female organs, endometriosis, vaginal

discharge, and during treatment following surgical procedures

- **Dental treatments**, after oral surgery and to support the excretion of toxins and other waste matter during and after holistic treatment

18.3

RTF and Medication

Patients often come to practices after having been prescribed various medicines, some of which cause undesirable side-effects.

As the patient's self-regulatory forces may be weakened by too many drugs or remedies, prescribed in an uncoordinated manner, the dosing of RTF as an additional therapy should be particularly carefully supervised.

As the complaints ease, the use of medications should be reviewed by the prescribing practitioner. The dosage can often be reduced or a particular medication replaced by a less harmful option.

18.4

Treatment of the Extremities

18.4.1 Nonspecific Treatment of Zones of the Extremities

As the representation of the whole person in the microsystem of the feet is essentially limited to the head, neck, and trunk, it has only been possible to treat the upper and lower extremities, above all in their distal regions, indirectly and nonspecifically via the zones of their nerve supply.

The treatment of the **upper extremities** is therefore performed via the zones of the lower cervical and upper thoracic spine (brachial plexus), as well as by mobilizing the metatarsophalangeal joints, especially those of the big toes.

Proceed very carefully when treating patients with whiplash, even if the trauma occurred a long time ago. Ortho-Bionomy is particularly suitable as the method of choice for treatment of the toes (see Chapter 10.2.4).

The **lower extremities** are treated via the zones of the lower spine from which the legs are innervated.

18.4.2 Collateral and Contralateral Treatments of the Extremities

However, collateral (same side) or contralateral (opposite side) treatment, also known as **consensual therapy,** can also be applied more specifically to the extremities. It is easy to incorporate into RTF.

Practical Rules

The following applies to the treatment of the **extremities:**

The other extremity in the assigned region is treated **collaterally**: arm on the leg and vice versa. The respective corresponding place is treated **contralaterally** on the extremity with the same name: left knee on the right and vice versa.

Reciprocal **collateral equivalents** are:

- Hip and shoulder joint
- Thigh and upper arm
- Knee and elbow
- Fibula and ulna
- Tibia and radius
- Medial/lateral ankle joint and medial/lateral wrist joint
- Big toe and thumb
- Four fingers and four toes
- Plantar side of the foot and palmar side of the hand.

The **contralateral** equivalents are obvious: the respective part of the upper or lower extremity **with the same name**.

This rule can also be applied to the **pelvic and shoulder girdles**: the scapula corresponds to the ilium and vice versa, the upper part of the scapula corresponds to the iliac crest and vice versa.

The collateral and the contralateral tissues are treated with massage grips which trigger good **hyperemia**, depending on the size of the section, using kneading or friction, for example. Smaller areas can also be treated with basic RTF grips.

Examples

- Strains in the **left** lower leg after fracture of the fibula are treated on the same anatomical site on the **right** lower leg (contralateral); Complaints in the left lower **leg** are treated at the related site on the left lower **arm** (ulna) (collateral).

This type of treatment has also proved suitable in the following situations:

- Patients with an **extension bandage or plaster cast** (extension treatment) after accidents. Intensive stimulation of the blood circulation on the collateral and contralateral sides can prevent atrophy of the tissue, and fractures will have a better chance of healing.
- Patients with a **crural ulcer**. In addition to the treatment of the zones concerned (Chapter 11), the open site on the lower leg can be treated at the same time via treatment of the lower **arm**.

  The crural ulcer usually only appears on one side, but the tissue at the same site on the other leg is often just as tender as at the site of the ulcer. For this reason we can usually only perform the collateral treatment and should avoid the contralateral side. There the precise site of the correspondence to the leg is revealed in the vicinity of the wrist by clearly defined pain on palpation and sometimes there is a reaction with clearly circumscribed mild or even intense reddening of the tissue.

Practical Advice

Sometimes, patients suffering from crural ulcer report that after treatment there is increased discharge of serous fluid from the wound, signifying cleansing and activation of the tissue. Simultaneously, itching is observed at the edge of the ulcer, indicating improved healing. Even if the crural ulcer initially becomes somewhat enlarged, this is not considered to be a negative reaction but an expression of self-regulation within the body.

The fact that the tissue on the **medial** side of the lower leg in the vicinity of the inner malleolus has the greatest tendency to form crural ulcers leads us to observe that, generally speaking, the patients affected are highly metabolically stressed: this is the point at which the **acupuncture** meridians of the liver, kidney, and spleen/pancreas meet.

Examination and alteration of dietary habits is essential if the patient seriously wants the crural ulcer to heal.

- Patients with **amputations** sometimes complain of intense neuralgic pain at the site of the amputation for months or even years. Apart from other options (e.g., neural therapy or visualization), treatment using contralateral or collateral measures has a good chance of easing aggressive phantom and residual limb pain.

When treating patients with amputated limbs at the appertaining collateral and/or contralateral site while stroking this area gently and attentively, it may be observed that this tissue has a different tone, usually involving reduced tension. It is **this precise spot** that should be treated. Patients can be involved in such treatment by showing them how to massage the corresponding site once or twice a day to promote good circulation.

18.4.3 Transferring Consensual Treatment to the Zones of the Feet

All areas which can be treated using the consensual rule in situ can be treated just as effectively on the **zones of the feet**. In addition, as the areas on the foot are smaller, far less time is required for treatment.

Example

Patient with epicondylitis on the right side.

Collateral treatment: the right knee **zone** is tonified; **contralateral**: the left elbow zone is also tonified. Naturally, the symptomatic **zone** of the **right** elbow can also be treated with a sedating grip, together with a series of other zones requiring treatment. As this is not a direct component of the aforementioned rule, however, it is not explored in more detail at this point.

18.5

Accompanying Measures

RTF may frequently be chosen as the **main treatment**. To motivate patients to support the course of treatment with their own activities, the following accompanying measures lend themselves:

Posture and movement. By giving patients support and encouragement to overcome the weaknesses and shortcomings of their own posture and to practice natural movements, they can learn to use their musculoskeletal system more economically than before in their personal and professional lives. In recent decades a number of special methods have been developed which offer constructive aid in this direction: **Eutonia, Feldenkrais, Alexander technique**, etc.

Nutrition. As many diseases are diet-related, examining and changing dietary habits is of great importance. If we are sufficiently patient and do not try to force our patients, they are usually more willing to cooperate.

Relying on one's own experience regarding nutrition always produces the best and most reliable outcome as it is always more realistic than other people's suggestions. This does not mean that patients should not get practical hints from relevant books on nutrition. These require critical analysis, however, as there is often fanaticism in the field of nutritional theories.

A common theme pervading all dietary and nutritional advice is that of **hyperacidity**. This is undoubtedly so topical because hyperacidity is not only a malfunction of the metabolic organs, but may also be deeply rooted in our fundamental attitude to life.

Respiration. Recommendations for healthy, functional respiration offered by experienced therapists are important not only for patients with respiratory problems, but also for those with psychosomatic difficulties and weaknesses.

Therapists who are able to teach their patients to become aware of their restricted or impeded respiration and to alter it through touch or exercises, create the best conditions for an improvement of their physical and emotional potential.

Heat regulation. Many people also tend to have cold feet in summer, even in warm climates. **Persistently cold feet** are an expression of the person's inability to make efficient use of their vital energy. There are many reasons for this, ranging from chronic constipation, spinal injuries, and disordered breathing to problems in the psychosocial environment.

Well-known measures such as **Kneipp** hydrotherapy and **Schiele** baths to improve sluggish circulation have produced convincing results for decades due to their circulation-enhancing effect.

Active exercising of the feet, vigorous brushing of the soles of the feet and above all, the natural stimuli of light, fresh air, and contact with the earth when **walking barefoot** can noticeably improve the patient's general condition.

Holistic tooth restoration. The most obvious function of our teeth is that of mastication of food. However, the teeth constitute a **microsystem** interconnected with the whole organism in just the same way as the ears, nasopharynx, eyes, hands, and feet, etc.

Like all other organs, teeth also provide clear signals in terms of body language and distinct emotional connections, as proved by expressions in many languages such as "to bare one's teeth," "to clench one's teeth," "to be fed up to the back teeth," or "to set one's teeth on edge." The designation of the eighth tooth as a **"wisdom" tooth** is also similar in many different languages.

Using electroacupuncture measurements, Dr. Reinhold Voll proved decades ago that each tooth correlates with a multitude of organs, tissues, and systems mostly through the energy flow of acupuncture meridians (see Chapter 26 for more details).

Although a reduction in dental caries as a result of significantly improved and intensified local oral hygiene and dental care is superficially encouraging, it is important to consider that gum inflammation in conditions such as **periodontal disease**, gingivitis, etc. is noticeably increasing. This is most likely due to the fact that eating habits have scarcely improved for centuries and metabolic stress has now shifted from the teeth to the mucous membranes and tissues (see Chapter 26 for more details).

Treatment of scars. As with teeth or chronically inflamed organs, scars may also constitute **interference fields**. A separate chapter is dedicated to this subject (Chapter 25).

Checks for geopathic stress and electrosmog. We advise examining where the patient sleeps, lives, and works for interference zones in the ground and environment, especially if he or she is chronically sick.

Beware of too many electrical appliances, for example microwave oven in the kitchen, working on computers for excessive amounts of time, halogen lighting, electrical underfloor heating, cell phones ("electrostress"), etc.

Caring for one's "inner health." One of the most important "support measures" for activating healing forces or even the **prerequisite**, strictly speaking, is a conscious awareness of one's inner life, in particular, if one has to cope with the difficult process of suffering as a result of illness.

Caring for one's personal inner health includes:
- the willingness to change fixed habits and attitudes;
- a kind and considerate approach to one's own weaknesses and those of others;
- the question of the sense and meaning of one's personal life;
- saying please and thank you at the right time;
- religious experiences in the literal sense of the word "religio," meaning the connection

with one's own spiritual sources as a means of renewal;

- forgiving and asking for forgiveness;
- respecting and tolerating the decisions and opinions of others, especially if they do not coincide with your own.

18.6

Reflexotherapy of the Hand

18.6.1 Hands and Feet: a Comparison

Hands and feet both have a direct relationship with the whole person, but in a different way.

Hands are linked to specific tasks and areas of life. They are usually open to the world and ready to maintain contact and are used literally to "handle" matters. Their radius of movement in the element of air is more comprehensive and many of their functions and activities are related to partnership and emotions.

On the other hand, the "partner" of the **feet** is the earth, which through its resistance helps us to assume an upright position and at the same time motivates us to move forward with determination.

Many people are made aware of the fact that the feet have a closer connection to our overall physical well-being than the hands on a daily basis. It is difficult to fall asleep with cold feet; mothers of today still know that their children should avoid getting cold, wet feet because getting too cold in this way is often directly related to the development of sore throats, bladder, and kidney infections, coughs, earache, and bronchitis.

Walking barefoot in meadows, forests, and on the seashore is valued highly by those in the know and should be practiced as often as possible. Natural stimulus has an invigorating effect, restorative effect, and promotes good circulation while also connecting us inwardly with "Mother Earth."

Compared with the hands, the feet are often more neglected and restricted, not least as a result of cultural and environmental conditions. Thus, we can observe that **pathological changes** are usually more obvious in **neglected areas** than in **well-cared for areas**.

18.6.2 Therapy of the Hand Zones

Treatment of the hands is not as widespread as that of the feet, although the hands would permit a freer approach to treatment because they are better looked after and more used to being touched than the feet.

Hand zones, though, have proved to be useful as a supplement or alternative to the zones of the feet, for example, for patients with amputated legs and those who have had accidents or suffered other trauma to the feet, or when the feet are in plaster.

Furthermore, we can use the zones of the hands in combination with those of the feet, integrating the symptomatic zones to reinforce the result, for instance. In addition, the hands provide a practical **homework assignment for treatment** in which patients themselves can make an active contribution to improving their health.

18.6.3 Performance of Therapy on the Hands

The 10 body zones of FitzGerald can largely be applied to the hands in the same way as the feet. A division of the hands into three areas is also possible:

1. The fingers are related to the **head/neck**.
2. The distal part of the palm corresponds to the **thorax** and **upper abdomen**.
3. The proximal part, including the carpal bones, corresponds to the **abdominal and pelvic region**.

The hand zones are treated with the grips known from RTF because here too the aim of therapy is to ensure a good supply of blood to the tissue.

18.6.4 Special Indications

Some zones of the hand are especially suitable for treatment in patients with **acute** symptoms or pain, for example:

- Vigorous stretching of the **zone of the stomach** in the interdigital fold between the thumb and index finger has proved successful in treating a feeling of fullness or heartburn.
- With **toothache**, the acute treatment of the zones of the teeth on the middle and proximal phalanges of the fingers usually has just as spontaneous an effect as on the toes and can help to bridge the hours and days when the dentist is unavailable in a relatively pain-free manner. The zones of the teeth are arranged in the same sequence and anatomical position as on the foot.

- With **menstrual pain**, vigorous rubbing of the wrist and thenar eminence (the zones of the pelvic organs) to promote the circulation of the blood provides rapid relief.
- Stretching the **interdigital folds** between all the fingers provides great relief at the onset of a cold and for hay fever and can also be employed by the patient as a preventive measure several times a day.

From My Practice

Time and again over the years I have seen in patients with foot or leg amputations how the hand zones on the same side responded better to treatment than the hand zones on the other side. The therapeutic stimulus triggered hyperemia in the tissue more quickly, and the tone of the painful zones normalized faster.

19 Self-treatment and Orthotic Foot Devices

19.1

Self-treatment

19.1.1 Possibilities

Treating oneself offers the **beginner** a good opportunity to gain experience in reflexotherapy of the feet without feeling self-conscious or under pressure to perform. But **patients** can also give themselves "first aid" treatment according to instructions, in particular, for acute pain.

> Self-treatment can also lead to good therapeutic results because no manual treatment is ever just about suppling external energy, but is also about freeing the obstructed and congested vitality in the patient's organism and of regulating its flow again.

Areas in which there is **often an obstruction of vitality** are, for example:
- Inflammation and spasms in the digestive tract
- Postural defects
- Interference fields such as chronically inflamed tonsils, devitalized (= "lifeless") teeth, scars
- Acute or chronic inflammation in the musculoskeletal and organic systems
- Congestion in the fluid systems of the kidneys, blood, and lymphatic channels
- Suppression of emotions to prevent pending life themes "resurfacing." A particularly significant amount of vitality is trapped in these areas.

The **focus** of self-treatment could be on health care (disease prevention) in particular. As too much emphasis is currently placed on the treatment of disease, prevention is no longer given the attention it actually deserves.

19.1.2 Limits

On the one hand, the limits of self-treatment can be seen in the patient and therapist being one and the same person. This renders a desirable balance impossible at an interpersonal level. In addition, the initial zeal to treat oneself soon wanes, and appointments are usually observed more punctually with a therapist than with oneself.

Moreover, when attempting to treat themselves some people notice that stiffness in their joints and muscles or their marked corpulence make it difficult for them to take hold of their own feet.

19.1.3 Good Indications for Self-Treatment

Acute situations such as toothache, ischialgia, indigestion, hay fever, menstrual pain, and diarrhea. It usually suffices to **sedate** the symptomatic zones.

Chronic diseases: Self-treatment is supportive here, especially for spinal and digestive complaints, sinusitis, etc.

For **acute** complaints short treatment sessions can be provided daily or several times a day, for **chronic** complaints once or twice a week.

19.1.4 Summary

Although the results of self-treatment can be very convincing, the optimum treatment effect can be achieved when the following participants combine to form a group of common interest:
- An open-minded **patient** who is prepared to actively cooperate;
- A well-informed and interested **physician** who is not only able to delegate but also to instruct the therapist;
- Well-trained **therapists** who accompany their patients through a series of treatments and know their capabilities and limits;
- An expert and conscientious **chiropodist** who takes **care** of the feet and knows how to provide the right professional support.

19.2

Mechanical Aids

Mechanical aids are very popular with health-conscious lay people (and persuasive salesmen). If used correctly, the various mats, plates, insoles (foot supports) and foot rollers made of wood, plastic, clay, or rubber certainly have a **generally** beneficial effect and may also be used to **support** manual treatment of the feet.

These aids are, for example, able to improve the **circulation** of the feet and legs, and can thus counter congestion and cold feet. Above all, if used regularly, they can convey a **better awareness** of one's feet. However, they should not replace any therapy but be used for approximately 10 to 15 minutes in the morning and evening as a supporting measure, or be used for a few weeks after completion of a course of treatment.

If, owing to ignorance of therapeutic correlations, special points on the feet are overemphasized and only treated with one of these aids or excessively strong and long-lasting stimuli are applied to them, complaints may **worsen** rather than improve. Therefore experience with these auxiliary measures that have been used for many years must be put into perspective and reviewed in the light of the more complicated illnesses of today's patients.

20 Diagnostic Possibilities and Limitations

20.1

General Information

There are only a few methods in which the therapeutic and diagnostic aspects are as closely related as in reflexotherapy of the feet (RTF). Where the focus of a treatment is placed is a question of professional background, personal approach, and favored priorities.

When I started teaching, I decided to emphasize the **therapeutic** (and not the diagnostic) side for two reasons. On the one hand, the vast majority of course participants come from manual auxiliary medical professions in which their therapeutic work has to be prescribed by a physician. On the other hand, the diagnostic approach alone does not come close to exhausting the possibilities offered by RTF and inevitably leads to the use of other methods (e.g., drugs, injections), which are at times unnecessary.

As a **differential diagnosis**, however, RTF can certainly be incorporated into other investigations but there some aspects to take into consideration in this regard:

- Diagnosis and therapy **combine** in RTF to form an indivisible unit. This characterizes the fluent transition typical of RTF, from findings to treatment: in each diagnosis the approach contains the therapy and each treatment session contains diagnostic statements.
- A reliable and comprehensive diagnosis cannot be arrived at from a number of abnormal zones on the foot because **any touch**, be it applied ever-so objectively, "touches" the whole person while at the same time altering their emotional state.

Therefore, diagnoses which are set for a longer period must be constantly called into question. We understand each diagnosis as a **fluid process**.

- A diagnostic conclusion about the **nature** and **duration** of the illness is not possible as abnormalities at the preclinical stage and functionally and organically manifested diseases both appear as irritation in the zones in the same way.

20.2

Differential Diagnostics

Statements may relate to both symptomatic and background zones.

Examples

- Patient with **acute abdomen**:
  Here the various zones on the foot potentially responsible for inflammation can be differentiated relatively easily because they are clearly separated from each other for the most part:
  - Gall bladder, in particular its dorsal site on the foot
  - Right kidney, ureter
  - Pylorus with duodenum
  - Appendix, ileocecal valve
  - Right ovary
  In addition, the **reactions** which occur during a series of treatments can help to clarify the background and connections with the disease.

- Patient with acute **lower back pain**:
  In addition to the zone of the lower spine, in a differential diagnosis the kidneys, genital organs and intestine must be examined as symptomatic zones. If neither the symptomatic zone nor the kidneys, genitals, or intestine respond to the treatment stimulus, **scar** zones, in particular in the lower abdomen, and zones of the **teeth** must be investigated (focus possibility).
  If the back pain is of **psychogenic** origin, in addition to the spinal column we can also cross-check the zones of the endocrine system, solar plexus, diaphragm (regulation of breathing), and the gastrointestinal tract ("digestion" of a problem).

- Patients with acute or chronic **headaches**:
  Here we can usually differentiate the various connections from each other fairly easily.
  In the background zones it is possible to differentiate between strains in the intestine, kidneys, liver, and gallbladder, upper and lower spine, stomach, and pancreas, genitals, tooth–jaw area, and autonomous nervous system.
  However, **several** zones almost always react simultaneously (Chapter 16).

20.3

Additional Information

As RTF combines therapeutic and diagnostic elements, uncertainty in beginners may give rise to a need to show the patient that one is well informed. This is sometimes expressed in ill-considered **diagnostic** statements which cannot be verified objectively when palpating zone abnormalities and which are more likely to call into question the therapist's credibility.

Examples:
- "What is wrong with your stomach then?" or
- "It feels like you have gallstones." or
- "You must have constant backache."

As already stressed in other chapters, it must be borne in mind that a painful point on the foot **cannot** provide any evidence as to the nature, duration, and background of the patient's present illness. The patient should therefore not be confronted with "half-baked" diagnoses but be encouraged to **experience** the treatment in practice, for example, with questions such as:
- "How does the grip feel on your foot?" or
- "What has changed during repeated treatment of the painful site?" or

- "It is important that you observe which reactions have occurred in response to the treatment before the next session."

In this way, the patient can become the therapist's attentive partner.

The following example may clarify the difference between **findings** and a **diagnosis**:

When a patient's stomach zone is painful, **no differentiation** is possible among
- a gastric ulcer,
- gastroptosis,
- a functional disorder, caused by agitation or stress,
- temporary strain on the stomach caused by a rather indigestible meal,
- chronic or acute gastritis, or
- a postoperative condition.

When the therapist encounters an abnormal zone, however, they know what is **essential: this point needs treatment**.

For the aforementioned reasons, a **great deal of caution** is recommended when formulating diagnostically useable indications.

21 Treatment Suggestions

21.1

General Information

> As illnesses, their symptoms, and origins are always of a personal nature, written suggestions for treatment can only provide general information. We do not treat the illness per se but rather the individual with their unique background.

Nowadays, a detailed initial assessment is quite often omitted in the **everyday practice** of reflexotherapy of the feet (RTF) due to time constraints. Often it also suffices if the essential, functionally assigned background zones are included with the symptomatic zones, that is, the central parts of the "submerged section of the iceberg" (= the afflicted area in which the symptoms were able to develop) are treated together with the "tip of the iceberg" (= symptom). However, **exclusive** treatment of the symptomatic zones is rarely promising for today's patients and can even exacerbate the symptoms.

For patients with **chronic diseases** or vague symptoms, however, it is appropriate and necessary to perform an **initial assessment** by thoroughly inspecting and palpating both feet. It is not possible to determine the areas causing a patient's symptoms until these results are obtained.

Generally speaking, at the **acute** stage of the illness or if the patient is suffering from acute pain, the **symptomatic zone** is initially treated with a soothing, **sedating grip** (Chapter 3). The **background zones** are **tonified**.

At the **chronic** stage of an illness, both the symptomatic zones and the background zones can usually be **tonified**. Here, as always, the patient's spontaneous reaction determines the intensity and duration of the treatment.

21.1.1 Tonifying and Sedating

The terms **tonifying** and **sedating,** which are frequently used in suggestions for treatment, are not binding in principle because the decision as to which zone requires what kind of treatment is sometimes only made "in situ." In all dysfunctional situations in which it is uncertain how patients will respond to therapeutic stimuli, initially observant,

gentle tonifying of a **neutral nature** aiming at **regulation** has proved successful.

After this neutral stage, it is often easier to decide whether to opt for more precise sedating or tonifying subsequently. Not infrequently, it is even possible to change from sedating to tonifying grips and vice versa during a **single** treatment session. In practical terms, patients are usually the best indicator because they spontaneously sense what is good for them. One of the most important questions during treatment is therefore **"How does it feel?"**

Furthermore, the reactions of the **autonomic nervous system** are a reliable benchmark of the patient's health. If signs of excessive stress become apparent (e.g., clammy hands, dry mouth, altered respiration rate and body temperature), under no circumstances is stimulation continued even if, subjectively speaking, the patient shows goodwill and encourages us to carry on working vigorously. A choice of stabilizing and/or Eutonic grips is always employed here.

Important note: Although laudable, the major challenge of locating and treating a zone on the foot as precisely as possible is unreliable in practical terms. We are often unable to decide accurately "from the outside" whether we are really treating the intended organ or tissue because the **location** of the organs and tissues may change both physiologically and pathologically; for example, the size of the stomach after fasting, lowering of the transverse colon, growth of the fetus in utero, nephroptosis, etc.

> However, we can be confident
> - that each selective stimulus has a "spreading width" so that it is not just of vital importance whether a zone is treated to the precise millimeter or not, and
> - that the intensity of the individual grips can also be offset "internally" by the healing and regulatory power of the person, provided they are not applied too roughly and for too long.

In our experience, the **quality of touch,** empathy, and seriousness with which we work has a decisive effect. Once again the advice which was formulated in previous chapters is worth repeating. Initially, an abnormal zone on the foot reveals **nothing** about the cause, nature, and duration of the illness.

However, it relays to us the important information that this point needs help. In the further course of treatment, the patient's reactions in each situation will provide a reliable indication of the zones requiring treatment and the therapeutic measures necessary.

Supplementary information about the following clinical pictures can be found in
- Chapter 5 "Indications and Contraindications"
- Chapter 14 "Reactions during Treatment Intervals"
- Chapter 16 "Management and Treatment of Pain in Acute Situations"
- Chapter 16.3 "Careful Treatment of Symptomatic Zones in Special Diseases"
- Chapter 22 "Pregnancy and Birth"
- Chapter 23 "Treatment of Babies and Children"
- Chapter 24 "Special Groups of Patients"
- Chapter 31 "Shared Practical Experience"

The following treatment suggestions are discussed in the order of the **seven groups of zones** already used in **Chapter 10**. I use the following colors for the illustrations:
- **Red** for symptomatic zones
- **Green** for possible background zones

For corresponding topics, there are some illustrations of **similarities in shape**.

> Similar anatomical shapes in the human body point to useful relationships for therapy, because they arise jointly from the internal plan of a previous energetic development level which was gradually condensed into matter (see Appendix, p. 243 Brochure 4 "Similarities in shape as the key to therapy").

21.2

Zones of the Head and Neck

21.2.1 General Information

There is seldom an indication group in which the background zones can occur as diversely, and at the same time as clearly, as in this group of zones, irrespective of whether "headache" manifests in its various forms, such as migraine, cluster headache, or trigeminal neuralgia.

In the **initial findings**, the symptomatic zones are always found in the head area, that is, in the toes. The background zones tend to be in the following areas, alone or linked to others:

- Intestinal tract, especially the small intestine
- Upper abdomen, including liver/gall bladder, stomach, and pancreas
- Spine and musculature, overall or in sections
- The genital organs, especially in women
- Kidneys and urinary tract
- Paranasal sinuses
- Teeth as an important microsystem
- Autonomic nervous system, which has a strong effect on the emotions
- Scars—not only in the head region

As the zones of the digestive tract are noticeable in 70 to 80% of all patients with headaches, it is important to point out the significance of regulation in **nutrition**. For strains on the digestive organs and inflammatory processes, **enemas** have proved their worth by helping, as they do, to rapidly excrete accumulated metabolic waste products and harmful substances. Unfortunately, this effective application is often overlooked these days.

The **similarity in shape** between the brain and intestine also points to therapeutically useful relationships (**Fig. 21.1**).

21.2.2 Treatment Suggestions

Headaches with Poor Digestion

Symptomatic zones: All head areas. At the acute stage, the symptomatic zones are first treated with a sedating grip. When they have been soothed (sometimes as early as the first treatment), they can be tonified, gently initially, and then more vigorously.

Possible background zones: Colon including hepatic and splenic flexure, sigmoid, rectum. Small intestine and ileocecal valve. Pelvic floor, especially anus. Lumbar spine—segmental correlations with the intestine. Diaphragm, as its up-and-down movement can be reduced by meteorism or the like, and the rhythmic "massage" of the abdominal organs is therefore no longer guaranteed. Autonomic

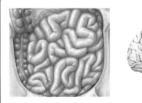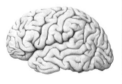

Fig. 21.1 Similarity in shape between intestinal and cerebral convolutions.

nervous system. Solar plexus, especially if there are emotional strains ("digestion" in the figurative sense), but also all other stabilizing grips.

Headaches as a Result of Upper Abdominal Complaints

Symptomatic zones: Liver, gall bladder. Stomach, cardia, and pylorus.

Possible background zones: Right shoulder girdle—segmental connections with the liver/gall bladder. Central and lower thoracic spine—innervation. Pancreas and spleen. Solar plexus and other stabilizing grips in order to stabilize the autonomic nervous system. Suggestions for a change of diet are often appropriate.

Headaches with Spinal Strains

Symptomatic zones: Head, in particular, base of the skull and the mastoid process. Cervical spine and the neck musculature.

Possible background zones: Lumbar spine as lumbar lordosis. Shoulder girdle, sternum, and sternoclavicular articulation.

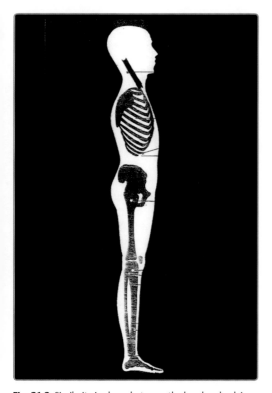

Fig. 21.2 Similarity in shape between the head and pelvis.

Sacrum and sacroiliac joint. Coccyx, especially after accidents.

Pelvic girdle—musculoskeletal relationship with the shoulder girdle.

Thyroid gland, as there may be calcium deficiency in the bones.

Solar plexus and/or other stabilizing grips.

Headaches as a Result of Lower Abdominal Complaints, Especially in Women

Symptomatic zones: The whole head, pituitary gland. Nasopharyngeal cavity—the mucous membranes are derived from the same germ layer as the lower abdomen. Eustachian tubes (which have the fallopian tubes, also called "tubes," as a counterpart).

Possible background zones: All the organs of the lesser pelvis, including the pelvic floor.

Lower neck and seventh cervical vertebra.

Lumbar spine, also sacrum and sacroiliac joint (innervation, segmental connections to the lesser pelvis).

All other glands with internal secretion. Lymphatic channels of the inguinal area for decongestion.

Autonomic nervous system: solar plexus and/or a choice of other stabilizing grips. (**Fig. 21.2**)

Headaches with Disorders of the Urinary Tract

Symptomatic zones: The whole head, especially eyes, calvaria, and occiput (the bladder meridian also supplies the eyes and the upper and rear parts of the head).

Important note: As headaches with a renal background are often associated with hypertension, the background zones may need treatment **before** the symptomatic zones. This may relieve the symptoms in advance. The zones of the head are first treated gently.

Possible background zones: Kidneys, ureter, bladder—also treat gently initially! Lumbar spine, especially sacrum (the segmental bladder zone in situ). Lymphatic channels of the inguinal area.

Tonifying of the lateral nail fold of the fifth toe (the final point of the bladder meridian which, inter alia, supplies the urinary tract with its energy. In pregnancy, only apply with corresponding expertise).

Spleen and other lymph organs, intestine (e.g., for cystitis without fever). Solar plexus and/or other stabilizing grips.

Headaches with Sinusitis

Symptomatic zones: Frontal and maxillary sinuses, also on the proximal halves of toe nails 2 to 4. Nasopharyngeal cavity and eustachian tubes. Upper lymphatics on the interdigital skin folds.

With **chronic** sinusitis (**Fig. 21.3**), the symptomatic zones are also tonified. Treatment should begin with the sedating grip at the **acute** stage, before subsequent tonifying to stimulate the excretion of secretions.

The four skin folds between the toes (upper lymphatics) are stretched carefully a number of times until stretching becomes easier. The intensity and repetition of the stretches can then be increased.

If **mycosis** (**athlete's foot**) is present: treat the interdigital skin folds between the hands.

Possible background zones: Intestine, especially small intestine: the quality of the intestinal mucosa influences the quality of all other organs and systems lined with mucosa.

Liver, spleen and thymus in all inflammatory and infectious conditions.

Tonsils and appendix as important lymph organs. Lymphatic channels of the inguinal area.

Organs of the lesser pelvis: "tubes" (both the eustachian tubes and the fallopian tubes) are derived from the same germ layer.

Autonomic nervous system: solar plexus and/or a range of other stabilizing grips.

Headaches with Allergies

Regarding allergies, see also Chapter 24.5.

Symptomatic zones: The whole head. Lymphatic areas of head and neck and tonsils. (If mycosis is present: treat interdigital skin folds on the hands and/or let the patients treat it themselves.)

Possible background zones: These are often difficult to ascertain as allergies can give rise to different symptoms. In general, however, the following are affected: intestine, especially small intestine and ileocecal valve. Spleen and liver.

Appendix (in holistic therapies also called the "tonsils of the abdomen"). Thymus to strengthen the immune system. Urinary tract.

Autonomic nervous system, which can be stabilized via solar plexus and/or other stabilizing grips. A series of RTF lymphatic treatments has proved successful both as a **preventive measure** and for treatment at the **acute** stage (Chapter 29).

Headaches as a Result of Scars after Operations and Accidents

Symptomatic zones: Head and neck overall. In general, treat gently until an individual reaction has been ascertained. Possibly start with the background zones, especially in patients who have had operations and accidents directly involving the head area.

Possible background zones: Scars, not only on the head. In particular, scars located centrally in the vertical median line (e.g., laparoscopy, cesarean section, abdominal and heart operations, perineal sutures), but others as well, can trigger headaches. RTF **scar treatment** is described in detail in Chapter 25.

Spine and/or joints which are affected by accidents and operations, for example, cervical spine and occipital region in whiplash (Chapter 16).

Kidneys/adrenal glands—adrenalin release in shock situations. Autonomic nervous system: solar plexus and/or other stabilizing grips.

Headaches as a Result of Devitalized Teeth

General: Usually these patients are treated by a dentist. However, when a clinical picture is viewed holistically, interactions may arise between the afflicted organ and the associated teeth (more information in Chapter 26), which can be used therapeutically.

The relevant teeth in situ are not always noticeable in terms of **symptoms**; that is, they are not painful but may react abnormally in their **associated zones**: teeth which are impacted or have undergone root canal treatment, teeth which are filled with silver amalgam or incompatible synthetic materials, cysts, crowns underneath which chronic inflammatory foci may develop, etc.

Symptomatic zones: The relevant teeth and their odonton (tooth root, tissue, nerve supply, bone parts). Nasopharyngeal cavity, in particular frontal and maxillary sinuses. Lymphatics of the head and neck.

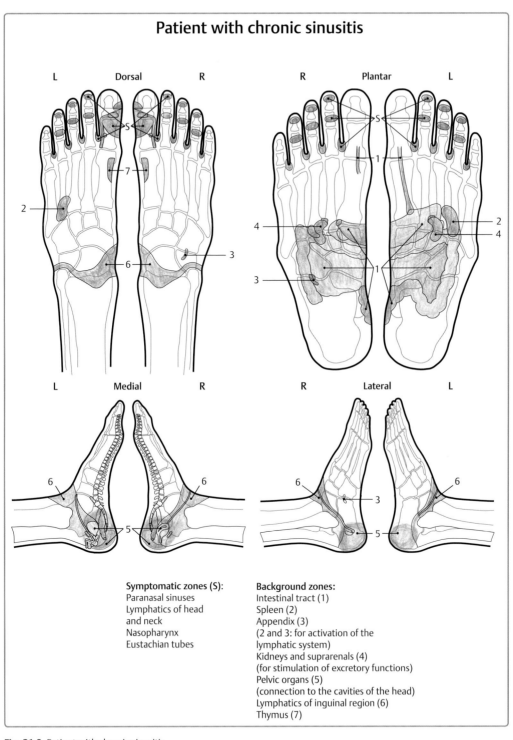

Fig. 21.3 Patient with chronic sinusitis.

Possible background zones: All organs and systems energetically associated with the devitalized tooth. In associated inflammatory processes in the oral cavity: intestine, liver, spleen, and lymphatic system.

To stabilize the autonomic nervous system: solar plexus and/or other stabilizing grips as often as necessary.

Acute Hearing Loss—Menière's disease

This also includes vertigo and tinnitus.

Symptomatic zones: Ears, base of skull, upper cervical spine and eustachian tubes. They are **always** treated with the sedating grip, even at the symptom-**free** stage—with tonifying there is a risk of deterioration. Even with **unilateral** symptoms, **both** sides are treated, initially on the symptom-**free** side. Lateral lymph chains: to reduce congestion they are stroked gently, but thoroughly, using fine movements until the tissue feels "permeable" (Chapter 29).

At the **acute** stage it is advisable not to start with the symptomatic zones but rather with the **background zones** concerned: even if no background cause is known, the zones which stabilize the **autonomic nervous system** are of great importance (the solar plexus and/or other stabilizing grips). They should be included as often as necessary before, during, and after treatment. An assortment of one or two grips is usually sufficient.

The whole spine from distal to proximal, especially the lower portion, sacrum and sacroiliac joint. Pelvis bony/muscular and organic. The zones of the pelvic ligaments (Froneberg) can also be differentiated and treated.

Diaphragm, because respiratory regulation likewise has a harmonizing effect on the autonomic nervous system.

Gall bladder and small intestine, as the meridian of the gall bladder and small intestine supplies the head laterally with their energy.

It is also worthwhile determining whether **interference fields** are present in the form of scars, devitalized teeth, or vertebral blockages. Good manual therapy or osteopathy may then be helpful as a complementary measure.

All in all, treatment of these patients is not easy. It requires patience, sensitivity, and experience. Beginners should not start with such patients.

More often than at first supposed and even if they occurred a long time ago, **traumatic experiences** or other kinds of severe emotional stress are associated with the development of impaired balance and vertigo. This is reflected in expressions such as "to lose one's balance." If, when, and how such topics can be addressed is dependent on various factors such as the patient's willingness to discuss such matters and the personal and professional skill of the therapist.

Acute Earache

See Chapter 16 "Management and Treatment of Pain in Acute Situations" and Chapter 23 "Treatment of Babies and Children."

Glaucoma

In particular, in patients suffering from primary glaucoma later in life, connected to overexertion, pronounced sensitivity to light or psychological strain; increased intraocular pressure can be significantly improved by one or two courses of RTF treatment.

Symptomatic zones: Eyes and visual center are initially treated with the sedating grip. Later, these areas can also be tonified. Stroke the lymphatic glands of the head and neck gently but thoroughly to discharge the increased pressure (Chapter 29).

Possible background zones: Nape of the neck—neuromuscular correlations are observed when "nodding off," when the eyes also close. Ears—together with the eyes, they are involved in balance.

Kidneys, ureter, bladder—the bladder meridian also supplies the eyes.

Pancreas—in the case of diabetics, treat the pancreas zone cautiously at first and monitor the blood sugar level carefully!

Thyroid gland (exophthalmus). Canine teeth—also known as "eye teeth." In accordance with energetic measurement according to Voll, they are associated with the eyes (Chapter 26). Possibly have teeth checked for interference field disorders.

Stomach as, inter alia, the stomach meridian also supplies the eyes energetically.

Solar plexus and/or other stabilizing grips which stabilize the autonomic nervous system.

Contact Lens Wearers

Sometimes patients suffer from watering and inflamed eyes, often associated with itching and/or severe dryness; frequently observed in allergy sufferers.

Symptomatic zones: Treat the eyes and visual center with sedating grips at first. The lymphatic glands of the head and neck. Draining, stroking movements until the tissue feels "permeable" (Chapter 29).

Possible background zones: Base of skull, nape of neck. Digestive organs, especially liver and small intestine. Kidneys, ureter, bladder. Spleen as the largest lymph organ. Appendix and thymus to strengthen the immune system. Solar plexus and/ or other stabilizing grips.

Vigorous stretching of the interdigital skin folds of both hands should be performed several times daily until the piercing feeling there has eased significantly; this exercise is suitable as "therapeutic homework" for patients.

21.3

Zones of the Spine, Shoulder, and Pelvic Girdle

21.3.1 General Information

For patients with disorders of the spine and joints, dynamic posture correction, which also includes inner bearing, always lends itself as an additional treatment (e.g., Alexander Technique, Eutony, Feldenkrais), thus making it easier for the person to go through life upright, to show some backbone where necessary, and to follow their life journey on the basis of inner motivation.

With all **transition joints**, like the elbow and knee, the joints above or below them should always be examined at the same time.

> As anatomical physical shapes always develop from a subtle energetic background, the therapeutic stimulus will always address the person **at all levels**, regardless of whether they are aware of it or not. The wisdom of self-healing decides which level of a respective treatment most gives rise to reactions.

The collective term "**rheumatic disorders**" covers a multitude of complaints such as polyarthritis, fibromyalgia, ankylosing spondylitis, osteochondrosis, arthrosis, neuromyopathies, epicondylitis, coxarthrosis, psoriasis–arthropathy, periarthritis humeroscapularis, carpal tunnel syndrome, gout, various connective tissue disorders such as systemic lupus erythematosus, etc.

Treatment of **rheumatics** should be gentle and gradual initially to avoid aggravating the condition. More important than the symptomatic zones of the individual joints and muscle groups are the zones which support the **metabolic system**, namely the intestine, urinary tract, liver, respiratory organs, and lymphatic system including the spleen.

The **autonomic nervous system** plays a major role (stabilizing grips, solar plexus) as often complex emotional issues also underlie the symptoms.

RTF has proved useful in combination with a consistent change of diet, fasting, homeopathy (e.g., with testing of noxious agents—all kinds of harmful substances), body-orientated psychotherapy, etc. The results are often more conclusive than those of symptom-oriented orthodox treatments.

RTF is ideally suited to preparation for **chiropractic** and **manual therapy** (Chapter 18.2) and follow-up treatment thereof.

Muscular overtension can be pretreated via the zones of the feet, enabling individual vertebrae to be repositioned far more gently and "fluidly." Now and then a vertebra even slides back into its normal position audibly and visibly during treatment, mainly in the neck and lumbar region, as a result of relaxation of relevant muscle groups and tendons achieved via the zones of the feet.

Abnormalities of the zones around the sacroiliac joint (lower spine, hip joint, posterior pubic symphysis, thigh and knee) often indicate an underlying **difference in leg length**. This should be assessed and, if a series of RTF treatments does not lead to the desired result, treated in addition using other methods.

As **transitions** typically and frequently prove to be weak points or sensitive areas, particularly on the spine, I should like to highlight the most important transitions in the spine:

- **Atlanto-occipital joint:** Be careful to avoid too rapid, manipulative movements of the big toe in trauma patients (craniocerebral trauma, whiplash injuries). See Chapter 16.3.
- **Cervicothoracic transition:** Where there are pathological changes, this point is known as **hallux valgus** (excessive lateral flexion of the big toe). The zones of the nape of the neck, the heart, and thyroid gland may be affected by the altered skeletal structure of the foot. Which connections are primary and which are secondary is irrelevant in terms of therapy; there are always **interactions** between skeletal structures and organ arrangements, which can show as weakness in the metatarsophalangeal joint.
- The **meridians of the spleen–pancreas** and **liver** run dorsally over the metatarsophalangeal

joint and their energy flow may be impaired by a pathological change in the position of this joint. **Scars** following a hallux valgus operation should be treated (Chapter 25) because they could become interference fields for zones and meridians. If the metatarsophalangeal joint is affected by stresses of this nature, movement and treatment should be cautious, possibly also including the option of Ortho-Bionomy.

- **Central thoracic spine:** This zone is often painful as a result of poor posture. Normally, the kyphosis of the upper thoracic spine should already assume a gentle lordosis at the level of the sixth and seventh thoracic vertebrae to ensure freedom of movement between the shoulder blades. The liver and stomach have their segmental correlation there.
- **Thoracic–lumbar transition:** Treatment at the level of the kidney zone is always started gently. As the nerve supply of the lower extremities originates from the lumbar plexus region, these zones are often painful in patients who suffer from complaints in the pelvic girdle and legs.
- **Lumbosacral transition at the promontorium:** Weakness and stress often occur as far as the sacroiliac joint and the skeletomuscular pelvic girdle as a result of the nonphysiological position of the pelvis. In combination with additional zones, these can be treated with RTF to achieve good, lasting results. In principle, we should not only approach blockages, weak points, and pain points in the skeletomuscular system from a pathological perspective, but concede that they also have **protective functions** which can prevent the organism from suffering greater damage until therapeutic intervention takes place.

21.3.2 Treatment Suggestions for the Spine

Lumbar Syndrome

(Fig. 21.4)

Symptomatic zones: Lumbar region of the spine. Lateral abdominal muscles.

Possible background zones: Cervical spine as upper physiological lordosis. Sacrum and sacroiliac joint. Sternum, which is involved in every movement of the sacrum. Symphysis, hip joint, gluteal muscles.

Intestine—especially important as a result of segmental connections with the lumbar spine. Kidneys with vague complaints in the lower back. Organs of the lesser pelvis with functional and/or organic abnormalities.

Teeth as potential interference fields (Chapter 26). Measurements in accordance with R. Voll show that 24 teeth interact with the lumbar spine. To stabilize the autonomic nervous system, the solar plexus and/or other stabilizing grips.

In an acute condition, the symptomatic zones are treated with the sedating grip. Pain can often be relieved more quickly if treatment starts on the lateral abdominal muscles, the antagonists to the lumbar spine. Depending on the patient's reaction, it may be possible to change from sedating to tonifying grips during pain management and acute treatment—at first cautiously and then more intensely in most situations. The Eutonic pelvis–leg grip provides additional relief (Chapter 6.4).

In patients with disk herniation or prolapse, treatment is similar to that for lumbar syndrome. Apart from posture correction, toxic loads on the intestine and clarification of any interference fields (e.g., scars, devitalized teeth) play an important role here.

> Many therapies overlook the following points: the front and back interact, as do the top and bottom, right and left, inside and outside. For example, a small scar resulting from laparoscopy (= front) may trigger severe disturbances in the lower spine (= back).

Cervical Syndrome

The treatment of patients with whiplash, even if it happened a long time ago, with craniocerebral trauma and operations in the ventral and dorsal neck region, should **always** be gentle and cautious; possibly, start with stabilizing grips and background zones.

Symptomatic zones: Cervical spine. Base of the skull and mastoid process. Neck muscles.

Possible background zones: Lumbar spine with sacrum, and sacroiliac joint. Upper edge of the trapezius and the shoulder girdle and joints. Sternum.

Heart, as the seventh cervical vertebra, has segmental correlations with the heart itself. Lymphatics of the head and neck. Thyroid gland.

Organs of the lesser pelvis. (The thyroid gland is opposite the seventh cervical vertebra, which

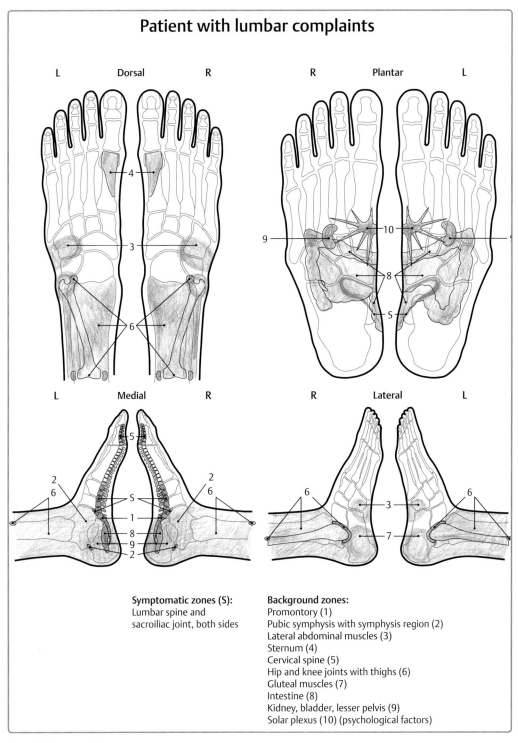

Patient with lumbar complaints

Dorsal — L / R

Plantar — R / L

Medial — L / R

Lateral — R / L

Symptomatic zones (S):
Lumbar spine and
sacroiliac joint, both sides

Background zones:
Promontory (1)
Pubic symphysis with symphysis region (2)
Lateral abdominal muscles (3)
Sternum (4)
Cervical spine (5)
Hip and knee joints with thighs (6)
Gluteal muscles (7)
Intestine (8)
Kidney, bladder, lesser pelvis (9)
Solar plexus (10) (psychological factors)

Fig. 21.4 Patient with lumbar complaints.

is referred to as the "third ovary" in holistic treatment methods.)

Solar plexus and/or stabilizing grips for overall stabilization.

In the course of treatment, cautious mobilization of the metatarsophalangeal joint may be offered. Avoid strong traction and rotation. The rules of Ortho-Bionomy have proved especially valuable here.

21.3.3 General Information about the Shoulder Girdle and Thorax

As the **sternoclavicular articulation** (transition from the sternum to the clavicle) is also always involved in the movement of the shoulder and can be impaired, it should be examined in all patients with shoulder symptoms and, if painful, treated at the same time. Mobilization in the region of the first and second metatarsal heads supports treatment.

Muscular tensions in the zones of the right side of the nape of neck, trapezius, and shoulder region are often associated with liver/gall bladder stresses, while on the left side they point to heart and stomach complaints.

The zone of the shoulder girdle often has **emotional associations** too: heavily strained metatarsophalangeal joints (MP joints) with little mobility not only constitute a structural deformity but may indicate a psychological burden which this person has to carry on their shoulders. It goes without saying that we should avoid interpreting or evaluating such aspects ourselves.

I regard the **sternum** as one of the most central zones in RTF. Multitudinous relationships are present which can be put to therapeutic use seeing that the **linea alba** constitutes a sinewy muscular connection from the sternum to the pubic symphysis. So, in patients with bony-muscular complaints in the **pelvic girdle,** the sternum should also be treated at the same time.

Treatment of the sternum also includes the **thymus** with its extraordinary importance for the immune system, blood formation, and bone metabolism.

As the zone of the sternum is in part identical to the zone of the heart, initially we treat this area gently in patients complaining of organic and functional disorders of the **heart** and respiratory organs, until their current reaction can be better assessed.

Blockage of the sternocostal joints is felt via the ribs as a painful restriction of movement in the thorax and thoracic spine. RTF treatment before and after manual therapies has often proved useful as an appropriate adjunctive therapy.

Structural misalignment of the sternum is a load on the whole person as far as the lower vertebral and pelvic region and the lower extremities.

As a flat bone, the sternum is involved in **blood formation** and should therefore be included in the treatment of patients with blood count anomalies, especially as it often proves painful.

Very introverted people often express their **introversion** by pulling in their shoulders and drawing back their sternum significantly. Here I should like to advise against superficial mechanical posture correction because changing external posture alone fails to get to the heart of the matter. Some people need periods of emotional withdrawal to protect themselves from excessive outward influences and this is expressed in a defensive posture in the true sense of the expression.

In our culture, the sternum is closely associated with **the self** because we instinctively touch it when we refer to ourselves as "I." In **religious ritual** gestures, people beat this region to confess their guilt to the Creator, while at the same time stimulating the activity of the thymus gland by means of this gesture.

The expressions used in connection with the **shoulder girdle** are also revealing.

Patients with chronic shoulder problems are often emotionally disturbed in addition to experiencing physical dysfunction:

- To carry a heavy burden on one's shoulders
- To be a pain in the neck
- To perceive oneself as a broken person
- To bear one's cross
- To demonstrate headstrong behavior, etc.

21.3.4 Treatment Suggestions for the Shoulder Girdle and Thorax

Shoulder–Arm Syndrome

Symptomatic zones: Shoulder girdle and musculature and joints, especially mastoid process. Lower cervical spine, upper cervical spine (brachial plexus as innervation for the upper extremity). Sternum and sternoclavicular articulation.

At the **acute** stage, the symptoms are treated with sedating grips. It is advisable to start on the complaint-**free** side. **Eutonic grips** in the shoulder girdle, applied before or after RTF, also relieve the complaints (Chapter 6.4).

Possible background zones: Central and lower spine. Pelvic girdle and pelvic ligaments. **Right**-sided pain: The liver and gall bladder—segmental connections. **Left**-sided pain: Stomach and heart—likewise segmental connections.

Intestine and gall bladder—inter alia, the two meridians supply the colon and gall bladder, arm, and shoulder with their energy.

Possible examination of interference fields in scars, for example, **smallpox vaccination scar** on the ventral part of the deltoid muscle (path of the colon meridian) in older patients. Depending on the therapist, – it can also be treated using neural therapy (= intracutaneous or subcutaneous injection with a neural therapeutic agent).

Devitalized teeth. The four wisdom teeth, in the maxilla the premolars, in the mandible the molars are energetically related to the shoulder girdle (Chapter 26).

Solar plexus and/or other stabilizing grips. **Collateral** and **contralateral** treatment (Chapter 18.4): **right** shoulder joint is assigned to **left** shoulder joint (contralaterally); **right** shoulder joint to the **right** hip joint (collaterally).

Epicondylitis

The **symptomatic** and **background zones** are similar to those of the shoulder–arm syndrome.

When applying the collateral and contralateral relationships, the **right** elbow is assigned to the **left** elbow (contralaterally), the right **elbow** to the right **knee** (collaterally).

Intercostal Neuralgia

The **symptomatic zones** are treated with the sedating grip, frequently interspersed with the solar plexus and/or other stabilizing grips, to alleviate the pain. Brief daily pain management at the **acute** stage (Chaper 16): the neuralgic points of the thorax, sternum with associated sternocostal joints, associated parts of the spine.

Possible background zones: At the **acute** stage, treat cautiously initially. For additional blockage of the ribs: thoracic spine overall.

Upper abdominal organs and intestine. Lymph organs, spleen, appendix.

Have **foci** such as devitalized teeth clarified. The organs in the vicinity of the inflammation in the thorax (e.g., the liver and spleen) are first sedated likewise.

In patients with **shingles** (herpes zoster) manifesting as viral intercostal neuralgia—which is accompanied by intense, stinging pain—significant relief can usually be achieved through the aforementioned pain management treatment.

At the **acute** stage of exanthema (the inflamed skin changes are usually in segmental paths) these zones are treated with **sedating** grips. Enemas, disposable or otherwise, are useful in counteracting the hyperacidity in the intestine with all the inflammation.

The **chronic** stage after the pustules and blisters have healed is usually characterized by intense neuralgic pain which is repeatedly classified as "resistant to therapy" and can last for weeks or months. Here too, the symptomatic zones are treated with sedating grips, whereby partial spontaneous pain reduction can be achieved.

The zones of the autonomic nervous system, digestive tract, and lymphatic system are particularly important. In addition **classical homeopathy** is a proven method of choice here. A strictly alkaline diet (potatoes, vegetables, avoidance of all unhealthy stimulants) supports the healing process.

21.3.5 General Information about the Pelvic Girdle to the Knee

The skeletomuscular pelvic girdle has functional connections with the shoulder girdle:
- Ventrally through the linea alba
- Dorsally through the spine
- As a diagonal connection from the top rear to the bottom front through the muscular movement spiral
- Through the clear functional relationship between the sternum and sacrum, which is also evident from the similarity in shape of the two bones (Appendix, p. 243 Brochure 4 "Similarities in shape as the key to therapy").

Apart from this, Consensual Therapy also points to connections (Chapter 18.4.2). Therefore, patients with disorders of the pelvic girdle should always be examined and, if necessary, treated in the zones of the shoulder girdle as well and vice versa.

It is now well known that therapeutically useful connections exist between the **hip** and **temporomandibular joint** not only in osteopathy and by holistic dentists but also by the rule of similarity in shape (**Fig. 21.5**). Those of us who employ RTF have been convinced for decades by the good results achieved by the practical implementation of these connections in the treatment of patients.

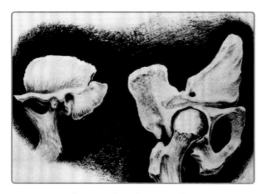

Fig. 21.5 Similarity in shape between the temporomandibular and hip joints.

From My Practice

A former patient of mine had been distressed in her professional and private life for a long time. I observed that speaking was very difficult for her and she could scarcely move her temporomandibular joint.

During a short course of pain management and acute treatment (Chapter 16), I sedated the zones of the temporomandibular joints, the base of the skull, and the mastoid process. I tonified the zones of the hip joint and the sacroiliac joint several times. As she displayed a strong reaction in autonomic nervous system (moist hands, increased respiratory rate), I often interspersed the sedation of the solar plexus zone among the other treated zones.

After only a few minutes I noticed her facial features relaxing, the pain in her temporomandibular joint eased significantly, and she was able to open her mouth almost normally. Then I carefully tonified the zone of the gall bladder (both the temporomandibular and the hip joint are supplied with energy by, inter alia, the gall bladder meridian), which proved to be very painful.

At the end of the 15-minute treatment session I re-examined the zone of the temporomandibular joint—it was now only slightly painful. In the following weeks, the woman came back a total of four times for rather more comprehensive treatments, which made her complaints disappear completely.

Fig. 10.1 shows the similarity between the temporomandibular joint and the hip joint.

The tissue surrounding the **external** and **internal malleoli** is more often congested in women than in men. Apart from known lymphatic and venous causes, there may also be other connections:

- In RTF these points are assigned to the pelvis and hip region with its frequent disturbances.
- In **meridian theory**, the bladder and gall bladder meridian supplies the lateral malleoli dorsally and ventrally, while the kidney meridian supplies the region surrounding the medial parts of the calcaneus and the inner malleoli.

As approximately a quarter to a third of the energy in the meridians is also supplied to the respective organs, the names of which they bear, we can treat the **zones** of these organs at the same time if they show abnormalities.

- At the point where the inner malleoli of both feet join, we can treat the zone of the front of the **pubic symphysis**. As part of the lesser pelvis, it often reflects not only functional but also emotional problems and should always be treated gently.

Significant pain points on the calcaneus and the malleoli are often found in patients with musculoskeletal irritations of the pelvis and/or with organic and functional complaints of the organs of the lesser pelvis. Here, inter alia, the zones of the **pelvic ligaments** are found, the treatment of which is indicated for many malfunctions. It is also highly valued in pregnancy and antenatal care (Chapter 27).

Practical experience with the site of the **gluteal muscle** zones: According to the rule of 'Similarity in Shape', the plantar-proximal tissue of the calcaneus (heel bone) corresponds to gluteal muscles. Due to the tougher and coarser tissue structure on this part of the sole, it is not always easy to treat effectively there, except on children's feet or small women's feet. Practice has shown though, that we can also reach the gluteal zones from the lateral sides of the calcaneus tissue. Overall, the treatment of these zones often brings about a **profound resolution** of excessive tensions in the entire pelvis and back because they are part of the stabilizing base of the torso.

21.3.6 Treatment Suggestions

Diseases of the Hip Joint

Symptomatic zones: Hip joint, ventrally and dorsally. For acute pain and restricted movement, the symptoms are first treated with sedating grips. Treatment can also be started on the opposite hip. Unless there is intense pain, that area is tonified, adjusted to the patient's reaction.

Possible background zones: Lower spine, sacrum, and sacroiliac joint. Pubic symphysis, gluteal and lateral abdominal muscles. Iliotibial tract (sinewy reinforcement on the outside of the thigh). Knee.

Temporomandibular joint. Canines (energetic measurements in accordance with Dr. Voll).

Digestive organs, liver/gall bladder. Urinary tract. Inguinal lymph channels. Spleen.

Collateral and contralateral treatment on the same-side shoulder and opposite hip, both in situ as well as in the zones (Chapter 18.4).

Scars (e.g., appendectomy scar), as the gall bladder meridian also supplies the hip region and the anterior superior iliac spine, at which the scar frequently begins.

Solar plexus and/or other stabilizing grips for stabilization of the autonomic nervous system.

> The gall bladder meridian, like all meridians, belongs to a pair. It supplies five joints on the lateral sides of the body: the temporomandibular, shoulder, hip, and knee joints, and the lateral malleolus. When complaints arise in **one** of these joints, the zones of the other four should be examined for abnormalities, likewise those of the gall bladder (Chapter 30).

Endoprosthetics of the Hip

The same treatment suggestions apply as for hip joint diseases. Treatment of the symptomatic zone should only be started cautiously after the wound has healed. Starting from the opposite hip joint may be preferable.

Again and again, in patients after implantation of an artificial hip joint, a more or less pronounced swelling occurs around the lateral malleolus on the side where the operation was performed. Gentle stroking in lateral to medial direction in the zones of the inguinal area not only relieves the local tissue, but also has a favorable effect on the overall healing process. A course of RTF lymphatic treatments (Chapter 29) has also proved valuable. Such swellings may, however, also indicate a disturbance in the energy flow of the gall bladder meridian (see above).

Knee Complaints of Various Kinds and Origins

> So-called regulatory therapies usually offer more options for patients with knee problems than conventional, usually symptom-oriented, treatments. With RTF especially many connections can be included.

Symptomatic zone: Affected knee.

Possible background zones: Entire muscular and bony pelvic girdle. Thigh and the muscles and fasciae. The opposite knee and the elbow on the same side, both in situ and as a zone (Chapter 18.4).

Lymphatic ducts and vessels of the inguinal area and thigh. All metabolic systems, especially in rheumatic complaints. Bladder, gall bladder, stomach, spleen, pancreas, liver and kidney, as inter alia, these meridians also supply the knee.

Scars, not only on the knee, but also remote ones.

Twenty teeth have energetic connections with the knees (Chapter 26). For stabilization of the autonomic nervous system, solar plexus, and/or other stabilizing grips.

21.4

Zones of the Urinary Tract

21.4.1 General Information

Relatively often the symptoms of kidney diseases are inconspicuous. Therefore, vague and ambiguous chronic back pain should be taken seriously and diagnosed. The zones of the kidneys are always tonified gently because their performance will be hampered rather than supported otherwise (exception: kidney stones). Kidney patients need **lots of sleep**.

- If **water retention** (retention of fluids in organs and tissues) occurs as a result of a renal disorder, the zones of the lymphatic system, in particular of the central collection vessels and the abdominal area, may be treated before those of the urinary tract.
- Gentle stimuli are then applied not only to the lymphatic system, but also to the kidneys, ureters, and bladder because they ensure normalization of the activity of the systems dealing with fluids far better than excessively vigorous stimuli.

- In **dialysis** patients, RTF and in particular lymphatic RTF, is highly appropriate as an adjunctive therapy. On the one hand, to alleviate the attendant symptoms associated with the disease, for example, circulatory disturbances, metabolic stresses in the pancreas, intestine and liver, lymph congestion, changes in sensory perception and emotional level. On the other hand, to support any residual function of the kidneys and to counter the fatigue induced by dialysis over a longer period.
- RTF, in particular lymphatic treatment, often results in good diuresis, both in patients with **edema of the leg** and in critically ill patients with **ascites** and **pleural effusions.** They obtain some relief from their symptoms with regard to the heart/circulation and respiration for at least a few hours. Short treatment times are important for critically ill patients.
- Previously, the **bladder** was only treated in the region of the zone of the sacrum, from where the function of the bladder can still be favorably influenced today. The effect cannot be explained, however, by the organ of the bladder, but by the segmental relationship of the sacrum to the bladder; the so-called bladder zone in the caudal part of the sacrum is known in connective tissue massage; it often manifests as a swelling or as a retracted area, both in situ and in the zone on the foot. In practice, the patient's reaction will decide which of the two options is the more crucial for bladder treatment; often both zones require treatment.
- In the case of frequent night-time urination, **cardiac insufficiency** should also be considered: clarify clinically.

21.4.2 Treatment Suggestions

Bladder Weakness, Incontinence

Symptomatic zones: Bladder, bladder sphincter, pelvic floor, pubic symphysis.

Initially, many patients react better to **sedating** treatment of the bladder sphincter and the bladder because the musculature tries to avoid over-frequent urination and involuntary passing of urine by means of increased tension. Later, the zone can be tonified.

Possible background zones: Lower spine, especially sacrum—innervation of the organs of the lesser pelvis. Pelvic ligaments (Chapter 27). All organs of the lesser pelvis. Nasopharyngeal cavity—derives from the same germ layer. All other sphincters (Chapter 6). Ureter and kidneys. Lymphatics of the inguinal area. Solar plexus and/or other stabilizing grips for harmonization of the autonomic nervous system.

R. Tanzberger formulates this condition thus, "Incontinence is a phenomenon involving tension, but it is not an illness."

Postoperative Urinary Retention

Initially, treatment can be offered several times a day as brief acute care: 8 to 10 minutes is sufficient.

Symptomatic zones: Bladder and bladder sphincter. Pelvic floor. Initially, treatment with sedating grips. After improvement of the symptoms, gentle tonifying is possible.

Frequently interspersed stabilizing grips, including solar plexus, are important to stabilize the autonomic nervous system.

Possible background zones: Lower spine, especially sacrum. Ureter and kidneys. All organs of the lesser pelvis. All other sphincters.

The lymphatic system of the pelvis and inguinal area can be added later. Some RTF lymphatic treatments (Chapter 29) support overall postoperative regeneration after the acute phase. Further information can be found in Chapter 16 "Management and Treatment of Pain in Acute Situations."

A one-year study conducted at a Swiss clinic in 1993 verified that of 56 patients with postoperative urinary retention, the symptoms of 41 disappeared without medication, usually after only two to three brief acute treatment sessions.

Bed Wetting (Nocturnal Enuresis)
(**Fig. 21.6**)

Symptomatic zones: Bladder, ureter, and kidneys.

Possible background zones: Solar plexus and/or other stabilizing grips, interspersed at frequent intervals throughout treatment, are particularly important.

Lower spine, especially sacrum—innervation of the organs of the lesser pelvis. The bony-muscular

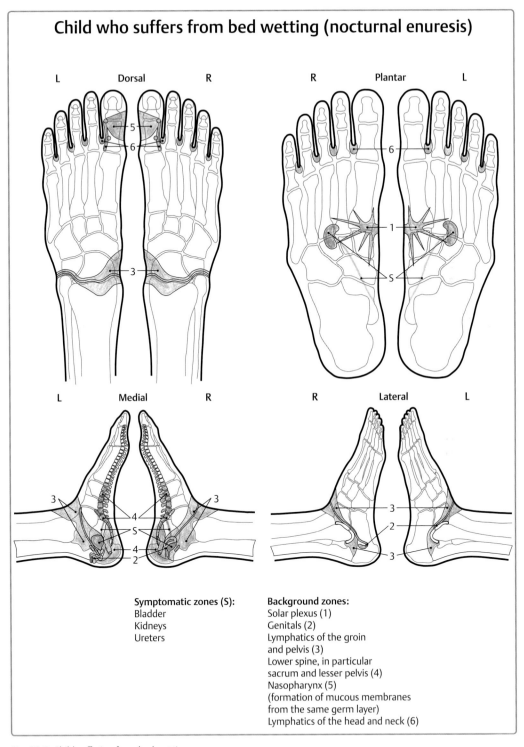

Child who suffers from bed wetting (nocturnal enuresis)

Symptomatic zones (S):
Bladder
Kidneys
Ureters

Background zones:
Solar plexus (1)
Genitals (2)
Lymphatics of the groin
and pelvis (3)
Lower spine, in particular
sacrum and lesser pelvis (4)
Nasopharynx (5)
(formation of mucous membranes
from the same germ layer)
Lymphatics of the head and neck (6)

Fig. 21.6 Child suffering from bed wetting.

pelvic girdle. The nasopharyngeal cavity—its mucous membrane develops from the same germ layer. Lymphatic tissue of pelvis, inguinal area, and thigh.

- As children suffering from bed wetting usually have functional disturbances and are seldom organically sick, symptomatic and background zones can be gently tonified from the outset.
- Apart from known links with any negative psychosocial environment, it should be diagnostically clarified whether the child has a hereditary organ malformation or disease of the urinary tract.
- A relationship of mutual trust between the therapist and patient is very important because, particularly with this clinical picture, it is evident that not only is the bladder sphincter weakened but that the child is suffering, even if he or she is not consciously aware of this.

  Apart from treatment of the aforementioned zones, the more successfully these patients can be helped to find their own **personal breathing rhythm**, the more they will be able to withstand the pressures of their environment, which often can only be changed marginally and gradually.

  As the effect of the **spleen** is wide-ranging and clearly also extends to the mind and emotions, it should be treated at the same time in all of these children (Chapter 21.8).
- In view of these closely-related links between family environment, respiration, the autonomic nervous system, organ function, and the endocrine glands, treatment of the **three diaphragms**—the floor of the buccal cavity, the diaphragm, and the pelvic floor—should also be included, as the normalization of their tone contributes significantly to the harmonization of overall vitality.
- **Scars**, which are found time and again in such children in the course of the bladder meridian on the eyebrows or forehead, should be examined for any interference field quality and if necessary, treated at the same time (Chapter 25).
- In addition to manual or breathing therapy or psychotherapy, changing the **location of the child's bed** (radiesthesia) may also be of major importance in improving the condition.
- Above all, relatives should be advised that punishment or the withdrawal of goodwill and loving care will help neither the child nor the adult.

- Frequently, the parents' irritation or resignation is so great that they would also benefit from some RTF treatment.

Renal and Ureteric Colic

Pain management and acute treatment are employed here (Chapter 16). If the kidney stone is too large to be excreted in the normal way, it is imperative that **both** kidney zones are only treated with gentle, sedating grips or not at all. Relatively prompt clarification by means of X-rays, ultrasound, computed tomography, etc. is important as kidney stones can enlarge fairly quickly.

The following treatments are suggested for kidney stones which are small enough to be excreted in the normal way.

Symptomatic zones: Bladder, ureter and kidney are tonified. This sequence has proven effective as preparation for the passing of kidney stones. Solar plexus and/or stabilizing grips.

Possible background zones: At the acute stage, stabilizing grips are sufficient. Once the colic has abated and in subsequent treatments, the lower spine and abdominal muscles, all organs of the lesser pelvis, the pelvic floor, and the intestine can often be added.

Tonifying can be relatively vigorous, adjusted to the patient's overall condition. The chances of the stone moving toward the ureter as a result are good. Any colic which occurs during or after these treatments is usually less painful and of shorter duration, and is usually well tolerated by the patient.

If the stone has already moved into the **ureter** (strong radiating pain in the bladder, pubic symphysis, genital organs, and medial side of the thighs), the path in the reverse direction of flow of the urine is cleared in turn: **at first** the bladder and then the ureter zone is gently tonified as far as the stone.

The site corresponding to the current location of the stone is easy to trace: the patient experiences a sharp, stinging pain spontaneously. From this site, vigorous stroking in the direction of the bladder is performed with the fingers. If we are fortunate, the stone will then begin to move and will be excreted in the coming hours or days. We advise the use of a sieve when urinating, in order to catch the stone.

It is beneficial for the patient to lie on a mud or heat pack during treatment to enable better relaxation of the back.

The release of **renal gravel** during treatment intervals is often observed within the general range of reactions and is relatively painless. Patients describe a slight dragging and ascertain a change in the color and consistency of their urine.

Ensure a de-acidified diet, significantly increased fluid intake (preferably hot water or mild herb teas), more exercise, and the avoidance of stimulants.

21.5

Zones of the Endocrine System

21.5.1 General Information

When treating complaints in the endocrine system, it is particularly important that, even if the symptoms seemingly only affect **one** of the endocrine glands, we always consider them in functional interaction with the other endocrine glands and the metabolic organs.

The zones which act on the autonomic nervous system—for example, the stabilizing/harmonizing grips and lymphatic zones—also form part of this functional range because the **endocrine system, autonomic nervous system**, and **emotional levels** are closely linked.

Despite the major significance and relief entailed in the discovery of artificial hormones (e.g., insulin, thyroxine), it is a fact that diseases involving this system are often the consequence of the unnatural lifestyle which has become the norm for decades in our overly civilized world. However much, for example, the contraceptive pill revolutionized the lives of women, it also has a downside.

> **The damaging effects** of electrosmog, in particular on the endocrine system, are still frequently ignored and many of our patients virtually take it for granted that we often consume artificial hormones and antibiotics when we eat meat.

The **treatment approach** for patients with hormonal dysfunctions should be cautious at first, especially in the symptomatic zones. Stabilizing and/or Eutonic grips together with a sufficiently long period of **subsequent rest** are sometimes the most important aspect during initial treatment.

21.5.2 Treatment Suggestions

Menstrual Complaints

(Fig. 21.7)

We offer a brief pain management and acute treatment course for **acute** menstrual pain and heavy bleeding (Chapter 16). Often the sedating grip in the region of the uterus and solar plexus is sufficient. The lower spine and the lumbar spine, sacrum, and sacroiliac joint can be gently tonified.

Disturbances of a **longer duration** such as chronic dysmenorrhea, milder forms of endometriosis (endometrium which extends outside the uterus), and changes of longer duration in the normal length of a menstrual cycle are treated as follows:

Symptomatic zones: Uterus and ovaries are first treated with sedating grips, likewise the pituitary gland. If stronger reactions do not occur, these areas may also be tonified in subsequent treatments.

Possible background zones: All other endocrine glands. Intestine, in particular in the lower region because of its direct proximity to the genital organs. Lower spine, especially sacrum and sacroiliac joint. Pelvic ligaments (Chapter 27) and pelvic floor.

Nasopharyngeal cavity—the mucous membranes of the organs of the lesser pelvis and the head cavity develop from the same germ layer. Lymphatic areas of the stomach and pelvis.

Devitalized teeth and scars—for example, in the course of the bladder meridian or the so-called conception vessel (Chapter 30).

Stabilizing- and/or Eutonic grips as often as necessary. Apart from the pelvic ligaments, all the regions can be **tonified**—cautiously at first.

If there is a **vaginal discharge** for a short time as a reaction, it should be understood as a clear sign of cleansing and stabilization of the pelvic organs. However, we frequently find that a discharge which may have existed for many years completely disappears after one or two menstrual cycles. For longer-lasting discharges which change in color, odor, and consistency, the causes must be ascertained by a gynecologist.

Fasting and other **cleansing cures** have an exceptionally regenerative effect on gynecological complaints because the frequent presence of fermentative dyspepsia or other imbalances in the acid–alkaline level of the digestive tract also have a debilitating and disruptive effect on all the other organs with mucous membranes.

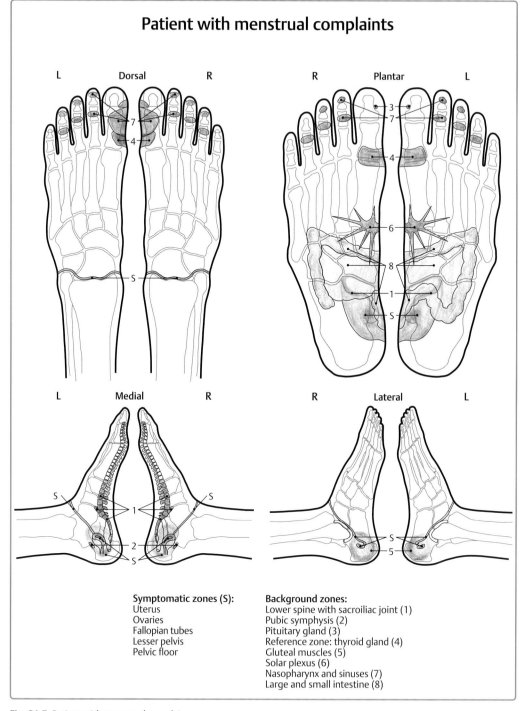

Patient with menstrual complaints

L Dorsal R

R Plantar L

L Medial R

R Lateral L

Symptomatic zones (S):
Uterus
Ovaries
Fallopian tubes
Lesser pelvis
Pelvic floor

Background zones:
Lower spine with sacroiliac joint (1)
Pubic symphysis (2)
Pituitary gland (3)
Reference zone: thyroid gland (4)
Gluteal muscles (5)
Solar plexus (6)
Nasopharynx and sinuses (7)
Large and small intestine (8)

Fig. 21.7 Patient with menstrual complaints.

From My Practice

A woman in her mid-50s came to my practice complaining of severe chronic pain in her lumbar vertebrae and sacral region as well as chronic fatigue. The initial findings revealed scarcely any complaints in the lumbar region, but the zones of the lesser pelvis, the sacroiliac joint, and the lateral abdominal wall were very painful. After only the second RTF session, she had a strong, malodorous discharge. She'd had her last period 8 years previously.

After the fourth treatment, she called me in the morning and reported that she'd been having heavy abdominal bleeding for several hours but the pain in her lower spine had disappeared. When I visited her at her home, I treated the zones of the uterus, ovaries, pelvic floor, sacrum, rectum, and spleen with the sedating grip. The bleeding decreased significantly after only 10 minutes. A gynecological examination (her last one was 10 years ago) revealed a myoma larger than a fist and she underwent surgery a few days later.

Afterward, I treated her once or twice a week for a month to stabilize her overall condition. In all probability, my treatment of the zones contributed to the chronic-progressive process in her abdomen becoming acute and identifiable as a result. Despite the drama of the acute situation, the patient was astonishingly relaxed and commented that she had sensed for a long time that "something crucial" was coming up for her.

Unfulfilled Desire to Have Children, Sterility, Infertility

Time and again the results of RTF are surprisingly good for troubles of this kind in women and men. This is probably due in large part to the fact that not only do the pelvic organs and the entire endocrine system attain an optimum state of equilibrium, but by applying RTF the overall emotional condition of the person stabilizes as well. Even if the desired outcome, pregnancy, is not always achieved, men and women find it easier to come to terms with the reality.

The **initial findings** will show, based on the disturbed zones, whether the treatment is more important for the woman or the man—from experience disturbances are more often found in women. The corresponding zones should be treated once or twice a week for two to three menstrual cycles.

Symptomatic zones: Organs of the lesser pelvis and endocrine glands, especially the pituitary gland.

Possible background zones: All the regions relating to the autonomic nervous system, stabilizing and Eutonic grips, also thymus and spleen. (Anthroposophical physicians and therapists refer to the spleen as the organ which is responsible for the coordination of all rhythmical processes within a person.)

Skeletomuscular system of the pelvic girdle, in particular, pelvic ligaments.

Nasopharyngeal cavity, larynx, and vocal cords. Intestine, especially the small intestine. Meridian courses which supply the pelvic organs with their energy and may be disturbed by scars, etc.

Teeth as possible interference fields (the incisors are assigned to the organs of the lesser pelvis in accordance with Voll's energetic measurements).

Radiesthetic aspects—disturbing factors within the earth, "electrosmog" disturbances affecting the workplace or bedroom (e.g., a cell phone which is permanently switched on, television in the bedroom, etc.) must also be taken into consideration.

Primary or Secondary Amenorrhea

As frequent triggers include trauma, various shock situations, and weight loss as a result of eating disorders (likewise usually of psychological origin), the zones which stabilize/harmonize the **autonomic nervous system** are paramount here:

- Regulation gets off to a good start via the **solar plexus** and additional stabilizing grips.
- The **sternum** (identical to that of the thymus) is also treated. It is directly related to our sense of self: when a person describes themselves, they touch this place. When one's sense of personal power is weakened, the sternum is retracted somewhat; when it is pushed too far forward, a person's body language may indicate that they give themselves too much importance.
- The **lymphatic system**, like other systems dealing with fluids, is also directly related to the autonomic nervous system and mood.
- If a patient feels comfortable with the close proximity to the therapist required for these grips, **Eutonic grips** and positions assist greatly in providing an awareness of one's own physical existence. A trusting relationship with the therapist is of fundamental importance.

RTF provides this group of patients in particular with significant and far-reaching back-up for psychotherapeutic methods and it would be beneficial if more professionals knew about this expertise.

The zones which are specified for "menstrual disorders" are suitable for the **specific** treatment of girls and young women.

Ovarian Cysts

These often recede of their own accord, especially in women entering the menopause. However, we have found that even in younger women, cysts respond unusually rapidly to RTF. Gynecologists confirmed by examination that cysts shrink significantly within only 3 to 4 weeks or are no longer detectable.

In order to achieve lasting results and to strengthen the organs of the lesser pelvis at the same time, we advise that reflexotherapy of the feet be continued once or twice a week for about two menstrual cycles.

The first assessment (Chapter 11) reveals chronic disorders of the **nasopharyngeal cavity** with great regularity, from chronic sinusitis to allergic symptoms, tonsillitis, middle ear suppurations and catarrh of the eustachian tubes.

Cryptorchidism, Retractile Testes

Whenever possible, parents must be informed that boys with cryptorchidism (invisible or nonpalpable testes) require treatment as early as possible. If the testes fail to descend into the scrotum in the first years of life, they can be severely damaged by the higher internal temperature of the pelvis, possibly resulting in sterility.

Before opting for either an operation or hormonal treatment, it is always worth conducting a course of RTF treatments. Even if this does not lead to the desired result, the child's overall condition stabilizes. Contact should always be approached cautiously because the inner trigger for the retraction of an organ is often related to emotional stress during pregnancy or birth, even if this is unconscious.

The younger the child, the shorter the treatment time. The parents may be instructed to perform some simple grips themselves in the morning and evening each day. Three to five minutes are sufficient initially.

Treatment time can be longer for children of two or three years old. **Warm feet** are very important. All children enjoy loving massage of their little feet and gentle "plucking" of their toes.

Symptomatic zones: Genital organs, inguinal area.

Possible background zones: All other endocrine glands. Autonomic nervous system, which can be stabilized with solar plexus and other stabilizing grips. Lower spine with sacrum and sacroiliac joint.

Inguinal area. **Note:** Here the clear, repeated stroking of the tendon of the tibialis anterior muscle (tibial tendon close to the inner malleolus) extending to the genital area has proven very effective. It is the normal path of the testes from the inguinal canal into the scrotum.

A sensitive therapist's hands detect a small hardening of the tissue which moves about in this path the more the testis is able to move in its intended direction. Parents can easily provide these stroking movements.

Prostate Adenoma

Enlargement of the prostate gland from epithelial tissue as a benign tumor is a relatively frequent disease in men over the age of 50 years. If treated in the early stages, troublesome attendant symptoms such as pollakiuria, dysuria, the urge to urinate more frequently and with greater difficulty but in only small amounts, can be expected to recede or disappear completely. Delayed micturition with a weak urinary stream can also be improved.

Symptomatic zones: Prostate gland, bladder, urethra, and scrotum.

Possible background zones: All endocrine glands. Pelvic ligaments. Lower spine with sacrum and sacroiliac joint. Kidneys, ureter. Intestine.

Scars in the **center** of the body. Teeth as possible interference fields (Chapter 26, section "Interference Field Review").

Stabilizing grips harmonize the often irritated mind.

Hyperthyroidism (Graves' Disease)

Symptomatic zones: Thyroid gland. Only treating it with sedating grips during initial RTF or not at all has proved effective. Nape of the neck. As there is a direct connection between the thyroid gland and the seventh cervical vertebra ("dowager's hump"), this area must also be treated cautiously. Rotation of the basal joints of the big toes is to be avoided completely at first.

Possible background zones: All other endocrine glands, especially pituitary gland and glands of the pelvis. (In holistic medicine, the thyroid gland is also called the "third ovary.") Heart, which frequently reacts to hyperthyroidism in the form of tachycardia.

Intestine, above all, the so-called small intestine. Scars, especially those which are located on the conception vessel in the vertical **center** of the body.

Solar plexus and other stabilizing grips. Eutonic shoulder–arm grip (Chapter 6) provides particular relief and release for the neck, nape of the neck, and shoulder girdle as well as the whole person.

Important note: Patients with hyperthyroidism should not be treated for longer than **20 minutes** initially. Treatment is most effective if performed in the first half of the day because when performed later, **nighttime sleep** may be disturbed.

Diabetes Mellitus

Although diabetes is not a contraindication, such patients, especially if insulin-dependent, should be treated by therapists with adequate RTF experience. As the regulatory possibilities of RTF can result in fluctuations in blood and urine sugar levels, accurate and frequent testing during a course of RTF treatment is particularly important.

Additional aspects:
- If treatment of the pancreas zone is performed too vigorously or unilaterally, this can trigger **hypoglycemia** (a fall in blood sugar with shaking, cold sweats, tachycardia, pallor, and apathy) as a spontaneous reaction.

The most effective treatment for hypoglycemia is the immediate consumption of glucose, for example, in the form of a sugar lump or a spoonful of honey (Chapter 16.3).

- It is quite possible to gradually **reduce** the **amount** of insulin. However, this requires particularly good cooperation between the physician, therapist, and patient.
- Generally speaking, even neutrally, RTF grips with a specific effect always achieve better **tissue perfusion** of the feet and can prevent long-term effects such as sensory disturbances, etc.
- As diabetes can cause **chronic kidney failure**, thorough but cautious treatment of the urinary tract is important for all diabetics.
- The best results are achieved in **elderly diabetics,** especially if they are not insulin dependent. In this group too, fluctuations in blood sugar level must be carefully monitored. In addition to a healthy diet, plenty of **exercise** in the fresh air plays a crucial role in the well-being of these patients.

With **juvenile** (childhood) diabetes, although the growth of the pancreas cannot be altered, overall

quality of life can be improved:
- Chronically cold hands and feet will receive a better blood supply.
- The tendency to infections in the respiratory and genitourinary tracts declines.
- There is a greater awareness of hunger and thirst and these are satisfied more sensibly.
- The children's emotional outlook is more balanced and they are more alert.
- Sleep is more restful.

General suggestions for treatment:

Symptomatic zone: Pancreas. Here too, similar to hyperthyroidism, it is advisable to treat the zone gently or not at all during the initial treatment sessions, until the patient's reactions can be evaluated rather more precisely.

Possible background zones: All other endocrine glands. Head, especially eyes (in long-term diabetics there is a risk of retinal opacity). Lower thoracic spine (innervation). Intestine, especially small intestine. Liver, spleen. Stabilizing/harmonizing grips as often as necessary. As the solar plexus zone cannot be distinguished from that of the pancreas, other stabilizing grips are preferable.

Interference fields in the form of devitalized teeth and/or scars. It should not be overlooked that even small scars can trigger major disturbances. For example: one of the two **micro-scars** resulting from surgical removal of the nail of the big toe is located precisely on the 1st point of the **spleen–pancreas meridian.** It may not only impair the energy flow in this meridian, but also put a considerable strain on the organs of the spleen and in particular, the pancreas. (The second small scar is usually on precisely the 1st point of the liver meridian and can also exert major strain on the metabolism.)

Here treatment of the small scar by an experienced professional using **neural therapy** would be the method of choice. The patient's condition must be carefully monitored as their **blood sugar level may change suddenly** and **significantly**.

21.5.3 The Thymus

As the thymus interacts not only with the endocrine system, but with the autonomic nervous and lymphatic systems as well, it could also be discussed elsewhere. The overall impact of this gland behind the sternum was long underestimated, perhaps partly due to its declining in size during the course of development from child to adult. (A similar trend is seen in the appendix.)

The thymus is of eminent significance for the human **immune system**. We can assume that it largely constitutes **a self-regulating system**. At the same time, it should be remembered that immunity not only involves smoothly functioning physical organs, but is also related to a person's ethical stance—toward themselves and their environment.

The zone of the thymus is an integral part of treatment for
- hormonal disorders in childhood, adolescence, and adulthood, also especially in the transition to the menopause,
- all disorders and irritations of the autonomic nervous system such as physical strain, emotional distress, lack of sleep, etc.,
- lymphatic abnormalities of any kind, for example, acute and chronic inflammation, cancer, and general metabolic inertia.

As this zone is located behind the zone of the sternum, the treatment technique can be varied according to the indication:
- If the **sternum** is interpreted as part of the musculoskeletal connections, we work with dynamic grips; usually the index finger is the most suitable, as in other zones on the **dorsum** of the foot.
- If the **thymus** is to be addressed as part of the immune system, flexible, gentle tapping with the tips of both index fingers has proved effective.

21.6

Zones of the Respiratory Organs and Heart

21.6.1 General Information—Respiration

The diaphragm as an important muscle for **respiratory and cardiac function:** In the past (according to Ingham) only the small point in the center of the proximal edge of the transverse arch was regarded as the diaphragm zone and at the same time corresponded to the "old" zone of the solar plexus. As this area continues to have a stabilizing effect on respiration—after all, according to current information it is at least **part** of the edge of the whole upper diaphragm—we have appreciated it as one of our stabilizing grips for decades (see **Fig. 6.3**).

Meanwhile, however, the zone of the diaphragm has expanded considerably, in accordance with the size of this muscle, and encompasses approximately the proximal half of the metatarsal bone on both feet as far as the Lisfranc's line (**Fig. 10.24**).

As the dynamic up-and-down movement of the diaphragm is not easy to portray, in practice, the anatomical position of this muscle changes in situ **and** in the zone with every respiratory movement. For this reason, the diaphragm zone can be expanded as far as the upper abdomen (i.e., as far as the start of the distal row of tarsal bones). It is easy to discern the cupola of the edge of the upper diaphragm in a similar shape on the feet: if the toes are bent toward the head, it is visible at the lower edge of the transverse arch.

The **pars lumbalis** of the diaphragm ("diaphragmatic lobe"): Many patients with respiratory diseases respond to treatment of the zones of the lumbar spine with improved respiratory capacity. There are various reasons for this:
- Parts of the origin of this large muscle are connected to the pars lumbalis and the ventral area of the first to third lumbar vertebrae, sometimes the fourth, as bundled tendons. In this way, the **lumbar spine is involved in every breath**.
- Via the skeletomuscular kinetic chain, the lumbar area also interacts with the thorax functionally.
- The obvious proximity of the lumbar spine to parts of the intestine and the overlapping of these zones frequently points to metabolic disorders where there is strain. As the quality of intestinal function and the numerous lymph nodes located there have a significant influence on all the other mucous membrane areas in the organism, treatment of the **intestine** is of **fundamental** importance for patients with respiratory diseases.

Important note: It is not possible to distinguish whether the lumbar spine, the pars lumbalis of the diaphragm, or rather parts of the intestine are addressed with the stimulus applied at this point—from a therapeutic perspective, it is irrelevant because all these areas are functionally interconnected.

The diaphragm **connects** the thorax and abdomen in a healthy individual, whereas it divides these areas in one who is sick. As a rhythmic "respiratory bridge" it moves and massages the organs of the abdomen–pelvis and those of the thorax, hence also the heart, lungs, and great vessels of the aorta and upper vena cava. Thus, when it is functioning correctly, it contributes to their normal activity. It should not be forgotten that the two other diaphragms of **the floor of the buccal cavity and the pelvic floor** are also addressed with every inhalation and exhalation.

The **heel stretch grip** (see Figs. 6.1, 6.2) and the **respiratory stabilizing grip** (see Fig. 6.3) are particularly suitable for supporting respiration. At the same time, they contribute to the autonomic stabilization of the patient. However, respiration should not be intentionally controlled by either the patients themselves or the therapist. If we initially support the existing respiratory rhythm without judgement (what is "wrong," what is "right") as it **is**, both grips are more likely to be able to "entice" it into a natural rhythm.

21.6.2 Treatment Suggestions for Respiratory Organs

(Fig. 21.8)

Acute Asthmatic Attack

Symptomatic zones: The lungs, bronchi, and diaphragm are not as important as theoretically assumed. Usually, an asthmatic attack can be arrested faster by vigorously tonifying the **background zones** of the intestine, especially the small intestine.

The adrenal glands (identical to the kidneys). The pelvic floor. Possibly the spleen. Afterward, the **symptomatic zones** of the larynx, trachea, bronchi and lungs, and diaphragm can be treated with the sedating grip as required, although it often becomes apparent that this is no longer necessary to a great extent.

For autonomic stabilization, the heel stretch grip and the respiration-regulating grip discussed in detail above, likewise the solar plexus, come into question.

Chronic Asthma

At the attack-**free** stage or with a chronic condition, a thorough initial assessment should be carried out in order to establish the most seriously afflicted zones individually. The **intestine** will undoubtedly play a decisive role in all patients because in asthmatics the issue of hyperacidity is always relevant. The intestine is often described as "the most extensive interference field" for good reason.

Important note: Psychogenic stresses are not always the cause of asthmatic complaints. Sometimes the effects of **harmful substances** (artificial additives in food, intolerance of medicines, allergenic factors in the home or the environment) are paramount and should be eliminated as far as possible.

In addition to the "Acute Asthmatic Attack" zones listed, further **background zones** come into question: the lymphatic system overall. The heart. The liver/gall bladder. The ileocecal valve. The urinary tract. The sphincters (Chapter 6). The thymus.

Possible interference fields in the form of devitalized teeth: eight teeth, after all, are energetically related to the respiratory tract.

Stabilizing grips (see above), but also Eutonic grips for general regulation of muscle tone and for mental support. The mind is always—whether primarily or secondarily—involved in disturbed respiration.

Chronic Bronchitis

The suggestions for the treatment of asthmatic patients are also applicable here. However, the **frontal and maxillary sinuses** must often be included in the treatment, as well as **the organs of the lesser pelvis** (the mucous membrane in the upper and lower area originates from the same germ layer).

21.6.3 General Information—The Heart

It is well known that there is a direct link between the various irritations of general living conditions today and the increase in cardiovascular disease.

Often, however, not enough notice is taken of the crucial role played by the **intestine,** the **lymphatics,** and all the other **excretion** and **incretion** involved in overall cardiovascular activity.

As early as 1928, the heart specialist and university professor **Martin Mendelsohn** said that
- "every disease has its origin in a disturbed metabolism and diseased organs (including the heart) are the **secondary consequence,** but never the cause,"
- "all the secretory glands in the body represent an enormous source of strength for the circulation of bodily fluids," and
- "metabolism occurs as an active movement of fluid for all living tissue," in which there is only secondary involvement of the heart.

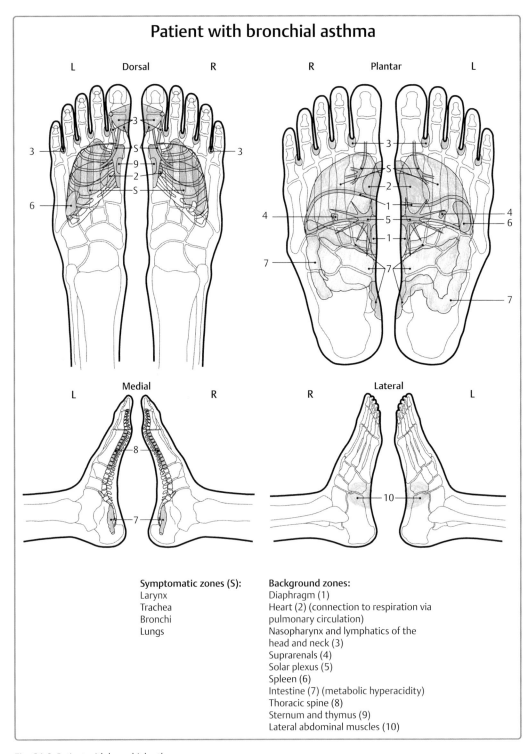

Patient with bronchial asthma

Symptomatic zones (S):
Larynx
Trachea
Bronchi
Lungs

Background zones:
Diaphragm (1)
Heart (2) (connection to respiration via pulmonary circulation)
Nasopharynx and lymphatics of the head and neck (3)
Suprarenals (4)
Solar plexus (5)
Spleen (6)
Intestine (7) (metabolic hyperacidity)
Thoracic spine (8)
Sternum and thymus (9)
Lateral abdominal muscles (10)

Fig. 21.8 Patient with bronchial asthma.

Our RTF experience with cardiac patients confirms this: overall, the **background zones** are in far greater need of treatment than the symptoms.

21.6.4 Treatment Suggestions for the Heart and Circulation

Angina Pectoris

(Fig. 21.9)
The name of the disease indicates the main symptoms of angina pectoris or coronary insufficiency: tightness in the chest. In principle, patients suffering from angina pectoris should be regarded as potential susceptible to cardiac infarction. It goes without saying that RTF only has the function of an **adjunctive therapy** but experience shows that patients benefit greatly from its regular application, especially because functional connections with other afflicted body systems respond well to treatment with RTF.

Symptomatic zones: The heart, lower cervical spine, and upper thoracic spine are first treated with slowly increasing doses. With too much emphasis on the symptomatic zones, the complaints may get worse rather than better because the afflicted terrain on which they have arisen has not been treated.

> **Important note:** As the meridians of the spleen and heart are closely connected and mutually influence one another (the spleen transfers its energy to the heart) in the energy circulation of the 12 pairs of meridians in acupuncture, it makes sense to treat the zone of the **spleen** before that of the heart. It usually reacts well to tonifying treatment. Likewise, it is also appropriate to tonify the zones of the **small intestine** vigorously **before** the symptomatic zone. Sine in many cardiac patients the intestine and its lymph nodes are overloaded with toxins and waste material, its volume is often enlarged, resulting in an inflexible and elevated diaphragm. As a result, the active movement of fluid throughout the whole torso and the rhythmic up-and-down movement of the diaphragm are unable to take place, which is of great importance for cardiac patients.

Possible background zones: The intestine, upper abdominal organs of the liver, and pancreas. The lymphatic system. The endocrine glands. The diaphragm. The shoulder girdle, left-hand side (segmental connections), the spine. The pelvic floor (lower "diaphragm").

A range of stabilizing and Eutonic grips. Scars, for example, in the course of the heart and/or circulation meridian.

The **metatarsophalangeal joint** should be carefully mobilized here because it is assigned to the zones of the heart, the lower cervical spine, the upper thoracic spine, and thyroid gland. **Orthobionomic** treatment according to A. Pauls is particularly suitable for this.

Cardiac Infarct

1. Call the doctor.
2. Keep calm.
3. **First Aid remedy:** 6 to 8 tablets of sodium bicarbonate, dissolved in a glass of warm water, provide immediate relief as they have a strongly alkaline effect and thus counteract the massive hyperacidity of the patient's heart tissue. Sodium bicarbonate also has the same effect for stroke patients as a First Aid remedy. Sodium bicarbonate tablets should be available in every practice for acute situations.
4. If it is possible to take the patient's feet in one's hands, stabilizing grips, especially the **solar plexus grip**, have a calming effect. The solar plexus zone on the hand also has a similar effect. The heart zone can be sedated. (In the early literature of E. Ingham, she suggests vigorous **tonifying**. Unfortunately, we lack in practical experience in this area. We therefore advise sedation of the heart zone until medical assistance can be provided.)
5. **Bach Flower Remedy No. 39**, known as Rescue Remedy: put a few drops on the tongue or in the center of the palm (= solar plexus hand zone). It is also beneficial for the therapist in such situations.

Functional Circulatory Disturbances

Often no organic cause can be found in these patients. As RTF, by its nature, is well able to treat **functional** complaints, it is particularly suitable for such disturbances.

Important note: In the zones on the foot, disorders are already apparent at the preclinical stage, hence before they manifest clinically. As a result, initial findings reveal an astonishing number of zones with abnormal reactions although the patient cannot confirm what is wrong with them, apart from circulatory lability.

Patient with angina pectoris

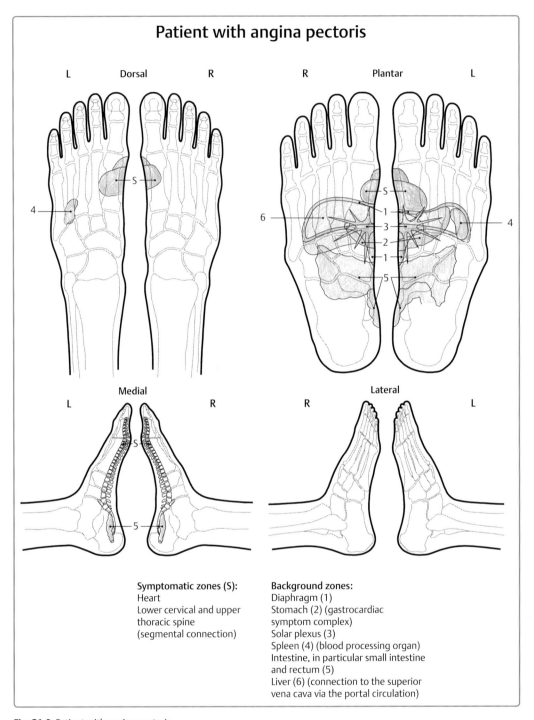

Symptomatic zones (S):
Heart
Lower cervical and upper
thoracic spine
(segmental connection)

Background zones:
Diaphragm (1)
Stomach (2) (gastrocardiac
symptom complex)
Solar plexus (3)
Spleen (4) (blood processing organ)
Intestine, in particular small intestine
and rectum (5)
Liver (6) (connection to the superior
vena cava via the portal circulation)

Fig. 21.9 Patient with angina pectoris.

Symptomatic zones: Autonomic nervous system, which can be satisfactorily stabilized via a range of stabilizing grips. The heart can initially be treated with a sedating grip and later tonified.

Possible background zones: They are usually more important than the symptomatic zones. The spleen. The intestine, especially the small intestine, the upper abdominal organs. The lymphatic system overall. The head. The diaphragm. The endocrine system. The spine. The organs of the lesser pelvis.

Interference fields in the tooth region and in scars. Stabilizing grips. The Eutonic **sacrum grip** (Chapter 6) has a highly harmonizing effect on all the organs as it develops its effect in the center of the abdomen.

If circulatory disturbances manifest as **hyperkinetic heart syndrome** (tachycardia, increased blood pressure amplitude, sudden coldness or perspiration, strong emotional fluctuations), the thyroid gland and seventh cervical vertebra (functional connection) are included in the treatment with sedating grips and all the other zones are treated cautiously initially.

Stabilizing and Eutonic grips/positions are paramount initially.

If **hypotension** associated with venous insufficiency develops as a result of serious illness or infection, a course of RTF lymphatic treatment is usually the method of choice. This both encourages the excretion of toxic loads in the organism and strengthens the heart/circulation and autonomic nervous system.

Dreams of all kinds underlie a functional or organic disease of the heart in more people than might be initially supposed. Unprocessed problems and constant stress in one's personal or professional life lead to complaints of this nature. They are often "forgotten" or not associated with the disease at all. We should be aware of these aspects when providing therapeutic support; whether this leads to a conversation or indications for further therapeutic measures will be seen if we are alert and compassionate in our support of the patient's reactions.

21.7

Zones of the Digestive Organs

21.7.1　General Information

It is widely recognized that the multiple functions of the gastrointestinal tract are severely impaired in most people today. The fundamental factors behind this are processed food and eating habits: food is eaten too quickly, in excess (or sometimes in inadequate amounts), at the wrong time, with too many distractions, and without appreciation.

> In principle, however, it is not **what** we eat that is crucial for our health, but what the organism is able to utilize and process from what is on offer.

It must be borne in mind that **metabolic problems** underlie almost all diseases, even if the connection is not apparent at first glance. That psychological factors also play a major role is revealed by the fact that constant distress has a negative impact on the composition of the intestinal flora because "digestion" is also an emotional process.

It is well known that patients with **impending** or **postoperative ileus** (bowel paralysis or intestinal obstruction) reinstate peristaltic movements after vigorous tonifying of the zone of the intestine. Brief symptomatic treatment can be performed several times a day. It is always worth trying because the treatment does no harm; "in the worst-case scenario" it does not produce the expected result. It would be good if this simple therapeutic measure were used more often in hospitals.

21.7.2　Treatment Suggestions

Chronic Constipation

Symptomatic zones: The whole intestine, cautiously at first, then tonifying more vigorously.

Possible background zones: All the sphincters. The lymphatic system. The upper abdominal organs and abdominal wall. The entire spine, especially the lumbar spine and sacrum. The pelvic ligaments. The endocrine glands. The interference fields (scars, teeth).

Stabilizing and/or Eutonic grips for autonomic reorganization.

Crohn's Disease, Ulcerative Colitis

(Fig. 21.10)

Symptomatic zone: The intestine. It is advisable to either leave out the zone of the intestine entirely during the initial treatment sessions or to treat it very gently until the patient's individual reaction can be properly evaluated. Astonishingly, however, some patients even react well to tonifying treatment.

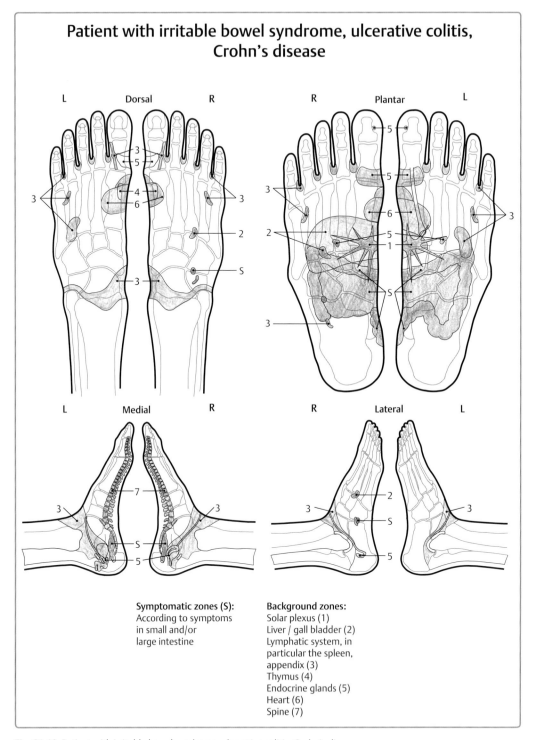

Patient with irritable bowel syndrome, ulcerative colitis, Crohn's disease

Symptomatic zones (S):
According to symptoms in small and/or large intestine

Background zones:
Solar plexus (1)
Liver / gall bladder (2)
Lymphatic system, in particular the spleen, appendix (3)
Thymus (4)
Endocrine glands (5)
Heart (6)
Spine (7)

Fig. 21.10 Patient with irritable bowel syndrome, ulcerative colitis, Crohn's disease.

Possible background zones: The lower spine (segmental connection with the intestine, see below, respiratory diseases: diaphragm). All the sphincters. The upper abdominal organs of the liver, stomach, pancreas. The lymph organs or the entire lymphatic system.

The head, similarity in shape between the brain and the intestine (**Fig. 21.1**). The endocrine system. The heart. The pelvic ligaments. Examination of interference fields in the form of scars or devitalized teeth.

As symptoms are often accompanied by primary or secondary, often psychological, stresses, autonomic balance is particularly important. Perhaps even at the outset, two or three reflexotherapy sessions **solely** for the purpose of stabilization are the method of choice. Eutonic and other stabilizing grips are highly suitable but employing too many at the same time should be avoided.

A precise analysis of **eating habits** is essential and the results must be implemented consistently. As diarrhea is often accompanied by **dehydration**, adequate fluid intake must be ensured, preferably by drinking water or mild herb tea.

Irritable Bowel Syndrome

(Fig. 21.10)
The aforementioned treatment suggestions apply here to a greater or lesser extent. As diarrhea and constipation alternate in this disease, general reactions should be carefully monitored. Experience shows that tonifying the symptomatic zone of the intestine is not always appropriate, even in phases of constipation.

If patients are taking anticoagulants (e.g., **phenprocoumon**), the **liver zone** should be treated with particular care. In Traditional Chinese Medicine (TCM) it is well known that digestive complaints of any kind respond well to **soothing** herbs, and RTF can also make use of this knowledge to provide gentle, soothing treatment of the liver zone.

Gastrocardiac Symptom Complex, Roemheld's Syndrome

It is usually men who suffer from these complaints as a result of distress of all kinds.

Symptomatic zones: The stomach and the cardia and pylorus, work with sedating grips initially. The liver/gall bladder, pancreas.

Possible background zones: All the other sphincters, in order to stabilize the autonomic nervous

system (Chapter 6). The intestine, especially the small intestine. The diaphragm and the large diaphragm muscle (pars lumbalis). The pelvic floor. The heart. The head and the temporomandibular joint and nape of the neck. The spine, especially the middle and lower cervical spine—segmental connection.

The **subsequent rest** period should be consistently adhered to in order to enable the treatment stimuli to abate gradually.

Hemorrhoids

Often this complaint is only regarded as an unwelcome disturbance. However, it should be clarified whether it is to be assessed as a symptom of serious, undetected illness. There is also always underlying severe hyperacidity of the metabolic organs which can be best remedied by a healthy diet and good metabolizing of food.

Symptomatic zones: The anus and pelvic floor. At the acute stage the sedating grip usually works very quickly. Stretching the entire pelvic floor in a ventral and dorsal direction also provides welcome relief.

Possible background zones: The oral cavity and lips are tonified vigorously as the "antithesis." The entire gastrointestinal tract and urinary tract for thorough metabolic reorganization. All the other sphincters (Chapter 6). The lymphatic system. The pelvic ligaments.

Stabilizing grips are particularly important because a harmonized emotional state normalizes the tone of all the sphincters. It is well known that **cheerful laughter** has a rhythmic effect on the large **and** small diaphragm, the pelvic floor—and as the beginning and the end are always coordinated, it is understandable that the lower sphincter reacts to the release of tension in the upper sphincter.

Rectal Prolapse

Symptomatic zones: The rectum, anus, and pelvic floor are first tonified gently, later more vigorously.

Possible background zones: The organs and muscles of the lesser pelvis. Initially treat the pelvic ligaments with sedating grips, then tonifying grips. The digestive tract. All the other sphincters.

The spine, in particular the sacrum–coccyx. The diaphragm, the floor of the buccal cavity. The lymphatic and endocrine system. Stabilizing grips which stimulate and deepen the breath (e.g., heel stretch grip).

21.8

Zones of the Lymphatic System

21.8.1 General Information

The functional interaction of the lymphatic, immune, digestive, autonomic nervous and endocrine systems can be observed in many diseases on the basis of abnormalities of the corresponding zones. The **lymphatic tonsillar ring** and the tonsils and the high density of **Peyer's Plaque** in the small intestine, together with the **appendix**, point to significant lymphatic foci inside the organism.

In our practical work we encounter direct and visible lymphatic abnormalities most often in inflammatory and congestive processes in the region of the nasopharyngeal cavity and the extremities, especially the arms and legs.

Generally, it appears that the lymphatic system plays an important role in stabilizing the patient's **emotional** state.

From My Practice

At the beginning of the developmental phase of the lymphatic zones approximately 30 years ago, a mother brought her two sons of 5 and 6 years old for treatment for chronic recurrent colds. In the fourth RTF session she said, "I scarcely dare say it, but since the last reflexotherapy session the boys have been playing with each other while before they only quarreled and were out of sorts all day. Now they are well-rested in the morning and ready for anything."

After 10 sessions of RTF, the enlarged adenoids of one of the boys had shrunk so much that he was able to breathe freely through his nose again, while the other's fever and inflamed throat had improved significantly, enabling him to attend kindergarten again regularly. Both of them stopped having malodorous diarrhea. However, what struck me most, because it was quite unexpected, was the lasting harmonization at an emotional level.

(Note that to avoid relapses, the children had to avoid eating too many sweets and certain types of cereal in the following months.)

At this time we also became aware of the importance of the **spleen**, to which we had not paid much attention before. The word "spleen" itself is linked to the emotions. The spleen requires attentive treatment far more often than was previously assumed. Although in medicine it has long been known that, as a blood reservoir and transformation organ, the

spleen plays a significant role in the breakdown of ageing erythrocytes and thrombocytes, it is also linked to other processes:

In TCM it is well known that the spleen tends to be weakened rather than overstrained during illness. Therefore food and herbs which **stimulate** the activity of the spleen are administered. In RTF we made a similar discovery: as a rule, patients respond well to gently tonifying of the spleen zone. However, we have observed that this area is not always painful initially and only "wakes up" after a few reflexotherapy sessions.

There are now significantly **more indications** for which the spleen is included in the treatment program:

- Blood count anomalies, **inflammations**, and **infections**. (Lymphocytes, which are responsible for dealing with infections, originate in the spleen.)
- **Allergies** of all kinds, including at the preclinical stage, for example, with hay fever, where the spleen is also treated at the symptom-free stage.
- **Heart disease**. Meridian theory starts from the principle that the energy in the spleen-meridian is transferred to the heart-meridian in a 24-hour cycle.
- All autonomic and emotional afflictions and irritations. In anthroposophical medicine, the coordination of all the **rhythmical processes** within a person are attributed to the spleen.

The **thymus**, which must likewise be included in the lymphatic system, was already discussed in detail in Chapter 21.5.3.

21.8.2 Treatment Suggestions

Acute and Chronic Inflammations in the Head and Neck Region

If the mucous membrane of the nasopharyngeal cavity and the head cavity is unable to excrete the accumulated secretions, the symptomatic zones are tonified according to the patient's respective reaction. In the case of the lateral lymph chains and tonsils, however, the alternating stroking movements specified in RTF lymphatic treatment should be employed in order to improve the flow of the lymphatic system.

As with other indications, here too the background zones are often more important in avoiding strengthening the overstrained and afflicted basic terrain of the symptoms. To foster successful reorganization, six to eight exclusive lymphatic treatments can be provided.

Symptomatic zones: The nasopharyngeal cavity and the sinus cavities and eustachian tubes, the tonsils, and lateral lymph chains on the neck. Interdigital skin folds between the toes (= lymphatics of the head and neck).

Stretching the interdigital skin folds of the fingers can also be recommended to patients as therapy homework: performed for a few minutes in the morning and evening, the piercing sensation in the tissue usually decreases after only a few self-treatments.

Possible background zones: The intestine, especially the small intestine. The appendix, the thymus. The organs of the lesser pelvis and the lymphatics of the inguinal area and the pelvis. The spleen. The suprarenals.

Stabilizing and/or Eutonic grips.

> **Important note:** A review of eating habits and changes to these where necessary is urgently recommended. Often lactose or fructose intolerances and/or allergic reactions to cereals (in particular, wheat) are a causative factor in the development of mucous membrane disorders.

Lymphatic Congestion in the Legs

There are many **reasons** for this: hereditary weakness of the connective tissue, severe metabolic disorders, especially of the intestine as a result of poor nutrition, inadequate fluid intake, lack of exercise, hormonal dysfunctions, etc.

Symptomatic zones: The lymphatic region of the inguinal area, the pelvis, and the thigh. Here alternating stroking movements have proved particularly effective, as described in Chapter 29.

Possible background zones: The entire intestine. The organs of the lesser pelvis. The upper abdomen, particularly the liver. The urinary tract. The heart, spleen. The appendix, thymus. The endocrine glands. The upper lymphatics.

Stabilizing and/or Eutonic grips. Examination of possible **interference fields** in the form of scars or devitalized teeth and their specialist treatment.

Mastectomy

(Fig. 21.11)

In women with breast cancer, whether or not they have undergone surgery, concomitant support with RTF has proved its worth for years.

> In our experience, it does not encourage metastasis but rather strengthens a woman's self-healing powers. A rule of all regulatory therapies and therefore of RTF too: with the right dose and acceptance of the contraindications, treatments of this kind cannot disrupt healthy processes but they can support weakened and diseased organs and systems within the framework of existing regenerative possibilities.

Symptomatic zones: Priority should be given to zones and grips which stabilize the patient's autonomic nervous system: the endocrine system, sphincter treatment, and a choice of stabilizing and/or Eutonic grips. Above all, this is so that women also regain their inner balance.

The zone of the operation scar is first touched gently, or gentle stroking movements are performed from the sternum in the direction of the axilla. After the wound has healed, **RTF scar treatment** can be offered (Chapter 25). A series of RTF lymphatic treatments has a preventive or dissipative effect—especially after partial or complete removal of the axillary lymph nodes—on all **lymph congestion in the arm**.

Possible background zones: The other side of the thoracic tissue. Cervical spine and shoulder girdle including sternoclavicular and sternocostal joints, initially sedating. The endocrine system and organs of the lesser pelvis (the female breast has clear connections with the endocrine system). All the other excretory and lymphatic organs.

Important note: During **radiotherapy** or **chemotherapy** no selective stimuli are applied. However, gentle, neutral grips which support the autonomic nervous system and the activity of the intestine, kidneys, and heart are also helpful in these phases.

Scar creams promote the healing process physically and emotionally. As women are not only affected physically, but above all, are "thrown off course" in the intimate and esthetic spheres after operations of this kind, the following short **pain management and acute treatment** has proved effective:

While the **zone** of the amputated breast is gently treated with the scar cream, the woman places her hand (over or under her clothing) on the scar, thus having the opportunity to process the effects of her shock more easily and without words. If her partner can be included in the care of the scar, this is particularly valuable for both parties. The Eutonic **shoulder–arm grip** has an exceptionally harmonizing effect and provides exceptional relief from musculoskeletal tensions in the back and entire thorax.

More information about lymphatic diseases can be found in Chapter 29 "Zones of the Lymphatic System" and in Chapter 23 "Treatment of Babies and Children."

Patient after left-sided mastectomy

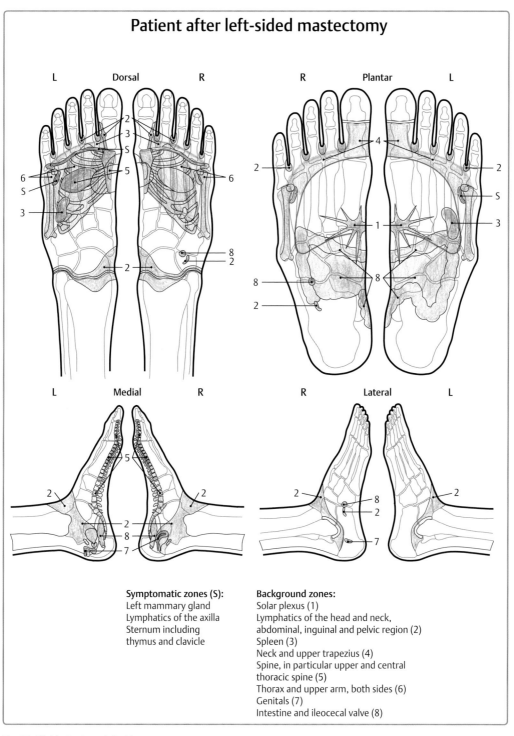

Symptomatic zones (S):
Left mammary gland
Lymphatics of the axilla
Sternum including
thymus and clavicle

Background zones:
Solar plexus (1)
Lymphatics of the head and neck,
abdominal, inguinal and pelvic region (2)
Spleen (3)
Neck and upper trapezius (4)
Spine, in particular upper and central
thoracic spine (5)
Thorax and upper arm, both sides (6)
Genitals (7)
Intestine and ileocecal valve (8)

Fig. 21.11 Mastectomy left side.

22 Pregnancy and Birth

22.1

General Information

Midwives and specialists from associated professions are able to integrate a great deal of practical and background information from reflexotherapy of the feet (RTF) into their work. This includes the care given to the pregnant woman from the time after conception to the care of the mother and baby in the postpartum period. Although pregnancy is a normal biological process, an increasing number of women suffer from a multitude of complaints during this special time.

Basically, we adhere to the rule that RTF support in pregnancy, during and after the birth, is experienced as extremely pleasant and **stabilizing** by the pregnant woman, even if she does not have any immediate complaints. At the beginning we advise regular care via the feet (roughly once a week) from the fourth month of pregnancy onward.

Frequently though, we observe that natural life processes nowadays are complicated by all kinds of irritations and increasing difficulties, and it is obvious that pregnant women often need help. It should be noted that for the most part the dosage of individual therapeutic grips for pregnant women is only **half the usual dosage**, at least at the beginning, until the personal threshold for the grips offered has been experienced.

Usually we make a **first assessment** as part of the normal care, in particular when the pregnant woman contacts the midwife at an **early** stage in the pregnancy. Then RFT can be a treasured accompanying measure throughout the following months. However, if there is little remaining time until the birth, situations involving **brief and acute treatment** often occur.

Under normal circumstances, mother and child collaborate in very finely coordinated symbiosis during delivery which should be carefully observed with all our professional skills but which should not be disturbed by hasty intervention.

22.2

Treatment during Pregnancy

22.2.1 Basic Treatment

In order to make the pregnancy easier for women, above all, between the sixth and seventh month of pregnancy, when the increasing weight of the baby results in a change in the woman's musculoskeletal system, the following "**basic formula**" has proved its worth:

- **Stabilizing grips** before, during, and after treatment, well adapted to the present condition of the woman.
- Gentle tonifying in the zones of the lower spine, gluteal, and abdominal muscles, intestine, kidneys and bladder, lymphatic system (alternating stroking movements), and diaphragm.
- The **zone of the uterus** can—but need not—be omitted during the first few treatments until the woman's general response has been reliably assessed.
  The spontaneous **reaction of the baby**, for example, in the form of greatly increased intrauterine movements, and the behavior of the mother-to-be provide a useful indication as to whether the dosage was correctly gauged. In the event of overdose, employ stabilizing grips.
- As a result of this treatment the bony and muscular area of the pelvis is gradually and evenly expanded and stretched and the baby obtains the natural space which it needs for development and movement.

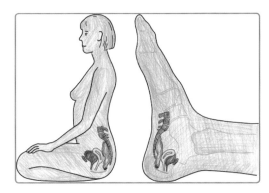

Fig. 22.1 Female pelvic organs in situ and as zones.

- The **diaphragm** can move freely up and down, thereby relieving the heart, circulation, and respiration.
- This basic "formula" for the proposed zones can either be incorporated into a normal course of treatment or offered as a short, self-contained treatment.
- The **subsequent phase of rest**, of at least 20 minutes' duration, is of special importance for pregnant women and should be consistently adhered to or even extended, according to individual requirements.

Additional Practical Advice

Highly irritated and overanxious women often have tiny drops of water spread over large areas of the inside of both heel bones (the zones of the pelvic organs) before beginning treatment.

- This indicates that they are unstable and initially need ample stabilizing grips. Specific treatment of the zones is only gradually built up in the course of a series of treatments according to the increasing stability of the autonomous nervous system.
- Every treatment session is interspersed with regularly repeated sedating grips, including in the zone of the solar plexus. Gentle, vibrant tonifying in the sense of **regulation** in this zone has a similar effect, in our experience.
- With these oversensitive women it has proved effective to initially treat them with their **feet covered** so that they do not feel directly "attacked."

22.2.2 Common Complaints

RTF treatment during pregnancy is usually greatly appreciated by most women as they experience its benefits in terms of improvement in their physical complaints and frame of mind.

The zones specified below can be supplemented or reduced, depending on the women's individual histories of complaints.

Important note: In most of the indications mentioned below, the lower medial and lateral edge of the calcaneus and lateral malleolus should be treated with the sedating grip as they include the zones of the **pelvic tendons and ligaments**. The **specific** treatment of these zones provides great relief and more space (Chapter 28).

Gentle, **alternating stroking movements**, especially in the zones of the thighs, are appreciated by all women as a very effective means of deconges-

tion, not only for the legs, but also for the entire abdomen and pelvis.

Vomiting and Nausea during Pregnancy (Hyperemesis gravidarum)

Stabilizing grips are the first choice.

Sedating grips in the zones of the stomach, including the cardia (often the most important) and pylorus, ileocecal valve, solar plexus, central thoracic spine, diaphragm and liver. After improvement of the symptoms these zones may be gently tonified.

Tonifying the zones of the small intestine and rectum/anus, including the pelvic floor and spleen, usually brings about spontaneous relief.

This short treatment may be performed several times a day, by a partner or another carer if appropriate, in particular in the zones of the stomach and solar plexus.

Backache

The more advanced the pregnancy, the more frequently many women complain of **backache**. With **acute** pain, we apply the rules of treatment in acute situations, as specified for patients with lumbar pain (Chapter 16 and Chapter 21.3.2, section on "Lumbar Syndrome").

Pregnant women with backache can decide for themselves **in which position** they are able to lie on the treatment table, for example, on one side or even almost seated. If they are starting to suffer from **inferior vena cava syndrome** (lying flat on their back, the baby causes compression of the inferior vena cava, possibly impairing the mother's circulation distinctly), we position them on their **left** side. In this position we can usually apply stabilizing grips quite easily and continue to work.

The zones of the **lateral abdominal muscles** (antagonists of the lumbar spine) are of special importance because as the girth expands

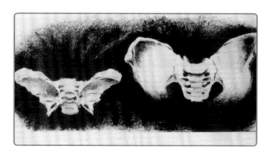

Fig. 22.2 Similarity in shape between the cuneiform bone (base of the skull) and the sacrum with the iliac bone.

increased excess tensions can arise. Sedating grips for the zones of the lower spine and sacroiliac joint are appropriate. Later, they can be gently tonified.

Pregnant women should check their sitting, standing, and walking posture and adapt these in accordance with the increasing ventral shift in weight as a result of the growing baby.

Due to the relocation of the organs and the enlargement of the uterus, **diaphragmatic elevation** often occurs. As the caudal dorsal part of the diaphragm, the **pars lumbalis**, is attached to the upper lumbar spine, these points are first treated with the sedating grip while those of the gluteal muscles and intestine are gently tonified.

A little local massage of the **occiput** and **nape of the neck** has a very relaxing effect on the pelvic organs. In craniosacral osteopathy therapeutic connections between the top and bottom are also known (**Fig. 22.2**).

Venous and Lymphatic Congestion of the Pelvis and Legs

As this situation is not acute, a normal **initial assessment** is indicated. This often results in a selection of zones requiring treatment:

The lower spine and abdominal muscles should be sedated first (frequent excess tensions). Tonify the liver, kidneys, spleen, and digestive tract with the appropriate dose. However, three or four exclusive RTF lymphatic treatments are usually the method of choice.

Often women already observe **increased diuresis** and subjective relief in the legs and pelvis after the first treatment.

Premature Labor

Here **stabilizing grips** are particularly appropriate for dispelling the woman's fear. In addition, **sedating grips** in the zones of the pituitary gland, uterus, ovaries, solar plexus, thyroid gland, suprarenals, lower spine, sacroiliac joint, pubic symphysis, and pelvic ligaments, or a selection of these zones.

The treatment can be performed daily or even several times a day for about 10 to 15 minutes until premature labor has stopped.

Cystitis

As long as there is no febrile condition indicating an ascending infection in the urinary tract we can use RTF and expect positive results:

We apply soft, gentle stroking movements in the zones of the lymphatics of the neck and alternating stroking movements in the zones of the

thighs and pelvis in order to include the lymphatic system ahead of the urinary tract.

Tonify the zones of the nasopharynx (representing a correlated mucous membrane area), and the spleen (to stabilize the irritation of the autonomic nervous system and increase the function of the lymphatic system).

Apply the **sedating grip** in the zones of the bladder and the lower sacrum (segmental connection with the bladder) and the sacroiliac joint. Optionally, the bladder zone can also be treated first.

In general: apply frequent **stabilizing grips**.

22.3

Complaints before, during, and after the Birth

Uterine Inertia, Insufficient Dilation of the Cervix

Tonifying of the zones of the uterus in the direction of the vagina, pubic symphysis, pituitary gland, suprarenals, thyroid gland, lower spine, and sacroiliac joint.

Cervix: **Sedating grip**, later tonifying.

Excessive Contractions

The same zones specified for uterine inertia are treated with the **sedating grip** in excessive contractions.

Stabilizing grips are most effective **at the start** of the interval between contractions. The sedating grip is more appropriate **at the end** of the interval between contractions, when the next phase of pain is starting.

Incomplete Separation of the Placenta

Tonify vigorously in the zones of the uterus, ovaries, pituitary gland, sacrum, sacroiliac joint, bladder, and pelvic floor, always adjusted to the woman's current reaction.

Usually, the remaining placenta is **expelled in full** after a few minutes, accompanied by a few weaker contractions. However, treatment should be continued until (usually 6 to 10 days) the uterine secretion (lochia) has normalized in color, odor, and consistency but there is no need to tonify as vigorously as before and other zones may also be included.

Stabilizing grips should be performed as often as necessary.

Excessive Afterpains

In **multipara** (women who have delivered several babies), the afterpains accompanying the involution of the organs are often as painful as the labor pains. Treating the feet for 10 to 15 minutes can result in these afterpains becoming far less aggressive, without impairing the physiologically significant contraction of the uterus.

The sedating grip is used in the zones of the uterus, ovaries, pituitary gland, sometimes also the lower spine, sacroiliac joint, and pubic symphysis. Interspersed stabilizing grips are important. This brief treatment can be performed several times a day.

Bladder Spasm after Delivery

Before, during, and after treatment, stabilizing grips are performed.

The **sedating grip** is applied to the zones of the bladder, sacrum, anus, pelvic floor, sacroiliac joint, and solar plexus.

Alternating stroking movements applied in the lymphatic tissue of the groin, pelvis, and thighs.

Tonifying the zones of the **nasopharynx** is important as they are correlated with the urogenital area. The practical experience of many midwives confirms the especially noticeable **interaction** between the mucous membranes of the head/throat and pelvis.

With this treatment, women can very often be **spared catheterization.**

Bladder Incontinence

First **sedate** and later **tonify** all the zones of the pelvis: bladder and bladder sphincter, pelvic floor, uterus, lower spine, anus, sacroiliac joint, pubic symphysis, gluteal and lateral abdominal muscles.

Stimulating (= tonifying) treatment is provided in the sense of the Arndt–Schulz rule: Weak impulses stimulate, strong ones retard, very strong ones paralyze.

Intersperse with **stabilizing grips** as often as appears necessary. **Active exercises** to stimulate the muscles of the pelvic floor should be recommended in addition.

Poor Lactation

- If the **flow of milk** is **inadequate**:
  We work with ample **stabilizing grips**, as all systems dealing with fluids can function more adequately if the autonomous nervous system is stable. The zones of the pituitary gland, neck, upper and central thoracic spine,

intestine as well as all other endocrine glands are gently **tonified.**

In the zone of the mammary gland we always work gently **in the direction of the axilla**, possibly also with "the velvet paw" grip (delicate treatment from medial to lateral with two opposing fingertips).

Here too, **RTF lymphatic treatment** (in parts or as a whole) has proved its worth. It can be offered daily.

- For abundant **lactogenesis, mastitis**:
  We first gently perform the **sedating grip** in the zone of the mamma, pituitary gland, and sternum.

  Gentle **tonifying** in the zones of the spleen and the intestine (cleansing of the intestinal environment that influences the quality of the mother's milk).

  As the flow of **normal lochia** may be disturbed at the same time in women with lactation difficulties, gently tonifying in the zones of the genital area often produces good results, both in terms of normalization of the lochia as well as lactation.

  After the acute phase it has proven effective to perform parts of the RTF **lymphatic treatment** in which the lymphatic collective grips and their interconnections are particularly important (Chapter 29).

  Traditional natural remedies such as **cabbage leaf** or **curdled milk compresses** on the breast provide additional relief fromsymptoms.

Aids to Involution of the Organs in the Post-Partum Period

The zones of the uterus, pituitary gland, bladder, intestine, sacroiliac joint, lower spine, and abdominal wall are **tonified** as firmly as the woman's condition allows. Perform frequent **stabilizing grips**.

Active exercises for the abdominal and pelvic muscles, especially those of the pelvic floor, should be recommended.

Painful Perineal Suture (Episiotomy)

Initially we perform the **sedating grip** in the zones of the pelvic floor and anus, on the right or left foot or on both sides, according to the site of the suture. Later the symptomatic zone can also be gently **tonified**, likewise the zones of the uterus and other zones of the pelvis. We perform **alternating stroking movements** in the lymphatic area of the pelvis and thighs.

In addition to the pelvic floor, the **diaphragm** and **floor of the buccal cavity** (likewise diaphragms) are also **tonified**.

22.4

Treatment of the Newborn

Every mother almost instinctively touches and holds the feet of her baby when it is with her.

Any existing or emerging disturbances in the neonate respond particularly well to RTF treatment immediately after the birth because RTF gently stimulates the baby's powers of self-regulation and supports weakened organs and systems in a natural manner.

Neonatal Jaundice

Newborn babies with jaundice, identified by strong yellowing of the skin or a blood test, should be treated once or even twice a day.

Brief gentle **tonifying** of the zones of the small intestine, spleen, pancreas, and heart usually suffices. The zone of the liver requires gentle treatment, initially even with a soft **sedating grip**, to strengthen and stabilize it.

Holding the little feet quietly for a few moments during and after the treatment appears to be a good **balance** to the tonifying stimuli. In particular, it should be ensured that there is a good supply of blood to the feet and that they **are always warm**.

"Sluggish/Feeble Babies"

A variety of aggravating circumstances make it difficult for some newborn babies to make the transition from the sheltered intrauterine element of water to the element of air without marked difficulties in adapting.

Multiple experiences confirm that brief RTF treatment can usually bring about an increase in vitality in the form of improved respiration, pulse rate, active movements, and normalization of skin color within the space of a few minutes.

We gently **tonify** the zones of the diaphragm and solar plexus and may include the zones of the lungs, heart, digestive system, and—with great care—head. The aim of these few minutes of constant treatment

is to **improve the blood supply** not only of both feet, but that of the whole baby. It is most satisfying to watch how quickly the baby takes possession of its previously weakened body.

This short treatment can be offered several times within the first few hours and days of the baby's life. It is of special importance that the child develops and maintains **warm feet** in the treatment intervals. Apart from the physical warmth, the natural warmth of the human hand also conveys the experience of being sheltered and safe.

Impaired Respiration

The respiratory tract of a newborn baby is usually aspirated with a tube immediately after delivery to prevent amniotic fluid reaching the lungs or remaining there. This unexpected and **drastic intervention** for the baby involving irritation of the upper airways can be compensated by treatment of the feet:

We perform tender **stroking** of the plantar and dorsal zones of the trachea and bronchi from distal to proximal and brief, gentle tonifying of the zones of the lungs, intestine, and diaphragm. If the expectoration of mucus is to be encouraged, stroking from proximal to distal, that is to say, in the opposite direction, is worth a try.

Apply **sedating grip** in the zone of the solar plexus. Furthermore, gently holding the baby's feet with warm hands regulates the baby's general tonus.

Practical Advice

The positive effects of RTF on newborn babies with the following complaints have been repeatedly endorsed by mothers, midwives, and therapists.

They noticed, for example, that many newborn babies and infants were startled and held their breath when touched around the **first metatarsophalangeal joint** (these are the zones of the throat and upper airways affected by the tube). Calm, gentle touching of these zones was often sufficient for the symptoms to visibly diminish. This treatment was equally successful in the case of newborn babies whose **umbilical cord** had been wrapped around their neck.

Similar reactions were ascertained in babies delivered with **forceps** or **ventouse** who likewise responded to delicate touch and very gentle treatment of the lateral or distal parts of the big toes (zones of the side of the head and cranium) with **less panic** and more balanced **respiration**.

Birth traumas of the kind mentioned or similar incisive experiences accompany some people into adulthood undetected. They can appear as a reaction to RTF at any age, rising from the subconscious to the tangible level of emotions and awareness, where they are able to be processed.

As a supplementary treatment to RTF, it has proven effective for newborn babies, in a traumatic birth, to apply the **Bach Flower Remedy No. 39** (Rescue Remedy) as an ointment or drops to the center of the palm or to the zone of the solar plexus. At the beginning, this can be repeated several times a day. Often it makes sense to give the mother this treatment simultaneously, or to also treat her with Classical Homeopathy.

In the 1990s the highly differentiated manual methods of **craniosacral osteopathy** also became more well-known in Europe. The constriction of the birth canal or the use of forceps or ventouse can displace the bones of the skull in many newborn babies (even fractions of a millimeter can lead to developmental disorders—even in later years). In these situations, craniosacral osteopathy can also be employed in the first weeks of life with very good results in terms of the child's later development.

22.4.1

Summary

Like the baby, the mother has also made remarkable efforts during birth. For midwives who have attended our courses it is perfectly natural to sit at the **mother's feet** for a few minutes after the birth or, if possible, to show the partner how to offer support and comfort just through touch or a simple stabilizing grip.

Apart from the therapeutic possibilities, every mother and father should be aware of the value of **natural touch** on babies' feet. Some babies have already had to process extreme trauma during pregnancy and birth and have lost "the solid ground under their feet" internally even before they experience it as a reality. Working with newborn babies and their health problems is one of the **most moving** and **satisfying** experiences in our profession.

The treatment of pregnant women, new mothers, and newborn babies should be performed with great **serenity, assurance**, and **sensitivity** as this time is special and unique for all concerned.

Practical Part

23 Treatment of Babies and Children

General Information

The pain triggered by the therapeutic grip in an afflicted zone is a distinct feature of RTF. This might give rise to the fear that RTF treatment is unsuitable for babies and young children but experience confirms the opposite.

In my experience, children have a more natural relationship to pain than adults and their sometimes over-anxious parents might have us believe. Probably they still have an innate knowledge of the positive significance and purpose of pain of this kind.

Babies and children have particularly rapid **powers of regeneration**, as their inner self-healing capacities are not yet, as often in later years, blocked and weakened by too many pharmaceutical medications.

In the treatment of babies and children the **interpersonal relationship** plays a particularly important role. Good personal contact is therefore crucial for the efficacy of the treatment. If the child likes the therapist, they will happily return for each treatment session even if they know that it may sometimes involve a certain amount of pain.

There is often a perception that such small zones cannot be palpated precisely. Practical experience will spontaneously convince the therapist otherwise, even one with large hands.

When treating children's feet we are often touchingly rewarded with affection, trust, and cheerfulness. This should convince us that it is worthwhile adopting a natural and impartial attitude to treatment of the feet early on, so that the **naturalness of touching the feet** can also be retained in adulthood.

It is not possible to perform an extensive initial assessment of babies and small children as they usually want to move about after a time. Depending on their age, they sometimes prefer to sit up and "help" with the treatment or to lie on their stomach, and should be granted this freedom.

Babies feel happiest when they are held and supported by their mother or another known caregiver. With **older children**, however, it is usually better if their relatives wait in the adjoining room because then the atmosphere becomes more neutral and the children are not distracted.

As the treatment of babies and small children usually only takes a few minutes to a quarter of an hour, it can be performed daily or, in acute situations, even several times daily.

The Correct Dosage

When treating children, the painful phases should be frequently alternated with playful and harmonizing ones. **Stabilizing grips** can be included more than usual.

As soon as children can express themselves verbally, at around 2 or 3 years, we should listen to their remarks with regard to the correct dosage.

With **babies,** above all, the symptoms of the **autonomic nervous system** (moist hands, restlessness, and discomfort) indicate the limits of grip intensity. Even if a baby starts crying, it can easily be calmed down again with a brief stabilizing grip and is rarely resentful.

Proven Indications

The following childhood illnesses can be successfully treated with RTF, in part exclusively and in part as an accompanying measure.

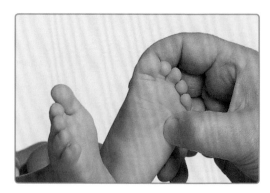

Fig. 23.1 A baby's feet in good hands.

Pyloric Spasm, "Three-month" or Umbilical Colic

These babies are usually tense and irritated. They respond very well to treatment when their little feet are first held with warm hands and gently mobilized. **Stabilizing grips** should be applied frequently.

Sedating grip in the zones of solar plexus, stomach including cardia and pylorus, liver, lower thoracic spine, and ileocecal valve. The anus, the important sphincter muscle at the end of the digestive tract, is also treated with the sedating grip initially.

Gentle tonifying of the diaphragm, spleen, and small intestine.

Constipation, Meteorism

Gentle **tonifying** of the stomach, intestine, and pancreas. **Sedating grip** in the solar plexus. As the anal sphincter is often very tense, the sedating grip is suitable in this zone initially. The zones of the cardia and pylorus should also be examined and, if necessary, likewise sedated.

All **sphincter muscles** have a direct relationship with the **autonomic nervous system**; regulating the tonus of these muscles has a harmonizing effect on the entire nervous system (Chapter 6).

The **oral cavity,** as the start of the digestive tract, should also be tonified, likewise the **teeth** on the individual toes. With babies' and children's feet, rubbing and stroking the toes on all sides suffices.

Teething Problems

These are usually accompanied by acute digestive disorders, pain, occasional fever, and disturbed sleep, which affects not only the baby but the whole family.

Due to the small size of babies' toes, it is not very easy to differentiate the zones of the teeth from each other and therefore **all the toes** are tonified gently or more vigorously, as described above. After a short time, a uniform slight reddening of the toes can be observed, indicating that the circulation has improved.

The **interdigital skin folds** are stretched to relieve congestion in the lymphatic system of the head and neck.

Initial application of the **sedating grip** in the gastrointestinal tract as far as the rectum and anus, also in the solar plexus. When there is an improvement, gentle tonifying can also be employed later on.

It is not uncommon for the pronounced **reddening of one of the child's cheeks** (in homeopathy this is known as "chamomile cheek," indicating the appropriate remedy) to assume the same, normal coloration as the other cheek within 5 to 8 minutes of treatment, and for the child to fall into a deep sleep for several hours and awake without pain.

This short treatment can be performed several times a day in the acute phase and mothers or other caregivers can be shown how to apply these grips.

Children with Lymphatic Problems

See also Chapter 21.8 "Zones of the Lymphatic System" and Chapter 31 "Taken from Practice—For Use in Practice."

In children with lymphatic disorders in the nasopharyngeal cavity, the lymphatic system generally regenerates particularly well.

With **chronic** disorders, the symptomatic zones of the head and neck are gently **tonified** in keeping with the child's resilience. In the **acute** stage the **sedating grip** is used in the nasopharyngeal cavity.

In both the acute and chronic stage, the lymphatics of the neck are gently treated.

One of the **most important background zones** is the gastrointestinal tract, often also other lymphatic zones such as appendix, thymus, and spleen, likewise solar plexus and the organs of the lesser pelvis. They can all be tonified together. The liver is treated gently and smoothly.

Improvement in the lymphatic system of children can be recognized by
- normalization of the digestion and the reduction of flatulence,
- decreased swelling of the tonsils and lymphatics of the neck,
- regression of polyps and unobstructed nasal breathing, especially during sleep,
- bright appearance of the eyes and the reduction in conjunctivitis,
- reduced inflammation of the middle and outer ear, associated with the normalization of neck tissue and improved hearing.

Remarkably often, these children's **mood** improves because the lymphatic system, the autonomic nervous system, and the endocrine system form a triad the harmonization which also affects the emotions.

Sometimes the improvement manifests as a **temporary reactivation** of complaints (intensified excretion of mucus via the nose, puffy tissue around the eyes, and greater querulousness) and should **not be interpreted as "deterioration."**

> It should be borne in mind that **any** inflammation, apart from subjective complaints, also represents a response of self-preservation by the organism. It is not a matter of fighting the symptoms, but rather of supporting the overall forces of self-healing.

Hyperactive Children

Hyperactive children, including children with poor concentration or similar difficulties (e.g., ADD = Attention Deficit Disorder) respond well to RTF as a rule. Here are some practical tips:

- **Lymphatic zones** (above all, the spleen, appendix, and tonsils) and digestive tract are usually paramount.
- Some children particularly appreciate calm, gentle **stretching of the toes**. The harmonizing effect can be observed in more even, deeper breathing.
- Often, more intensive treatment of the zones of the head only lends itself later in the course of treatment. In addition to the head, including the **pelvis** and the **endocrine glands** has proved worthwhile.
- Of the **stabilizing grips**, the heel stretch and palm-sole grip are particularly appreciated by most children. Gentle holding of the solar plexus at the beginning and end of the treatment has also proved effective.
- Treatment should not last longer than about **10 to 15 minutes** initially. The duration of treatment is gradually increased (two to three times a week, later once a week) in keeping with the child's condition.
- At the beginning of a course of treatment it is sometimes wiser **not** to insist on subsequent rest but this should always be offered.
- If the child associates the treatment with a **pleasant** experience (it only hurts a little; someone is taking care of me), they will be more inclined to come willingly than if they feel they "have" to.
- The child need not always lie still either—they can **sit up** now and again and if appropriate, even "help."
- Sometimes a few treatment sessions for the stressed mother **before** the course of

treatment for the child provide relief for both sides.
- In hyperactive children, the existence of **food intolerances** (e.g., including to phosphates) must be investigated as a matter of urgency.
- The **evening ritual** of a warm footbath, after which the child's feet are rubbed with a pleasant-smelling natural ointment, helps them to feel that even when they are asleep at night time, they have the "ground under their feet."
- It is well known that **overstimulation** (television or computer games which affect the child for too long) increases irritation and should be kept under control as far as possible.
- It is sometimes overlooked that fidgety children may be **highly gifted** children who are not receiving enough individual support.

Croup

If possible, children who suffer from this constriction of the respiratory tract and larynx, usually caused by allergies, should be treated at a stage when they are **free** from attacks.

- Use frequent **stabilizing grips**. Correctly dosed tonifying of the zone of the suprarenals, digestive tract, and possibly the lesser pelvis to improve the central mucous membrane environment of the metabolic organs.
- The **sphincters**, the cardia, pylorus and above all, anus are sedated, the liver is treated gently.
- Additional **tonifying** of the thymus, spleen, and diaphragm as far as the lumbar part of the spine, likewise the nasopharyngeal cavity, tracheae and bronchi. At the **acute** stage the sedating grip is employed.
- Gentle treatment in the region of the lymphatics on the neck and gentle stretching of the interdigital skin folds to **stimulate the flow of lymph** from the head and neck contribute to relief of the symptoms.
- It can be of great comfort to parents of children with croup if they are shown how to treat the essential zones. This enables them to give their child First Aid **treatment themselves** in the event of an attack during the night to bridge the time until therapeutic or medical help is available.
- Wherever possible, parents or caregivers should hold the child's feet in their hands every evening because loving touch has a calming and harmonizing effect.

- **Important note:** In children with a strong **aversion to touch**, the caregiver, usually the mother, can initially touch the child's feet while they are asleep, perhaps even through a blanket. When awake, stockings or socks provide initial protection in order to be able to better tolerate the personal proximity of touch. Such children also allow their feet to be touched more readily in the water when being **bathed**.

Any child who shows a certain aversion to or fear of touch in general, and especially on the feet, has suffered experiences which have deeply injured their sense of basic trust (e.g., birth traumas, blood samples from the heels directly after birth, operations, isolation from the mother, shock during pregnancy).

From My Practice
When beginning my work on the feet, more by accident than intention, I made some interesting observations.
Even relatively healthy and symptom-free children had painful zones on their feet in places that I had not expected at all. A comparison with the findings on the feet of the mother or father provided an explanation: the parents' painful zones and those of their children displayed an astonishing correlation, except that the children's abnormal zones returned to normal within three or four treatment sessions while those of their parents often required a longer period of treatment to become symptom-free.

The obvious conclusion is that children's feet show a **latent constitutional tendency** which is manifested in the parents in tangible symptoms and diseases as the result of a corresponding disposition.
By constitution we mean the sum of all physical, emotional, and mental qualities which we have inherited; the term disposition means the susceptibility and sensitivity to diseases resulting from internal and externally acquired factors.
Constitution and **disposition** form the actual basis of the patient's present disease.

23.4

Summary

The treatment of babies and children can be supplemented very effectively by appropriate **accompanying measures**, for example, a change in eating habits and homeopathy. It should **not be restricted to times of illness**. The treatment of the feet is also highly appropriate in times of health as a useful means of support at the start of life because it can help to ensure that the person has a firm foundation on which to start their journey through life.

Part III
Special Topics and Further Developments

24 Special Groups of Patients

24.1

Chronically Sick and Bed-Ridden Patients

24.1.1 General Information

Reflexotherapy of the Feet (RTF) has proved its worth as a form of long-term, supplementary care for improving the quality of life, easing severe pain, and maintaining interpersonal contact.

Depending on the patient's regenerative capacity, the **basic functions** of the intestine, kidneys, respiratory, and cardiovascular systems may be expected to improve.

In patients with impaired sensibilities of various kinds and origins, **body awareness** can be developed and promoted through conscious, watchful experiencing of the treated areas of the feet.

Many of these patients also suffer from very **cold** and **lifeless** feet and are grateful for human touch and an increased body temperature. It is often useful to instruct friends and relatives how to move and massage the patient's feet. The application of a good skin oil or cream is always found to be particularly beneficial.

In patients suffering from **chronic pain**, harmonizing the autonomic nervous system by stabilizing grips is of major importance in breaking the spirals of tension, pain, and anxiety which are constantly re-establishing themselves.

Individual symptoms of pain can be recorded in a brief course of **Treatment in Acute Situations** (Chapter 16). In addition, the zones of the excretory and metabolic organs (intestine, urinary tract, lymphatic system including the spleen and thymus, nasopharyngeal cavity and lungs) and those of the endocrine system, tailored to the patient's response, are tonified.

24.1.2 Special Chronic Diseases

Multiple Sclerosis

In patients in the early stages of the disease, we can usually perform an initial assessment which indicates the zones in need of treatment. If the disease is already more advanced, an initial assessment is of little use as impaired sensibilities, paresis (partial paralysis), and the restriction and slowing down of all movement prevent the finding of reliable information.

Practical Advice

- Therapy focuses on the symptoms which have arisen as a result of cerebral and spinal impairment and afflict the patient the most. However, during the first few sessions the feet should be treated in their entirety, not according to specific stimuli, and in combination with ample stabilizing grips in order to obtain a better understanding of the patient's current response.
- In the **acute phase** it is preferable to perform stabilizing grips and to avoid strong stimuli. The symptomatic zones of the brain and the spinal column should be treated sensitively using the sedating grip, avoiding the application of excessive pressure.
- **Symptomatic** relief can be expected in:
  - **Evacuation of the bladder and intestine:** Sometimes spontaneous evacuation occurs immediately after treatment, sometimes the function of these systems improves as a result of a longer course of treatment.
  - Within the urinary and the digestive tracts, the **sphincters** are treated using the sedating grip (neurovegetative balance).
  - **Spastic paresis:** The rules of first-aid treatment are applied in the zones of the partially or completely paralyzed spastic muscle groups, provided they can be treated as zones. As a result of relatively vigorous treatment with the sedating grip, the acute spasm is often increased slightly for a brief period, before entering a phase of distinct relaxation of the muscles and joints which lasts a few hours.
  - **Difficulties in swallowing:** First the sedating grip is applied gently, later the following zones can be gently tonified: ventral and dorsal neck region, above all, in the region of the larynx, as well as the diaphragm and pelvic floor (corresponding to the base of the mouth), gastrointestinal tract, and all sphincter zones, especially the anus. Treat the lateral lymphatics of the neck gently and carefully.
  - Stabilizing grips, above all of the solar plexus, should be frequently interspersed. Eutonic positions (Chapter 6) have proved particularly effective.

Geriatric Patients

There is often the misconception that ageing is synonymous with being ill. In therapeutic circles, however, we are confronted, almost without exception, with **sick** elderly people. RTF offers a wide range of possibilities for alleviating such people's condition:

- A frequent sense of **isolation** can be alleviated by the remedy of touch alone. Touching the feet, including in the form of neutral massage and footbaths, has a particularly powerful effect on the whole person and constitutes a kind of "care for one's roots." After all, there is an intrinsic "memory" in everyone's feet documenting how they have literally carried the whole person through their life. For these reasons too, we have been training geriatric nurses for a long time.
- As **basic metabolic functions** (both anabolic and catabolic) are naturally slower in the elderly, they can be supported by gently tonifying the zones of the brain, heart, respiration, digestion, kidneys, skin, immune and lymphatic systems.
- **Dehydration in the elderly**, unfortunately often not sufficiently recognized, cannot be counteracted by RTF alone. First and foremost, fluid intake should be increased in this case.

Parkinson's Disease

In these patients, nonspecific treatment of all zones is well suited; the brain and the spinal column (symptomatic zones) should be treated gently at first and they can gradually also be tonified if the patient responds positively. RTF of the lymphatic system has also proved effective (Chapter 10.8.4).

The following partial **improvements** can be expected:

- The markedly slower muscle movements observed with hypokinetic symptoms, including those of the **mimic** musculature, become more pronounced and lively again.
- The abrupt release of normal muscle tension, above all, during passive movements, known as the **cogwheel phenomenon**, may occur less often and/or in an attenuated form.
- **Rest tremor** may diminish in extent and frequency.
- Above all, **mood lability**, which is often significant, is stabilized.

Bechterew's Disease (Ankylosing Spondylitis)

The treatment can be performed at any stage of the disease; even in the final stage it has a good palliative effect.

The following symptomatic and functional relief can be sought and obtained for the patient:

- It is possible, for example, to delay progressive skeletal and capsular **ankylosis** and to counteract the threat of complete immobility. Therefore, treatment of the zones of the spinal column and joints, including the pubic symphysis, sacroiliac joint, and sternum and their articulated connections with the thorax is paramount, initially with sedating grips and later possibly using gentle tonification.
- As the normal function and movement of the thorax and abdominal organs is greatly restricted by incipient or existing thoracolumbar **kyphosis**, tonifying treatment of the heart, respiratory organs, and digestive tract is particularly useful and can provide marked relief.
- A course of treatment of the lymphatic zones on the foot has also proved effective as it has a harmonizing effect on the emotional level of the person.
- Eutonic grips and positions bring relief for hours.

Hemiplegia, Paraplegia, and Tetraplegia

What all patients with these conditions have in common is paralysis of areas of organs or parts of the body as a result of complete (-plegia) or partial (paresis) failure of the sensorimotor supply from the spinal cord or damage to the central nervous system (CNS). Usually, accidents or diseases of the CNS are the triggers for these diseases.

As normal sensation transmitted by the neural supply is partially or completely impaired in these patients, not only the feet, but all the paralyzed parts of the body should be **touched as often as possible** to stimulate and activate other, more subtle qualities of perception and to prevent the patient from rejecting, isolating, or becoming indifferent toward the impaired areas.

Practical Advice

- In incomplete paraplegics, above all, the disturbing attendant symptoms of a lack of control of bladder and intestinal function must be treated by means of gentle tonifying of these groups of organs. Again and again during RTF, patients hear bowel sounds and feel peristaltic movements which may also result in the spontaneous evacuation of the bowels. Albeit with individually differing results, deliberate control of the evacuation of the bowels can be supported. Above all, chronic recurrent ascending urinary tract infections decline.

- The area of the spinal column where the lesion occurred should first be treated gently with sedating grips (Chapter 16.3). Later, in accordance with the vegetative response, it can also be tonified, possibly even somewhat more vigorously. Treatment begins **distal** to the impaired zone, but also includes the proximal part of the spinal column extending beyond the lesion. Intense pain can often be relieved by this means.

- Treatment of the heart and respiratory organs improves the circulation as far as the peripheral areas and can prevent bronchial and pulmonary infections at the same time.

- Initially, it is preferable to begin treating patients afflicted by cerebrovascular accident (CVA: apoplexy, stroke) on the foot that is **not** affected by paralysis. Stimuli may also be cautiously applied to the paralyzed foot, but here the dose limit should be carefully observed in order to avoid additional spasms. Particular caution should be exercised when treating the head, representing the symptomatic zones, to avoid overreactions.
  After one or two courses of RTF, patients with CVA usually show improvements in
  - basic functions of their metabolic and excretory organs,
  - verbal articulation, and
  - mobility of the paralyzed side of the body;
  - above all, their mood becomes more stable. Treatment is also indicated if a disease is long standing.

- When treating patients with pareses or plegia, particular attention must be paid to the symptoms of the **autonomic nervous system** (Chapter 4.2) as these indicate the appropriate dose, especially as patients do not **feel** the therapeutic grips, as a result of the disease, and often think the therapist should treat them

with firmer and more intense grips. Treatment should be interspersed with gentle tonifying of the solar plexus at repeated intervals.
By touching the paralyzed parts of the body, at the same time the therapist imparts the unspoken knowledge that the severe trauma involving the spinal column and head region always deeply affects the patient's personality as well, regardless of whether they are aware of this or not.

The keen nature of emphatic touch on the sensorily impaired parts of the person thus has a special quality.

Cancer

In general, RTF is highly appreciated by patients with cancer as a reliable concomitant therapy.

- As a result of our extensive experience, we advise that **during** chemotherapy or radiotherapy patients are treated **nonspecifically**, that is, with ample stabilizing grips and cautious, gentle grips in the zones of the heart, spinal column, lymphatic system, digestive tract, and endocrine system. Approximately 2 to 3 weeks **after** radiotherapy or chemotherapy has ended, stimuli can again be applied in the zones, depending on the response, more vigorously and with more emphasis on the organs. This primarily concerns the symptomatic zones, even if the organs have been surgically removed. From our observations, the patient's physical and mental condition stabilizes faster than usual as a result of the additional offer of RTF. The patient's quality of life improves within the framework of their overall condition.

- Cancer patients in intense **pain** due to the severity of their disease respond to first-aid treatment in the symptomatic zone (Chapter 16) with a reduction of pain lasting several hours, and recover somewhat in a relatively undisturbed sleep phase.

24.1.3 Summary

Treating the chronically sick can be very exhausting, partly due to the physical strain, partly because of the absorption of subtle irritations and stresses, particularly because the fate of this person also touches and affects us emotionally.

We should therefore take care of ourselves and be sure to find enough time for recovery and relaxation. Washing our hands under running water, remaining adequately hydrated, and airing the room help to neutralize our own energy field.

If therapists take on the pains and symptoms
of their patients after a treatment session,
that is, feel them physically and emotionally in
themselves, although such experiences indicate
that they are very sensitive, they also reflect the
need to conserve their own energy.

In spite of all our well-meaning empathy for the
patient, it should be remembered that the disease
and its complex background always belongs to the
patient and that all we can do is support and accompany them.

24.2

Care of Patients in Palliative Medicine

There is often a strong taboo surrounding the transition between life and death. Many are uncertain
and fearful about how they should deal with it,
particularly when it involves friends and relatives.

I should like to encourage all those who are
involved with patients in the final stages of their
life to touch their feet as often as possible. Even if
no improvement in their overall condition can be
expected, this kind of **noninvasive, interpersonal**
contact is particularly beneficial: which part of a
person would be better suited to support them on
the journey from this life into the next than the
feet with which they have actually passed through
life hitherto? In addition, touching the feet is often
easier for the patient to accept than areas closer to
the trunk.

24.2.1 Professional Support from Caregivers

- Daily care need only take **a few minutes** as a
  couple of appropriately selected grips usually
  suffice to make the patient's condition more
  bearable. Stabilizing grips (Chapter 6) are the
  best suited as they harmonize the **autonomic
  nervous system** and are therefore also able to
  calm the mood. Many patients in the terminal stage find the lemniscate (the symbol of
  infinity), applied on the soles of their feet
  particularly effective (see **Fig. 6.8**).
- Patients in very **severe pain** are treated with
  the sedating grip in the symptomatic zones,
  at first cautiously and then later rather more
  vigorously. **Examples:** In patients in the terminal stage of stomach cancer, the stomach is

sedated and in those with brain tumors, the
head, together with ample stabilizing grips.
- The vital centers of the **respiratory** and
  cardiovascular systems are supported in their
  function by "stretching" and widening the
  zone of the diaphragm and gently tonifying
  the zone of the heart.
- Excretion via the **intestine** can be improved
  as far as possible by treating the intestine.
  In patients with **ileus** vigorous tonifying has
  proved its worth, also postoperatively. This is
  performed for a few minutes several times a
  day and can help to prevent further surgical
  intervention!
- With **heavy fluid retention** in the tissue, for
  example, in the legs and feet and in the trunk
  in the case of ascites, performing alternating
  strokes in the lymphatic zones and carefully
  tonifying the heart and kidneys can bring
  relief, at least for a few hours. This is usually
  reflected in improved diuresis.
- Treatment with specific grips should frequently include the central zone of the **solar
  plexus**; this can be gently tonified or sedated
  depending on its condition. As a result, the
  person is more at ease and their sleep phases
  are more refreshing.
- **Eutonic grips** (Chapter 6) provide particular
  relief because they enable the entire person to
  relax for a few hours.

24.2.2 Care Provided by Friends and Relatives

- After a brief introduction, most of the aforementioned grips can also be performed by
  friends and **relatives**. The "remedy of touch"
  is important for both parties because many
  issues can still be broached and possibly
  resolved nonverbally via this bridge where
  words are no longer appropriate.
- Friendly, affectionate **stroking** of the feet and
  legs is soothing on its own, while simultaneously removing the sense of helplessness and
  creating a healthy distance as well as an inner
  closeness. A natural oil with a pleasant fra-
  grance or a good ointment supports this effect.
- A short treatment of the feet with the
  heel-stretching or palm-sole grip, for example,
  lends stability and support. For patients, it is
  a major relief when they feel that they are not
  held back in spite of all their relatives' sorrow
  and concern.

- Most grips are also suitable for **comatose** patients. Although the patient is unaware of them on a conscious level, they nonetheless provide relief. This is objectively confirmed by the change in the curve on the **monitors**.

24.3

Sleep Disturbances

In many people healthy alternation between waking and sleeping can be impaired by a number of disturbances. During the first assessment various connections are revealed by corresponding background zones.

Practical Advice

Frequently, the following zones require treatment:
- The **digestive tract**, as there is too much fermentation in the intestine, impairing the function of the metabolic organs during the night (e.g., as a result of eating raw fruit and vegetables in the evening, which a weakened digestive tract is unable to process adequately).
- The **head** often reacts with many painful sites (interference fields of decaying and devitalized teeth, or the presence of silver amalgam and other incompatible metals in the oral cavity; lymphatic congestion in the nasopharynx, racing thoughts).
- If **musculoskeletal** blocks exist, many people are unable to have a relaxing night's sleep. They often think the blame for their inability to relax lies with a bed that is too hard or too soft. However, it is rather their own tensions which are disturbing them.
- **Dysfunctions in the endocrine system** can alter the quality and quantity of sleep. Apart from the endocrine glands with their internal secretions, the lymphatic areas must be considered as an expression of an important flow system. As hyperacidity of the intestinal environment also influences hormonal regulation, additional intensive treatment of the digestive organs is often necessary.
- **Menopausal symptoms,** including frequently troubling hot flushes and periods of depression or aggression in menopausal women are one of the **best indications** for RTF. The solar plexus and other stabilizing grips must be included in any treatment from time to time. Carefully obtained initial findings will reveal the areas requiring treatment.

- In patients with sleep disorders, factors which can be **radiesthetically** determined may also have to be taken into account, for example, disturbing influences on the patient's sleeping location.
  Beware of electrostress in the form of electric alarm clocks and radios in the direct vicinity of the head, televisions in the bedroom and electric blankets on the bed. With disorders of this kind, patients report that their complaints primarily occur at night and in the morning and they do not feel refreshed. Consistently switching off these devices and removing them from the bedroom for approximately 10 to 14 nights is more convincing than any theoretical argument.
  - Sometimes the mere **thought** of possibly lying awake again for one or more hours at night causes so much additional anxiety and tension that this alone prevents healthy sleep. A change of attitude with regard to a nocturnal phase of waking can help to produce completely new insights and understanding.
  - With the customary sensory overload and overexposure of our outdoor life, it is particularly important to end the day **consciously** and **with gratitude** and to entrust ourselves to the healing and constructive forces within and around us for the night.

24.4

Anorexia Nervosa and Bulimia Nervosa

These illnesses almost exclusively affect young girls. A disturbed eating pattern has its roots in deep disturbances in the process of personality development and is often triggered by stress-inducing events.

RTF is a proven complement to well-known therapeutic approaches including psychotherapy and breathing therapy. Perhaps even providing an important basis for RTF is the anatomical fact that these patients do indeed need their **feet** to take daring new steps through their uncertain life in order to find their personal way.

Experiences from my own practice have taught me that support from the feet can be fundamental in helping the patient to gain more **confidence** and courage for the transition to adulthood and to becoming a woman.

Language offers a number of examples demonstrating the importance of the feet in general, aside from the fact that certain groups and systems of organs can be specifically treated with RTF. Familiar expressions such as the following indicate this:

- Having solid ground under one's feet again
- No longer being "up in the air"
- Things are going better
- Standing on one's own two feet, etc.

Anorexic patients can experience physical and emotional support through the therapist's attentive contact with their feet, without the need to talk much about it. In addition, the feet are at a "safe distance" from the overall person and for this reason treatment can usually be accepted.

Practical Advice

- At the beginning of a course of treatment neutral stroking, stabilizing grips and differentiated gentle stimuli help to gradually regain body awareness, which has to a great extent been lost. It is sometimes appreciated if we keep the feet covered when beginning treatment in this way.
- The **Arndt–Schulz Rule** (German psychiatrist, 1835–1900) as a basic biological principle also applies here: light stimuli kindle the life force, moderate stimuli encourage it, strong stimuli inhibit it and very strong stimuli paralyze it.
- Such patients may also be treated for approximately 15 to 20 minutes daily for a week but great care should be taken to find the right dosage and to ensure that the patient has a sufficiently long rest after each treatment.
- After a few treatments, according to the patient's level of vitality, more precise grips in the zones of the gastrointestinal tract, endocrine system, head, spinal column, and kidneys may be offered. As soon as it is possible to work more vigorously, however, an interval of one to two—or even more—days between individual treatments is necessary.
  In these patients, the **kidneys** are at particular risk and require careful treatment. An adequate intake of fluids, possibly combined with vitamin and mineral supplementation, must also be ensured. Treatment in the kidney zones is cautious initially ("moderate stimuli encourage the life force"). Warm or hot water, drunk in small sips, is ideal for ensuring an adequate

intake since the body does not have to use its own limited heat to warm up the fluid.
- My experience with anorexic patients has shown me that simply discussing their problems is usually not enough to bring about any real change but that the **concrete experience** of an **awareness of one's own body** is also necessary.

Only the vital experience of becoming and being touched can open up a new and healthier quality of life which is not stuck in intellectualization and discussion, but is tangible and perceptible. Touch has a more profound quality than eye contact and speech!

24.5

Allergies

Allergies are indicators of weakened or congested vital forces. The term allergy is usually restricted to the following symptoms: hay fever, asthma, and skin irritations of all kinds. However, an allergic component or intolerance may also lie behind a series of other symptoms our patients may have, for example:

- Migraine
- Rheumatism
- Hypotension and hypertension
- Depression
- Digestive problems of various kinds
- Susceptibility to infections, etc.

"To **whom** or **what** are you allergic?" is a justified question because—apart from allergenic triggers and causes in food, the environment, and medication—some people are allergic to other people and their behavior. This too is documented by language as an expression of human experience, for example:

- "I can't breathe," say asthmatic persons who are experiencing personal difficulties in their surroundings.
- "I don't have a thick enough skin," report many sensitive people who are having difficulty coping in their professional or family life and who come for treatment of skin problems of all kinds.
- "I can't talk about the problem," say patients who are chronically hoarse or whose voice is husky.

Often it is not possible to change our patients' difficult situations in life from outside because these are usually associated with factors of a very personal nature and have to be worked out by the patients themselves. The allergy is simply the **driving force** which very intrusively and insistently indicates the **opportunity and necessity for change**.

However, with RTF we can offer therapeutic assistance which has a stabilizing effect and enables marked oversensitivity to be transformed into healthy sensitivity.

As a discipline of holistic medicine, RTF provides a good opportunity to activate a person's self-healing powers and reduce their susceptibility to troubling factors which give rise to disease. In particular, our special **treatment** of the **lymph system** has its place here. As an exclusive or concomitant therapy used in various forms of natural medicine, it has often proved its worth.

Patients with allergies require a therapist with a great deal of sympathetic understanding and inner stability. We can support the therapeutic process by taking small, patient steps.

Practical Advice

- As with other groups of patients, an initial assessment is performed when treating patients with allergic symptoms. Experience has shown that with allergies of whatever nature, similar zones of organs and systems are frequently afflicted:
- **Digestive tract** including the upper abdominal organs, small intestine, rectum, and anus: At the start of the course of treatment we should work with gentle tonifying grips, the intensity of which can be increased with increasing stabilization. The liver frequently responds better to **gentle** treatment.
  Exceptions are patients suffering from a chronically inflamed intestine; here only sedating grips are used initially in the intestine. At the start of the course of treatment these grips are also applied more gently. The significance of the digestive tract is indicated by **Pischinger**, who describes the digestive tract as "the most extensive interference field".

Clinical studies have proved that psychological stress has a negative effect on the quality of the intestinal flora.

- **Autonomic nervous system:** Solar plexus and sphincters, above all cardia, pylorus, and anus are initially treated with the sedating grip. Later they can be tonified. The sphincter muscles are directly connected to the autonomic nervous system and in patients with allergy they are very often excessively tense. All the stabilizing and Eutonic grips also have a harmonizing effect on the autonomic nervous system.
- **Lymphatic system:** Tonsils, lateral lymphatics, pelvis, and lymphatics of the groin are treated gently but thoroughly. Thymus, appendix, and spleen can be tonified. The specific RTF treatment of the lymphatic system has proved effective as a regulator for processing waste matter and toxins in all patients with allergies.
- **Endocrine system**, preferably suprarenals and thyroid, but also pituitary gland and genitals. The suprarenals usually tolerate rather more vigorous tonifying while with the other endocrine glands, attention should be paid to the autonomic response.
- When patients with allegies in an **acute phase** come for treatment, First-Aid is provided (Chapter 16). Besides the symptomatic zones, primarily the background zones of the kidneys/suprarenals, spleen, and small intestine should be treated and many stabilizing/harmonizing grips employed.
- The **background** zones are often more important than the symptomatic zones because the afflicted environment can be improved via them and the acute complaints regulated as a result.
- In patients with **neurodermatitis** and **psoriasis**, I regard RTF as an important, comprehensive concomitant therapy. However, classical homeopathy has proved to be an effective instrument for detecting and treating deep-rooted and unrecognized hereditary disorders which lie behind existing symptoms. Furthermore, the often extremely distressing symptoms (itching, mental irritation, esthetic aspects) can be significantly alleviated by exact compliance with **dietary** instructions. The same rules apply to the treatment of this group of patients as to those with allergies.

The **period of subsequent rest** should be particularly generous for all the aforementioned groups of patients.

25 Treatment of Scars with Reflexotherapy of the Feet

25.1 General Information

Almost everyone has scars, but many injuries and wounds heal naturally, leaving no particularly disturbing impressions at either a physical or emotional level. Nevertheless, time and again we find that sooner or later scars may become **interference fields** in relation to various functions in a person. In these cases they may, for example, adhere to the surrounding tissue so tightly that they cause congestion, local circulatory disturbances, and restriction of movement.

In **acupuncture** it is also known that scars inhibit the flow of energy in the affected meridians.

As more people nowadays are open to connections of this kind and themselves notice that scars can impair health, a series of effective methods has been developed, for example:

- Connective tissue massage
- Traditional scar massage
- Neural therapy
- Manual lymphatic drainage
- Various meridian therapies
- Light, color, and gemstone therapy, etc.

The method used depends upon the therapist's professional background and the special disposition of the patient. However, we should consider the possibility of the "**interference field scar**" during the first assessment and ask specific questions in that direction.

When questioned, patients do not always remember their scars spontaneously. It is therefore advisable to briefly mention the most common events resulting in scars:

Operations, dog bites, cycling accidents, barbed wire, kitchen knives, pieces of broken glass, war injuries, stones being thrown, perineal sutures, vaccination scars, work or sports accidents, boil excision, injuries from spades or lawnmowers, burns, road traffic accidents, etc. With a weakened constitution and troublesome current disposition, scars from **piercings** can also become interference fields.

Any scar may develop into an interference field sooner or later, regardless of whether it is fresh or old, large or small, painful or not.

An "**interference field scar**" can be recognized by the following means:

- The development of complaints which did not exist previously and which coincide with the appearance of the scar, whether far from the scar, in its immediate vicinity, or in the surrounding area
- Energetic measurements of the tissue tension of the scar and its surrounding area
- Spontaneous description of unpleasant or painful sensations in the region of the scar
- Noticeable emotional reactions if the patient is asked about the scar or if it is touched
- Reactions in the **zone** to which the scar is assigned. This can manifest itself as
  - pain in the zone of the scar,
  - symptoms of autonomic irritation during treatment of the zone, and/or
  - unexpected emotions triggered by treatment of the zone corresponding to the scar in situ. **Memories** of how the scar was acquired are frequently evoked as a result.

If treatment of the scar zone does not trigger any physical or emotional reactions at the time or before the next treatment session, we can safely presume that the scar does **not** constitute an interference field.

25.2 Performance

25.2.1 Choice of Scars for Reflexotherapy of the feet

Above all, **larger** scars on the head, neck, and trunk are suitable for zone treatment.

Scars on the **extremities** can be treated as far as the region of the elbow and knee. However, collateral and/or contralateral therapy lends itself on the extremities (Chapter 18.4), especially on the lower legs and feet and lower arms and hands.

Small scars are usually treated more effectively with other methods, for example, neural therapy, etc.

Important note: It should be pointed out to the patient that not only physical but also emotional blocks may be released during scar treatment and that they can and should express the thoughts and feelings arising as a result.

25.2.2 Localization of Scar Zones

(**Fig. 25.1**)

Experience shows that zones of scars are usually found in the **dorsal** part of the feet as most incisions during an operation are performed **ventrally** in the thorax and abdomen.

Locating the zone of the scar is easiest when applying the guiding principle of the method: a seated person corresponds in shape to the feet. Therefore, scar zones of the

- head and neck are found in the region of the toes,
- thorax and upper abdomen on the metatarsal bones,
- abdomen and pelvis on the tarsal bones, and
- thigh and knee in the distal part of the lower legs.

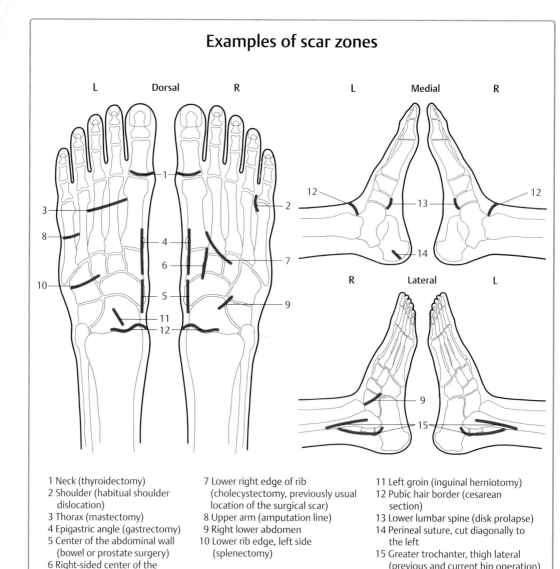

Examples of scar zones

1 Neck (thyroidectomy)
2 Shoulder (habitual shoulder dislocation)
3 Thorax (mastectomy)
4 Epigastric angle (gastrectomy)
5 Center of the abdominal wall (bowel or prostate surgery)
6 Right-sided center of the abdomen (cholecystectomy)

7 Lower right edge of rib (cholecystectomy, previously usual location of the surgical scar)
8 Upper arm (amputation line)
9 Right lower abdomen
10 Lower rib edge, left side (splenectomy)

11 Left groin (inguinal herniotomy)
12 Pubic hair border (cesarean section)
13 Lower lumbar spine (disk prolapse)
14 Perineal suture, cut diagonally to the left
15 Greater trochanter, thigh lateral (previous and current hip operation)

Fig. 25.1 Examples of scar zones.

25.2.3 Treatment Technique for Scar Zones

The obvious aim of treating scars with RTF is to normalize the assigned zone of the foot. As both physically and emotionally troublesome experiences may be stored at these points, the **sedating grip** is chosen first. After improvement of the complaints in the zone, it can also be tonified.

In **resilient** patients, the zone of the scar tissue is then vigorously "scratched" with the finger**nail** in a grid pattern. If this is too painful, only the finger**tips** vigorously stroke the tissue of the scar zone. This stimulates blood circulation over a wide area.

Whether the physical or emotional side reacts more decisively is demonstrated by the patient's **reactions** occurring during and after scar treatment with RTF. Further care is structured according to the current situation.

- When reactions appear more clearly on the **physical** level (e.g., easing of the pain and general complaints in the scar in situ, in assigned muscle groups or organs), a lengthy subsequent rest period usually suffices.
- Marked **emotional** reactions may require longer care and support, as described in Chapter 17.

The use of **scar creams** or ointments is recommended at the end of treatment, both in the zone of the feet and in the scar itself. For example, Bach Flower 39 as an ointment is very effective.

The patient should continue to apply the ointment once or twice a day for several weeks due to

- the physiological effect of bridging interrupted energy lines (usually segments, meridians, or reflex zones of various kinds), and
- the psychological effect, because **gentle touch always has a healing effect**.
- If and when scar zones should be treated more frequently depends on the

- condition of the scar in situ and its zone on the foot,
- subjective improvement of the complaints after treatment,
- duration of the improvement.

The **intervals** between scar treatments may vary from days to weeks and months. Usually, after two to three standard treatment sessions with RTF the condition of the scar zone is checked again in order to decide whether treatment should be repeated. Sometimes a single scar treatment session releases so much tension and (usually subconsciously) suppressed emotion that a second session is unnecessary or might even be excessive.

Important note: Treatments of this nature require tranquility and time. As it only becomes clear during the course of treatment whether the patient requires our support for longer than usual, it is advisable to allow for more time or to give the patient the last appointment in the evening.

25.3 Summary

From our experience of scar treatment, we can see that many scars are associated with "life-changing" experiences, not only on a physical but also an emotional level. They can leave traces of an external and internal nature, and, even if they do not change the person completely, they often change the person's relationship to themselves and their surroundings. Decades of experience and providing support for patients with troublesome scars have shown me that by treating the scars, enormous potential for **vitality** and **zest for life** can be released.

26 Zones of the Teeth and Their Energetic Interrelationships

General Information

The zones of the teeth have already been described in a neutral way in the section "The Tooth–Jaw Region" in Chapter 10.2.3 and their arrangement on the individual toes is shown in **Figs. 10.2** and **10.3**. Furthermore, however, the teeth also constitute a **microsystem** which has long been used in holistic dentistry.

Dr. Reinhold Voll discovered the significance of the interaction between the tooth–jaw region and the whole organism in the middle of the last century. He ascertained his numerous measurement results by means of electroacupuncture diagnosis (EAP). The present chart was configured by **Dr. Fritz Kramer**. It is intended "to help make diagnosis easier in patients with suspected or actual disease and to improve therapy."

As I was able to make Dr. Voll's acquaintance in person during my initial trials with reflexotherapy of the feet (RTF), as far back as the early 1970s, consideration was given to
- whether the individual teeth can be found and treated as **zones on the feet**, and also
- whether the numerous energetic connections in situ that were well-known to dental specialists are also reflected in the zones.

Both of these considerations were confirmed. Thus, we have long had the option of treating the microsystem of the teeth and at the same time, their energetic relationships with organs and systems as well via the zones of the feet—**a therapeutic treasure trove!** Although there are also diagrams with differing assignments, we have retained the dental chart of Voll/Kramer because it has proved its worth in the context of our work.

Our patients virtually never consult us primarily on account of dental problems, but by combining both methods, we can both influence the courses of certain diseases and contribute to clarification as well as determining
- whether a certain tooth is linked to corresponding complaints in the patient,
- whether specific treatment by a holistic dentist makes sense and is necessary. This can be established by examining the zones of the interrelationships with the aid of the dental chart.

That we are able to treat patients with acute toothache **in an emergency** and how we do so until further dental care can be provided are described as Example 1 in Chapter 16.2.2.

The Dental Chart

(Fig. 26.1)
Explained by Dr. Kramer (according to Voll EAP measurements) for RTF therapists in a practice-oriented manner. In the horizontal center of the diagram the maxillary and mandibular teeth and their odonton (functional circuit of mandibular part, surrounding tissue, mucus membrane, and nerves) are numbered from 1 to 8 respectively:

The **maxillary** teeth on the right-hand side are prefixed by the number 1, those on the left-hand side by the number 2, the **mandibular** teeth on the left-hand side by the number 3, those on the right-hand side by the number 4. Thus, the four quadrants, starting at the top right-hand side, are arranged clockwise from 1 to 4.
- All the tissue and organ assignments **above** the first numerical series listed in quadrants 1 and 2 have energetic links to the **maxillary** teeth.
- All those **below** the second numerical series listed in quadrants 3 and 4 are energetically linked to the **mandibular** teeth.

As the dental chart was primarily created for holistic dentists (and not for manual therapists!), for quite a number of assignments there are no zones on the feet, for example, ulnar and radial part of the hand, foot, big toe, arteries, etc.

26.2.1 Practical Application

Patients with Acute Toothache

The following guide is an extension of the options which are described in Chapter 16.2.2.

In the corresponding tooth zone the sedating grip is used for treatment, likewise in the adjacent tooth zones on the right and left hand sides. The right–left interchangeability of the zones must be borne in mind in the process (Chapter 15). All the organs and tissues assigned to this tooth according to Voll are tonified, apart from those which are very close to the symptomatic zone.

Example: With acutely painful wisdom teeth, the zone of the ears is not tonified but likewise treated with sedating grips.

The zones of the lymphlymphatic nodules and chains of the head/neck, digestive organs, spleen, and appropriate stabilizing/harmonizing grips are included. The zones of the teeth on the **hand**, which are briefly sedated several times a day, are suitable for emergency **self-treatment**. They must be translated to the fingers from their anatomical position on the toes.

In **infants with teething problems**, usually a "problem which runs in the whole family," RTF has long proved its value and can also be performed by relatives: Good circulation in all the toes is encouraged using appropriate grips (discernible from a delicate pink coloration of the toes) and the interdigital skin folds are stretched, at first cautiously, then also more intensely. To this end, the zones of the intestine and pelvic floor including the anus are sedated or gently tonified. Diarrhea and soreness around the lower sphincter point to the relationship with the teeth.

Diseases Not Located in the Tooth–Jaw Region

With almost every clinical picture, tooth relationships can be found in the Voll dental chart. Whether they must be included as background zones in RTF can be clarified immediately in each patient.

Example: In patients with hip problems, the tooth zones 13, 23, 33, 43 assigned to the hip are examined; in stomach complaints, those assigned to the stomach: In the maxilla the molars/rear molars (16, 17 and 26, 27), in the mandible the premolars/anterior molars (34, 35 and 44, 45). If the corresponding tooth zones are painful, they are included in the treatment, in severe pain with sedating grips, otherwise with tonifying grips. In addition, all the Voll relationships with the respective tooth can be treated, in particular, in chronic diseases.

Note: From a subjective perspective, the respective teeth in situ are not always afflicted. However, as they form part of the functional circuit of the present disease, their **zones** may quite possible react abnormally.

Interference Field Examination

The following may prove to be interference fields:
- Endodontically treated (dead, devitalized) teeth

- Impacted (firmly embedded in the jaw) teeth
- Chronic and acute inflammations, suppurations
- Material intolerances (frequently silver amalgam)
- Scars from surgical procedures in the oral cavity, cysts

The affected tooth zone is first tonified but if the tooth and its odonton are acutely painful, sedating grips are employed. Then, all the assignments shown in the Voll chart are examined by means of tonification grips. If **more than half** of these tooth assignments react painfully and also **remain** affected after several treatment sessions, it is obvious that the tooth has the quality of an interference field. To confirm this, a holistic dentist should carry out a more precise examination.

As a corollary: the **primary** focus of the affliction need not always be in a tooth but may also be in one of the organs or tissues which are assigned to this tooth energetically.

Example: Persistent complaints in the right-hand side of the sacroiliac joint can over time contribute to irritation of the teeth **and** tooth **zones** 18 and 48. If the complaints in the sacroiliac joint have improved, the assigned teeth and zones can also be restored, thus inflammations in situ may abate and dental fistulas recede.

Note: Every afflicted tooth may have a disturbing effect on any constitutionally weak areas of the person, regardless of the Voll chart. The measurement results of holistic dentists are the method of choice here.

Adjunctive Therapy during Holistic Dental Restoration

Holistic dental restoration involves implementation of the results of energetic measurements and various conventional examinations. It may relate to
- Removal of incompatible materials such as silver amalgam or plastics of various kinds
- Tooth extractions and, if necessary, the use of bridges, etc.
- Checking whether dead or displaced teeth represent interference fields
- Surgical removal of impacted teeth, etc.

The corresponding zones can already be treated a few weeks **before** the start of restoration as a supportive measure—usually with sedating grips in the tooth zones and tonifying in the assigned zones (Voll dental chart).

Energetic interrelationships between the tooth–jaw region and the rest of the body

Interrelationships of the odontons of the maxilla with the rest of the body

		18	17	16	15	14	13	12	11
SENSORY ORGANS		Inner ear	Maxillary sinus		Ethmoidal cells		Eye	Frontal sinus cavity	
JOINTS		Shoulder/elbow		Jaw	Shoulder/Elbow		Knee, rear		
							Hip	Sacrum/coccyx	
		Hand, ulnar Foot plantar Toes and SI*		Knee, front		Hand, radial Foot Big toe		Foot	
SPINAL CORD SEGMENTS		C8 T1 T7 T6 T5 S3 S2 S1		T12 T11 L1	C7 C6 C5 T4 T3 T2 L5 L4		T8 T9 T10	L3 L2 co S5 S4	
VERTEBRAE		CS7 TS1 TS6 TS5 S2 S1		TS 12 TS 11 L 1	CS7 CS 6 CS 5 TS 4 TS 3 L5 L4		TS 9 TS 10	L3 L2 co S5 S4 S3	
ORGANS	Yin	Heart, right side		Pancreas	Lung, right side		Liver, right side	Kidney, right side	
	Yang	Duodenum		Stomach, right side	Colon, right side		Gall bladder	Bladder, right side urogenital region	
ENDOCRINE GLANDS		Anterior lobe of pituitary gland	Para-thyroid gland	Thyroid gland	Thymus	Posterior lobe of the pituitary gland		Pineal gland	
MISCELLANEOUS		Central nervous system Psyche	Mammary gland, right side						
NEW NOMENCLATURE FOR MAXILLARY TEETH		18	17	16	15	14	13	12	11
NEW NOMENCLATURE FOR MANDIBULAR TEETH		48	47	46	45	44	43	42	41

Interrelationships of the odontons of the mandible with the rest of the body

		48	47	46	45	44	43	42	41
MISCELLANEOUS		Energy management			Mammary gland, right side				
ENDOCRINE GLANDS, VESSELS		Peripheral nerves	Arteries	Veins	Lymphatic vessels	Gonads		Suprarenals	
ORGANS	Yang	Ileum, right side	Colon, right side		Stomach, right side Pylorus		Gall bladder	Bladder, right side urogenital region	
		Ileocecal, region							
	Yin	Heart, right side	Lung, right side		Pancreas		Liver, right side	Kidney, right side	
VERTEBRAE		CS7 TS1 TS6 TS5 S2 S1	CS7 CS6 TS5 TS4 TS3 L5 L4		TS 12 TS 11 L 1		TS 9 TS 10	L 3, L 2 co S 5, S 4, S 3	
SPINAL CORD SEGMENTS		C8 T1 T7 T6 T5 S3 S2 S1	C7 C6 C5 T4 T3 T2 L5 L4		T12 T11 L1		T8 T9 T10	L3 L2 co S5 S4	
JOINTS		Shoulder/Elbow			Knee, front		Knee, rear		
		Hand, ulnar Foot, plantar Toes and SI	Hand, radial Foot Big toe				Hip	Sacrum/coccyx	
					Jaw			Foot	
SENSORY ORGANS		Ear	Ethmoidal cells		Maxillary sinus		Eye	Frontal sinus cavity	

Fig. 26.1 Tooth relationships.

Frontal sinus cavity	Eye	Ethmoidal cells	Maxillary sinus		Inner ear			SENSORY ORGANS
Knee rear		Shoulder Elbow	Jaw		Shoulder Elbow			JOINTS
Sacrum/coccyx	Hip	Hand, radial Foot Big toe	Knee, front		Hand, ulnar Foot plantar Toes and SI*			
Foot								
L2 L3 S4 S5 co	L2 L3 S4 S5 co	C5 C6 C7 T2 TS3 TS4 L4 L5	T11 T12 L1		C8 T1 T5 T6 T7 S1 S2 S3			SPINAL CORD SEGMENT
L2 L3 S3 S4 S5 co	TS9 TS10	CS5 CS6 CS7 TS3 TS4 L4 L5	TS11 TS12 L1		CS7 TS1 TS5 TS6 S1 S2			VERTEBRAE
Kidney, left side	Liver, left side	Lung, left side	Spleen		Heart, left side		Yin	ORGANS
Bladder, left side urogenital region	Bile ducts, left side	Colon, left side	Stomach left side		Jejunum Ileum, left side		Yang	
Pineal gland	Posterior lobe of the pituitary gland	Thymus	Thyroid gland	Para-thyroid gland	Anterior lobe of the pituitary gland			ENDOCRINE GLANDS
			Mammary gland, left side		Central nervous system Psyche			MISCELLANEOUS
21	22	23	24	25	26	27	28	NEW NOMENCLATURE FOR MAXILLARY TEETH
31	32	33	34	35	36	37	38	NEW NOMENCLATURE FOR MANDIBULAR TEETH
		Mammary gland, left side			Energy management			MISCELLANEOUS
Suprarenals	Gonads		Lymphatic vessels	Veins	Arteries	Peripheral nerves		ENDOCRINE GLANDS, VESSELS
Bladder, left side urogenital region	Bile ducts left side	Stomach left side	Colon left side		Jejunum Ileum, left side		Yang	ORGANS
Kidney, left side	Liver, left side	Spleen	Lung, left side		Heart, left side		Yin	
L2 L3 S3 S4 S5 co	TS9 TS10	TS11 TS12 L1	CS5 CS6 CS7 TS3 TS4 L4 L5		CS7 TS1 TS5 TS6 S1 S2			VERTEBRAE
L2 L3 S4 S5 co	T8 T9 T10	T11 T12 L1	C5 C6 C7 T2 T3 T4 L4 L5		C8 T1 T5 T6 T7 S1 S2 S3			SPINAL CORD SEGMENTS
Knee, rear		Knee, front	Shoulder-Elbow					JOINTS
Sacrum/coccyx	Hip		Hand, radial Foot Big toe		Hand, ulnar Foot, plantar Toes and SI			
Foot		Jaw						
Frontal sinus cavity	Eye	Maxillary sinus	Ethmoidal cells		Ear			SENSORY ORGANS

Interrelationships of the odontons of the maxilla with the rest of the body

Interrelationships of the odontons of the mandible with the rest of the body

Special Topics and Further Developments

Abbreviations: SI: Sacroiliac joint, C: spinal cord segments of the cervical spine, CS: cervical spine, T: thoracic segments, TS: thoracic spine; S: Sacral spine; L: Lumbar spine; co: coccyx

Strong reactions can be significantly attenuated if the affected tooth zones are briefly sedated immediately after the dental appointment and over the following days. To support the healing process, patients can briefly sedate these zones on the hand several times a day as **self-treatment**.

Important note: Women must ensure that they do not receive silver amalgam fillings or have them removed during pregnancy and lactation.

For the **release of toxins and harmful substances,** gentle tonifying of the lymphatic zones of the head/neck, intestine, liver, spleen, and kidneys is included. If there is no specific adjunctive or detoxification therapy with homeopathic remedies, taking **Coffeae carbo** (formulation: Dr. Heisler's Carbo Königsfeld, Müller Göppingen) has also proved effective: insalivate one teaspoon thoroughly twice a day in the mouth. For decades Coffeae carbo has been used as an **absorption medium** for toxins in the gastrointestinal tract and lymphatic system, including for children. Furthermore, it can be rubbed into the gums locally in the morning and evening for periodontal disease.

Support in Correcting the Positioning of Teeth

This relates to those who wear braces (often young people), patients whose normal occlusion (correct meeting of the teeth) is being restored, etc.

It should be noted that vegetative and/or organic **irritations** frequently occur during tooth correction:

- Increased nervousness
- Reduced physical resilience
- Disturbed sleep
- Greater emotional instability
- Increased sweating or shivering
- Reduced powers of concentration

Knowledge of the interrelationships between teeth and the whole organism makes these reactions understandable.

Here RTF presents itself as an adjunctive treatment throughout the entire period of correction. It can result in stabilization of the desired normalization of the tooth position, and the teeth being better able to retain their intended position.

RTF is particularly effective for management and treatment of pain in acute situations involving **difficulties** adjusting to the **brace**. The zones of the teeth are all gently tonified, including the relationships according to Voll where there are particular tensions in the oral cavity. The zones of the upper lymphatics, occiput, cervical spine, intestine, and pelvic ligaments are treated at the same time, likewise the solar plexus and/or a range of other stabilizing grips. The same proposed therapy applies to patients who—usually at night—**grind their teeth** and therefore often wear a splint.

Special tooth–jaw regulation involves **bionator therapy** in accordance with **Prof. Balters**. This is a functional orthodontic therapy in which a small plastic plate with metal brackets is placed under the tongue for an extended period. It may result in reshaping of the dental arches and changes in the tooth and jaw position by way of the muscular forces in the jaw region.

26.3

Summary

Any dental intervention in the "intimate area of the mouth" may also trigger **mood** disturbances. With tooth extractions, it must be borne in mind that they always constitute a loss which may sometimes be reflected unexpectedly and spontaneously in feelings of irritation. The term "wisdom tooth," which according to Voll energetic measurements is also connected to—among other things—the mind and psyche, points to this. The tooth commonly referred to in this way has a similar name in many other languages.

It is strongly recommended that more extensive restorations in the oral cavity (the removal of silver amalgam, the selection of new filling materials) are only carried out after **expert measurements** have been performed, for example, EAP (electroacupuncture according to Voll), bioresonance and kinesiology, and that a second opinion is obtained. Holistic dentists provide comprehensive clarification of the options available.

Important note: Nowadays many patients cannot cope with the extraction of more than **one** tooth at a time during a dental appointment. Patients should be thoroughly informed about this.

From My Practice

Report from an RTF therapist: "Three days ago a 16-year-old girl had all four of her wisdom teeth removed in one session with resulting complications such as heavy postoperative bleeding, severe swelling of the whole face, severe pain.

RTF treatment: For 3 consecutive days cautious pain management and treatment for acute situations involving sedation of the four tooth zones and treatment of the energetic relationships according to Voll. Frequently interspersed with stabilizing grips. At the end of the respective treatment lymphatic zones of the head, neck, and thorax. Ample subsequent rest.

Therapeutic 'homework': Three to four times a day brief self-treatment of the four tooth zones on the little fingers with the sedating grip, stretching of the interdigital skin folds between the fingers to stimulate the flow of lymph.

Result: Already significant reduction of swelling of the face and pain after the first treatment session. More peaceful sleep, the patient 'feels as if she is back in the land of the living.' After three treatment sessions further reduction of swelling and stabilization of overall condition."

27 Zones of the Pelvic Ligaments

Pelvic ligaments, like fasciae, cartilage and bone, mainly comprise collagenic connective tissue and are for the **connection, stabilization,** and **mobility** of the skeletal and organic structures of the pelvis.

Walter Froneberg (**Fig. 27.1**) developed the zones of the pelvic ligaments in the early 1980s based on the principles of our courses. They were later supplemented and modified by personal experiences. At the beginning their use was limited to skeletomuscular stresses on the pelvis, but it soon became apparent that they had a much broader range of indications.

27.1

Indications

- Skeletomuscular strains such as pelvic misalignment, lumbago, complaints of the cervical spine, slipped disk, scoliosis, coxarthrosis and gonarthrosis, shoulder-arm syndrome, epicondylitis
- Chronically cold feet, venous, arterial, or lymphatic congestion of the legs and pelvis

- After operations in the abdominal area and pelvis, on the legs once wound healing is complete
- Functional and organic disturbances of the organs of the lesser pelvis such as menstrual and menopausal symptoms, fallopian tube adhesions, prolapse complaints; prostate problems, sterility, impotence
- Physical imbalance, mental and emotional instability
- Migraine, tension headache, tinnitus
- Jaw and temporomandibular problems, for example, in those who wear braces or have malocclusion, nocturnal tooth-grinding (see **Fig. 21.5** similarity in shape between jaw and hip joint).

27.2

Contraindications

- Recent operations in the pelvic-abdominal area
- Inflammations in the pelvic-abdominal area

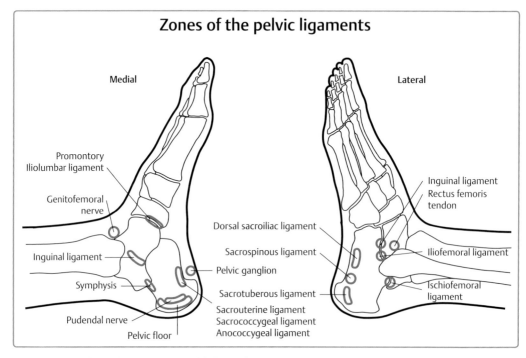

Fig. 27.1 Zones of the pelvic ligaments (modified according to W. Froneberg).

- Until approximately fourth month of pregnancy
- Extremely pronounced lymphatic congestion of the legs and feet (e.g., elephantiasis) and varicose veins which extend to the zones of the feet
- All other contraindications of the basic courses.

27.3

Treatment Technique

Location and performance of the treatment requires precise, practical instruction because although the technique resembles the sedating grip, it requires practice. Working with the correct angle in the direction of the periosteum is crucial for accurate treatment of the zones of the pelvic ligaments.

As the individual zones are usually located on the periosteum of the inner and outer heel, as a rule they are rather painful. An **affliction** is present if the pain in a zone lasts longer than about five seconds. The grip is maintained there until the intensity of the pain significantly recedes but not longer than approximately 15 to 20 seconds. Even if only isolated zones are painful, a brief examination of **all** the respective zones is indicated.

In **preparation** for treatment of the zones of the pelvic ligaments, the entire lesser pelvis and the lower spine including the sacrum and sacroiliac joint are treated with gentle grips to loosen them up. Usually, a choice of one or two stabilizing grips is also indicated for general tone regulation.

Depending on the symptoms, it also makes sense to include in treatment the zones of organs and systems pertaining to the patient's complaints, for example, the endocrine system in women with menstrual complaints and the upper spine including the neck in of headaches of various kinds and geneses.

28 Zones of the Face and Neck

28.1

General Information

A person's individuality is reflected particularly clearly in their face. Furthermore, facial diagnosis and pathophysiognomy provide detailed information. But the functional relationships between the individual face–neck zones and the whole organism can also be put to therapeutic use. They can be explained via various routes:

- Nervous system
- Development history
- Meridians
- Similarities in shape
- Empirical experiences and observations

Interrelationships are always involved: for example, a disease of the kidneys may affect the eyes while an eye disease may also affect the function of the kidneys.

28.2

The Relationships in Detail

The respective facial zones are shown in **Fig. 28.1**.

1. **Interrelationships** between the **eyes** and:
   - **Pancreas:** Deterioration of the retina is a known long-term effect in diabetics.
   - **Thyroid gland:** If the thyroid gland is hyperactive, an exophthalmus (significant protrusion of the eyeball) may develop.
   - **Kidneys:** Both the eyes and the kidneys are paired organs and are both found in the same FitzGerald longitudinal zones. Both are involved in the transport of fluids ("solutions").
   - **Liver** and **gall bladder:** Jaundice (transfer of bile components into the blood and into other body tissue) can be identified earliest in the sclera as a result of the white background of the conjunctiva.
   - **Neck:** Muscular tensions are relatively common in severely visually impaired individuals. With whiplash injuries in the region of the cervical spine, the eyes are also adversely affected. Neurophysiological: when tired, the eyelids close and the person "nods off."

   - **Stomach:** The eyes "eat too," that is, the secretion of saliva and gastric juices are coordinated in their reactions. The stomach meridian supplies the eyes, among other things, and ends in the zones of the eyes on the feet.
   - **Inner ear** and eyes jointly enable the coordination of movement (balance). Both develop from the same germ layer (ectoderm).

2. **Interrelationships** between **eyebrows** and **bladder meridian**: Its first point is located medially on both eyebrows. In its course to the little toes, it supplies, among other areas, the back muscles, kidneys, bladder, organs of the lesser pelvis, and the dorsal regions of the legs with its energy.

3. **Interrelationships** between the **mouth** and **nasopharyngeal space** and:
   - **Bladder–genital area:** The mucous membrane develops from the same germ layer respectively (entoderm).
   - **Abdominal organs:** Changes in the mucous membrane in the genital area (e.g., in pregnancy) are accompanied by physiological and pathological changes in the mouth and nasopharynx.
   - **Metabolic system:** Thrush in the oral cavity and herpes on the lips can arise as a result of bacterial disturbance in the intestine.

4. **Interrelationships** between the **lips** and:
   - **Sphincters:** Infants with teething problems are sore around the anus. Hurried drinking with pyloric spasm, etc.
   - **Cervix:** The tonus of the lips and cervix is coordinated—frequent confirmation as a result of observations by midwives.
   - **Digestive organs:** Dry, very wrinkled and chapped lips, rhagades, and herpes labialis often occur with gastrointestinal problems.

5. **Interrelationships** between **vocal cords** and **genitals:**
   - **Voice** and mood changes are associated with pregnancy, the monthly cycle, puberty ("breaking of the voice"), and the menopause. Famous singers are allowed to rest their voice during menstruation.

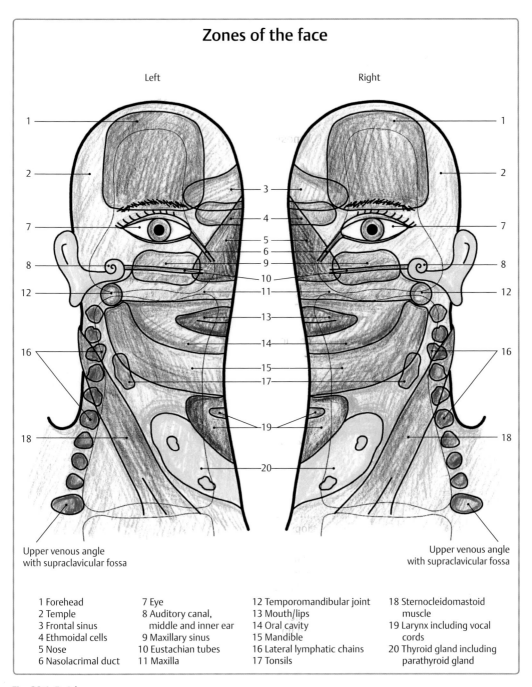

Zones of the face

Left

Right

Upper venous angle with supraclavicular fossa

Upper venous angle with supraclavicular fossa

1 Forehead	7 Eye	12 Temporomandibular joint	18 Sternocleidomastoid
2 Temple	8 Auditory canal,	13 Mouth/lips	muscle
3 Frontal sinus	middle and inner ear	14 Oral cavity	19 Larynx including vocal
4 Ethmoidal cells	9 Maxillary sinus	15 Mandible	cords
5 Nose	10 Eustachian tubes	16 Lateral lymphatic chains	20 Thyroid gland including
6 Nasolacrimal duct	11 Maxilla	17 Tonsils	parathyroid gland

Fig. 28.1 Facial zones.

- Abdominal disorders and operations may change the pitch and range of the voice.

6. **Interrelationships** between the **eustachian tubes and fallopian tubes or spermatic cord:**
   - Tissue structure, form and function are similar to the Eustachian tubes.

7. **Interrelationships** between the **temporomandibular joint** and:
   - **Hip joint:** Both the temporomandibular and the hip joint are supplied by the gall bladder meridian. Hip patients have relatively frequent gall bladder disorders and vice versa. **Similarity in shape** between the jaw and hip joint (**Fig. 21.5**).
   - **Autonomic nervous system:** The temporomandibar joint and the assigned muscles are frequently tense if there are emotional difficulties.

8. **Interrelationships** between **ears** and:
   - **Intestine:** Germ layer connection—the entoderm forms the epithelium of the tympanic cavity and the gastrointestinal tract.
   - The **small intestine meridian** ends at the earlobe.
   - **Genitals:** The pinna and the gonads both develop from the mesoderm. Ears belong to the erogenous zones. With mumps, complications may occur in the form of orchitis (testicle inflammation) and sterility.
   - **Kidneys:** The ears and kidneys are paired, both are partner organs. Both develop from the mesoderm.
   - **Tonsils:** They are directly adjacent to the ears and they also perform their filter function for the ear region. Both the ears and tonsils develop from the ectoderm.

9. **Interrelationships** between the **teeth and digestive tract:**
   - Here, after the comminution of food, **digestion** starts—the salivary enzyme ptyalin brings about the preliminary digestion of carbohydrates.
   - **24 teeth** are assigned to the digestive tract by way of Voll's energetic measurements.
   - **Intestinal disorders** often arise in infants with teething problems.
   - **Emotional state:** We describe problems which we have difficulty "digesting" as being "hard to get your teeth into."

10. **Interrelationships** between the **thyroid gland** and:
    - **Genitals:** In holistic therapies the thyroid gland is referred to as the "third ovary." In girls and women thyroid problems are common in puberty and the menopause.
    - **Heart:** Thyroid hormones influence, among other things, cardiac rhythm (paroxysmal tachycardia).
    - **Eyes:** Hyperfunction of the thyroid gland, see above.
    - **Seventh cervical vertebra:** Connective tissue thickening in this region, so-called "dowager's hump," is well-known after major abdominal operations—it also occurs in the menopause.
    - **All the endocrine glands:** They are interrelated.

11. **Interrelationships** between **tonsils** and:
    - **Ears:** Filter function of the tonsils, see above.
    - **Kidneys:** Both are paired organs, both have filter functions and are similar in shape.
    - **Joints:** Chronically inflamed tonsils may be involved in the development of rheumatic (and other) diseases.
    - **Heart:** Bacterial tonsillitis may result in myocarditis.
    - **Liver:** Both develop from the same germ layer (entoderm), both are important organs of detoxification.

Treatment method: Usually the index finger is the most suitable for selective treatment of these zones. With lymph congestion in the region of the face and neck, alternating stroking movements from RTF lymphatic treatment lend themselves.

Use of the zones of the face: For a better understanding, as already described in Chapter 10.2.3, the zones of the head and neck can all be treated on the plantar, dorsal, medial, and lateral sides of all the toes. However, in **Figs. 10.2** and **10.3** the zones of the face are only treated **generally** on both the big toes.

They are not shown extensively and **in detail** until this chapter and in **Fig. 28.1** because the localization of all the zones of the face in a concentrated form on both the big toes has only been achieved through decades of practical experience. It may perhaps be understood in the sense of a microsystem reduced still further in size.

In **everyday practice** the following applies:

- The detailed zones of the face on the big toes simplify **initial assessment** because all the zones can be checked in a short time on the small surface.
- In the course of **follow-up treatment**, however, it is important that the afflicted zones in the region of all the other toes are also treated at the same time.
- Experience shows, for example, that both the zones of the ears on both big toes as well as those on fourth and fifth toes frequently require treatment.
- Of particular therapeutic interest are the **functional relationships** mentioned in this chapter which can be produced between the zones of the face and many of the person's organs. They enable comprehensive treatment of the patient's complaints.

From My Practice

In the late 1970s three patients came to me for treatment within the space of a few weeks, whose lacrimal fluid was only able to drain negligibly into the nasopharyngeal space via the tear duct any longer. Two women were suffering from chronic inflammations and allergies in the head region while, in the third patient, all their facial bones had been smashed as a result of a serious accident.

As E. Ingham had already established the existence of the zones of the forehead on the nails of the big toes as well as those of the nasopharyngeal space, my idea was that it might be possible to locate the zones of the tear duct precisely. Palpation revealed a millimeter-sized, hard and very painful swelling proximal to the nails (= part of the nasopharyngeal space) in the two women. In the third patient, the region was highly sensitive over a wide area.

To the extent that, in the course of several treatment sessions the hard thickening of tissue was reduced in both the female patients, the secretions found their normal route inward again. In the third patient, the lacrimal fluid continued to drain outward but he had significantly less facial pain. In addition to the symptomatic zones, other zones were also included in all the patients' treatment and in particular, frequent stabilizing grips were necessary.

From this impressive experience, together with the experiences of therapists and course participants, today's detailed facial zones were developed.

29 Zones of the Lymphatic System

General Information

*Just as it is not possible to learn an instrument by reading about it, learning about the specific therapy for the zones of the lymphatic system cannot be done simply by reading either.
To really be able to work with this therapy, "head" knowledge must be transformed into practical, "hand" knowledge by means of practical training and experience.*

In my opinion, the emergence of the specific zones of the lymphatic system nowadays is one of the **principal developments** in reflexotherapy of the feet (RTF). Experience of previous decades had shown that increasingly we could rely on the feet as a "self-image of the whole person," making extraordinarily precise treatment possible.

Thus, it was only logical for me to also start trying to assign the flow system of the lymphatics to the corresponding areas on the feet as early as the mid-1980s. After a few years of personal experience, and observation of the effects in corresponding groups of patients, in 1993 the zones of the lymphatic system were officially included at all our training centers.

Admittedly, a few lymphatic zones had already been identified by W. FitzGerald and E. Ingham: the tonsils, appendix, spleen, and lymphatic areas of the inguinal region. But it was evident that the selective treatment technique developed hitherto would have to be changed in order to do justice to the principle of the lymphatic system in its entirety. Thus, a **new treatment technique** with gentle, targeted stroking movements guided by the physiological direction of flow of the lymph was developed.

Of interest: When it is considered that all the organs apart from the brain are supplied with lymphatic vessels, it is understandable that even **before** comprehensive lymphatic treatment we also achieved good results with traditional RTF, above all, in patients with **general** lymphatic disorders. Nonetheless, it has been demonstrated that the results with the new way of treating the lymphatic system **selectively** have been significantly improved for specific **lymphatic indications**.

Advantages of RTF Lymphatic Treatment

- It is **not painful**. Nowadays, an increasing number of patients come for treatment who, for a variety of reasons, are unable to tolerate pain any more. They discover with relief how the gentle, stroking quality of RTF lymphatic treatment can set stagnating processes in motion again.
- It has a significant impact on an **emotional level**. Although initially the positive effects were more evident on the physical level, it soon became clear that patients were also more stable emotionally. (Tip: another word for fluid is solution. As lymph is also a fluid, the double meaning of the word "solutions" confirms our decades of experience.)
- It can be combined with **manual lymphatic drainage**, both during treatment and on an alternating basis during a course of treatment.
- It is **economical in terms of time** because the treatment is concentrated on the small surface area of the feet.

Indications and Contraindications

The following are **indicated**:
- Lymphatic diseases of all kinds, also postoperatively
- Chronic infections of the sinus cavities and ears
- Allergies, in particular, in children, general lowered resistance
- All skeletomuscular afflictions, restricted movement of the joints (apart from in the acute stage of inflammation)
- Sports injuries of various kinds, accident after-care
- Insufficiencies in the transport of various body fluids, for example, congested veins, circulatory disorders, reduced diuresis, premenstrual syndrome, lactation difficulties in nursing mothers, etc.
- Chronic diseases such as multiple sclerosis, Parkinson's disease, apoplexy

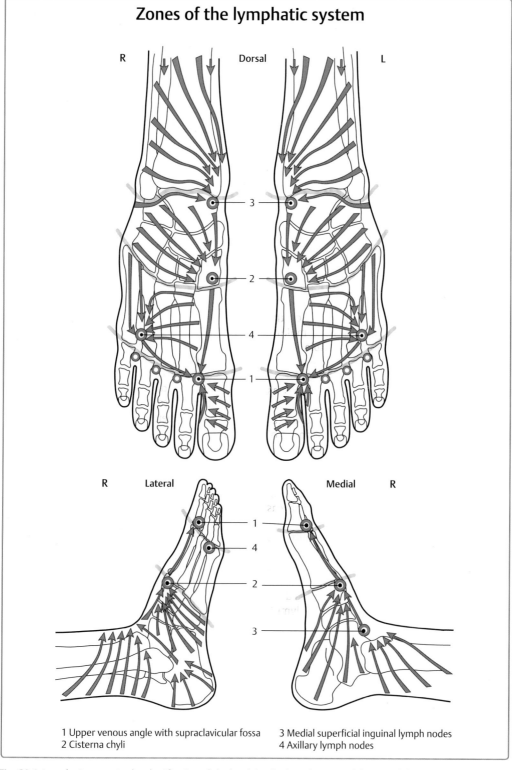

Zones of the lymphatic system

1 Upper venous angle with supraclavicular fossa
2 Cisterna chyli
3 Medial superficial inguinal lymph nodes
4 Axillary lymph nodes

Fig. 29.1 Lymphatic zones in the classification of the head (neck, thorax), upper abdomen, abdominal area (pelvis, and thigh to knee).

- Psychovegetative irritations such as restlessness, depression
- Problems falling asleep and sleeping through the night, hyperactivity, ADHD in children and adults
- Pregnancy-related problems of various kinds from approximately the fourth month, including emotional instability
- Support during fasting and detoxification cures and holistic dental restoration to assist the release of toxins
- Care at the end of life as a short treatment providing relief.

The following are **contraindicated**:
- Severe infections (e.g., high-fever viral influenza, acute tonsillitis, acute hepatitis)
- Inflammations in the lymphatic and venous systems such as lymphangitis and phlebitis
- Phlegmons (diffuse inflammation in the connective tissue with local, severe signs of inflammation)
- Cardiac edema and other serious heart disease
- Degenerative kidney diseases, pulmonary emphysema
- Chronic high blood pressure of unknown origin, above all, in the elderly.

In addition, all the contraindications described in Chapter 5.2 are applicable.

29.4

Practical Application of RTF Lymphatic Treatment

The three parts of RTF lymphatic treatment:
1. **Preparation:** It is performed in the zones which are in direct contact with the lymphatic system:
   - Urinary tract
   - Intestine, liver
   - Spleen, heart
   - Thymus

The zones are tonified with the well-known grips. Preparation is completed by one or two stabilizing grips because the lymph achieves equilibrium more readily if the autonomic nervous system is stable.
2. **Targeted treatment in the lymphatic zones:**
   We distinguish two different grip techniques:
   - The treatment of the areas of the four **collecting vessels**: Upper venous angle on the supraclavicular fossa, cisterna chyli,

medial inguinal lymph nodes, and axillary lymph nodes. They are treated selectively with gentle circular movements leading deep into the tissue in order to ensure the drainage of lymph at these central points.
   - Treatment of the **lymph vessels** in their direction of flow: this is performed with so-called "alternating stroking movements": the flat fingertip of one hand gently strokes along the specified path toward the assigned collecting vessel. Before it finishes stroking, the fingertip of the other hand follows the same path in order to evenly stimulate the flow of lymph. Depending on the size of the area for treatment and the patient's feet, two or three fingertips are used. The whole RTF lymphatic treatment is divided into **five groups of zones**:
     - Head and neck
     - Thorax and upper abdomen
     - Abdominal area and pelvis
     - Inguinal area and gluteal muscles
     - Thigh to knee.

Each alternating stroking movement is repeated in the corresponding zone until any tissue congestion present has improved. Usually four or five stroking movements are sufficient—depending on the findings sometimes fewer, sometimes more, are required. Improvement is demonstrated by the fingertips being able to stroke through the tissue in a uniform flow and without interruption. After each group, the assigned collecting vessels must be treated again. To make the **transition** to the next group of zones, the zones of the heart, kidneys, and intestine are tonified, respectively.
3. The **conclusion** follows the same pattern as preparation. **Subsequent rest** to initiate the regenerative process is particularly important, likewise increased fluid intake—preferably water or a light herbal infusion.

29.5

Possible Reactions

Although RTF lymphatic treatment is performed gently, the possible occurrence of **stronger reactions** should not be underestimated. They always relate to the background to the disease and the patient's capacity for regeneration. All the usual reactions of the autonomic nervous system, as listed in Chapter 4.2, also apply here.

a) Special reactions **during** lymphatic treatment:
- Pressure and congestion on the sternum, heart, head and neck
- Eye pressure, dry or burning eyes, in particular, in allergy sufferers
- Reduced salivation, dry mouth
- Persistent dizziness when lying down or standing up
- Temporary nausea emanating from the stomach or circulatory system
- Restlessness
- Increased pressure in the kidney region

Dealing with reactions during lymphatic treatment:
- Tonifying of the zone of the heart for better absorption of lymphatic fluid into the bloodstream and/or
- Slight tonification of the zones of the kidneys, which are almost identical to the zones of the suprarenals (adrenaline release) and/or
- Inclusion of a stabilizing or Eutonic grip and/or
- Treatment of the zone of the solar plexus (Chapter 10.8.4)
- Ample subsequent rest and encouragement to increase fluid intake

One or two of the suggested grips is sufficient.

b) **Reactions during treatment intervals:**
- Increased diuresis. During the initial treatment sessions additional slight congestion may also occur temporarily but will ease as treatment progresses.
- Less fluid retention in the hands and arms, feet and legs as well as in the trunk, for example, in patients with ascites. These are indications that metabolic processes are being stimulated.
- Pronounced sensation of thirst, from time to time a healthy appetite as well.
- Increased positive attitude to life as an indication of psychovegetative harmonization.

- More vivid dreams as a sign that current life issues are appearing by way of internal images.
- Copious yawning points to a profound resolution of tensions, distress can be relieved. At the same time, breathing becomes deeper and calmer.
- Borborygmus ("grumbling" noises in the intestines) as an indicator that subconscious or suppressed emotional blocks are being released.

In lymphedema in the extremities, for example, in women after a mastectomy or in severe congestion in the legs, **circumference measurements** should be performed at various points of the affected extremity in order to objectify the changes before, during, and after a course of RTF lymphatic treatments.

- Changes in skin texture: slacker or firmer tissue tone (e.g., in the face), reduced or sometimes temporarily increased itching, altered perspiration.

c) **Treatment duration and intervals:**
Average length of a **single** treatment session: 25 to 30 minutes. **Caution:** in severely weakened patients, initially 15 minutes suffice during which, in particular, the central collecting vessels are treated, combined with stabilizing grips. Stable patients may also be treated for longer depending on the indication. As a **course**, depending on the disease, 6 to 8 or 10 treatment sessions are indicated. Initially they are offered twice or three times a week while subsequently intervals may be extended to weekly, fortnightly, or once a month. In **long-term patients** it can clearly be observed when the retuning effect of RTF lymphatic treatment is declining. Treatment can be interspersed with manual lymphatic drainage or other appropriate treatment if need be.

After RTF lymphatic treatment, therapists should also increase their fluid intake and wash their hands thoroughly to **neutralize** themselves energetically before the next treatment starts.

30 Interrelationships between Zones of the Feet and Meridians

30.1

General Information

All the systems comprising a person, those which are visible and those which are invisible, are interactively linked. Their interaction ensures the harmonious operation of all the vital functions. Among many others, the energetic principles of the meridians and the zones of the feet may also be combined.

There is a therapeutic **"bridge"** between the two methods. Approximately a quarter to a third of the life force which flows in a meridian is also available to the organ or tissue after which it is named. As there are organ zones on the feet for most of the names of the meridians, where there is strain these zones can be treated at the same time.

30.2

What Are Meridians?

The term meridian comes from Chinese Medicine and denotes specific paths of an energetic flow system which runs through the person. The acupuncture points are arranged on them. The principle is comparable to an underground railway network in which these points correspond to the underground stations. **Dr. Reinhold Voll** was one of the first people to measure this energy using an electroacupuncture device (EAV) he developed in the middle of the last century.

The flow of energy in the meridians forms a dynamic cycle which is known as the **"Chinese organ clock."** Within a 24-hour period, each of the 12 main meridians is active for 2 hours and in a recovery phase for the same time. After the two-hour peak period of the meridian, it transfers its energy to the next meridian. After 24 hours the cycle begins again.

The **12 main meridians** are arranged in pairs and run symmetrically to the midline. Six meridians are each assigned to the Yin and Yang principle. Both these complementary "forces of the universe" were already known in the natural philosophy of ancient China and are roughly comparable to the functions of the sympathetic and parasympathetic nervous system.

The **Yin meridians** are the kidney, liver, and spleen–pancreas meridians and supply their energy ventrally from the feet into the trunk. In **Fig. 30.1** they are marked in blue. The **Yang meridians** are the bladder, gall bladder, and stomach meridians and their energy flows from the head to the feet. They are marked in red in the diagram.

In addition to the 12 main meridians, there is a meridian in the anterior and posterior vertical median line respectively: the anterior central Yin meridian is called the **Conception vessel** while the mainly posterior central Yang meridian is called the **Governing vessel**. Together they form an ellipse which, among others, W. Penzel has described as a "Small energy cycle" (Chapter 6).

In connection with reflexotherapy of the feet (RTF), only the meridians which affect the **feet** are discussed accordingly. They are also paired there.

30.3

Practical Application

Three Yin and three Yang meridian pairs also supply the feet in situ (**Fig. 30.1**). Therefore with presumed afflictions in the **zones**, knowledge about the path of the **meridians** should be included at the same time.

Examples:

1. **Yin Meridians:**
The **kidney meridian** passes through, inter alia, the zones of the organs of the lesser pelvis on the medial side of the heel. Swelling, significant cold or warmth, spider veins, or pain at these points may therefore also be seen as energy flow disturbances in the kidney meridian. Therapeutic consequence: check the **zone** of the kidneys and if affected include in treatment.

Spleen–**pancreas** and **liver meridians** start medially and laterally on the nail of the big toe. Scars such as those which arise, for example, during surgical removal of a nail or a Hallux valgus operation may disturb the energy flow of both these meridians. The three organ **zones** concerned are examined and included in the treatment if affected.

The aforementioned **three Yin meridians** intersect approximately four finger-widths above

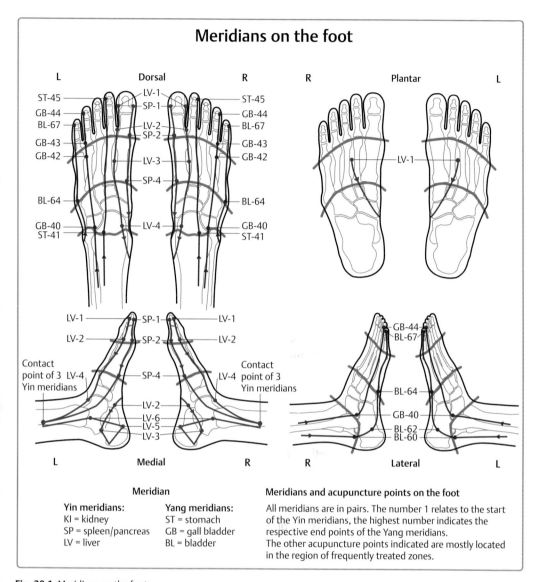

Meridians on the foot

Meridian

Yin meridians:
KI = kidney
SP = spleen/pancreas
LV = liver

Yang meridians:
ST = stomach
GB = gall bladder
BL = bladder

Meridians and acupuncture points on the foot

All meridians are in pairs. The number 1 relates to the start of the Yin meridians, the highest number indicates the respective end points of the Yang meridians.
The other acupuncture points indicated are mostly located in the region of frequently treated zones.

Fig. 30.1 Meridians on the foot.

the inner malleolus. If congestion, pain, changes in temperature, varicosis and/or a crural ulcer (ulcus cruris) occur here, this indicates weaknesses in the metabolic system. The four **zones** of the kidneys, spleen, pancreas, and liver are included in the treatment if affected.

2. **Yang Meridians:**
Toward its end, the **bladder meridian** runs laterally/dorsally on the foot to the nail of the fifth toe. If swelling and/or scars are present in the **posterior,** external malleolus region, as well as marked deformities of the little toe, this may indicate a weakness in this meridian. The zone of the bladder is therefore examined and included in the treatment if affected.

The **gall bladder meridian** ends on the nail of the fourth toe. With congestion, scars, and injuries around the **anterior** part of the outer malleolus and/or disorders of the fourth toe, the **zone** of the gall bladder should be examined and included in the treatment, if painful.

The **stomach meridian** runs to the second toe. As a result of its rather often marked length, it is the most frequently affected by the orthopedic deformity of hammer toes. If disturbances of this kind are observed, it is useful to examine the **zone** of the stomach and include it in the treatment if affected.

30.4

Meridian Afflictions in situ

The aforementioned relates to energy flow disturbances of the meridians in the region of the **feet**. When considering the therapeutic "bridge"

between both systems, however, with knowledge of the meridians, afflictions over the **entire** path of the meridians must also be considered. Scars, inflammation, or static-muscular deformities, for example, frequently cause disturbances of all kinds there.

Examples:

- The **gall bladder meridian** supplies energy to five joint regions in the **lateral** part of the body: the temporomandibular, shoulder, hip, knee joint, and outer malleolus. With disturbances at any point in the path of this meridian, for example, as a result of scars from operations and/or accidents, apart from the zones of the joints, those of the gall bladder must also be examined and, if necessary, included in treatment.
- The meridian connections are particularly relevant in patients with **knee complaints**. When it is considered that three Yin and three Yang meridians respectively supply the knee with their energy, this results in the possibility of including all seven organs, the names of which the meridians bear, as **zones of the feet** in the treatment.
- Furthermore, relationships to the microsystem of the **teeth** can be established both from the meridians and the zones of the feet. **Example:** The bladder meridian supplies the sacroiliac joint with its energy **in situ**; the wisdom teeth, inter alia, interact energetically with the sacroiliac joint (measurements according to Dr. Voll). As the sacroiliac joint **and** the wisdom teeth and their energetic relationships can be treated with RTF, this produces another possible combination of interest.

31 Shared Practical Experience

The following brief descriptions of treatment processes for reflexotherapy of the feet (RTF) are excerpts from well over 1,500 reports, which course participants have kindly been sending us for decades. They have proved their worth as a practical "reference work" in day-to-day RTF treatment.

Here are a few examples, each from **23 indications**, in part somewhat abridged.

> Here too, as mentioned in Chapter 21, individual practical experience cannot automatically be transferred to patients simply on the basis of their symptoms. Although symptoms may be the same, or similar, we have to realize that the background against which they developed differs, always depending on a patient's **personal** medical history, and any treatment should reflect this.

31.1

Management and Treatment of Pain in Acute Situations

31.1.1 Threatening Ileus

I work at a rehabilitation clinic for metabolic disorders and colorectal cancer aftercare.

An 82-year-old male patient with colorectal cancer had suffered severe spasms with pain and vomiting for 1 day. Medical diagnosis: Incipient ileus. Infusions, enemas and medication brought no relief.

Treatment: Relatively strong tonifying in the symptomatic zone of the intestine for approximately 10 minutes, stabilizing grips.

Result: After an hour the patient had a bowel movement. He and his wife were very relieved because this meant that he did not have to be transferred to another hospital.

31.1.2 Restricted Mobility of the Left Shoulder Joint

Apart from the above complaint, the 43-year-old female patient had inflammatory changes in the sternoclavicular articulation and was in great pain.

Preliminary treatment: Ten weeks of psychotherapy, 12 PNF (proprioceptive neuromuscular facilitation) treatment sessions, and leeches, as a result of which the complaints had eased somewhat but by no means disappeared.

Treated zones: Sternoclavicular articulation and shoulder girdle, frequent stabilizing grips as the zones were very painful. Patient mentioned in passing that she had had a capsular injury involving her left second toe a few years ago (zone of the sternoclavicular articulation). As a result, I sedated this area carefully and treated the aforementioned zones again gently and softly.

Result: To our surprise and joy, her left shoulder was free of pain and as mobile as her right shoulder immediately after RTF.

Interesting point: Furthermore, the stomach meridian which, among other things also supplies the sternoclavicular articulation with its energy, ends at the second toe.

31.1.3 Acute Tonsillitis

A 14-year-old girl, diagnosed with acute tonsillitis by an ENT specialist. Antibiotics were prescribed but not taken.

Treated zones: Approximately 30 minutes' treatment of the intestine, lymphatics of head, neck, and thorax. Frequent stabilizing grips which relaxed the girl wonderfully.

Reactions: Patient is very tired, sleeps deeply in broad daylight. Footbath in the evening with bath salts, deep sleep again throughout the night.

Result: The next morning her sore throat had gone, she was even able to take part in a class test and felt completely well again.

31.2

Skeletomuscular Diseases

31.2.1 Ischialgia

A 31-year-old neighbor had given birth 2 months previously. Severe back pain radiating into the buttocks, hip, and thigh for the last 5 days. Analgesics and manual forms of therapy without effect.

Treated zones: Three days in succession: lower spine and pelvic ligaments, shoulder girdle. Lymphatics of head/neck and pelvis/thigh. Frequent stabilizing grips, in particular, heel stretching grip to stabilize the autonomic nervous system.

Result: The woman was symptom-free afterward. Repetition of RTF for the same complaints a year later. The next day the pain had already eased by 70%.

31.2.2 Bursitis of Left Elbow

A 62-year-old male patient, athletic, slim, used a computer for his work, right-handed. During treatment of a ganglion on the right wrist, he was advised to operate the computer mouse with his **left** hand.

Treated zones: Both elbows (interestingly the symptomatic zone was inconspicuous), shoulder, temporomandibular and hip joints, excretory organs, and heart. Lymphatic treatment every second RTF session, many stabilizing grips. At the point at which the bladder meridian runs through the elbow **zone**, tonified particularly vigorously on both sides.

Reactions and outcome: Patient has a "cold" after the third RTF session but does not feel ill. After the fourth RTF session brief swelling on the **right** elbow; increased and significantly darker urine, although he had not increased his fluid intake. After seven RTF sessions all the symptoms have disappeared.

31.2.3 Severe Pain in Thigh and Hip on Right Side

A 65-year-old female patient with total hip replacement on both sides, various knee operations and scoliosis. Presented with severe pain in the right thigh and hip. Mood swings.

Conspicuous and treated zones: Hip joint, thigh, knee, bony and muscular pelvis, as well as pelvic ligaments and lateral abdominal muscles and entire spine. Inguinal region, intestine, and kidneys/bladder. Alternate tonifying and sedating grips. Six RTF sessions, twice a week.

Result: The patient is free of pain at the end of the course of treatment and can walk for long distances again. This is also emotionally beneficial for her. She is delighted with the result because she had not believed she could be helped further after having resorted to many options in orthodox medicine. It was a great pleasure for me to see her radiant smile!

31.3

Sports Injuries

31.3.1 Calcaneal Fracture after Accident

A 47-year-old male athlete, complicated calcaneal fracture a year ago, underwent several subsequent operations due to repeated infections. Transfer of the microsystem to the macrosystem:

First treatment on pelvis and buttocks in situ at the points corresponding to the injury of the heel (= **zone** of the pelvis). Tonified relatively vigorously.

Visual inspection: 17 cm long accident scar on the lateral calcaneal border above the ankle (in the pathway of the bladder meridian), elevated and not painful. The whole foot is bluish and swollen.

Zones treated subsequently: Pelvic ligaments, lower spine, bladder, associated teeth, shoulder/nape of the neck with sedating or tonifying grips depending on the quality of the pain. Surprisingly, RTF lymphatic treatment does not alleviate congestion at all.

Therapy homework: Rub cream into the scar daily, treat contralaterally on the other foot, and ensure wrist on same side is well supplied with blood using tonifying grips.

Result: After third RTF session, no more "warm-up" pain when walking, which he had not reported initially. Foot significantly softer, barely congested any more, no longer blue. Patient cycles to work again after having been incapable of work for a year.

31.3.2 Fall during the Tour de France, Fracture of the Clavicle

In addition, hairline fracture on the scapula. Operation including fixation, titanium plate, start of RTF during rehabilitation.

Treated zones: In addition to the symptoms of the pelvic ligaments, spine, intestine, urinary tract, and genitals. Gall bladder and bladder meridian on the feet very painful. Subsequent RTF scar treatment.

Result: Elevation, retroversion, abduction, adduction significantly improved. Better kidney and intestinal function, deeper, more restful sleep, less muscular pain, patient also feels mentally fortified.

General observations: I look after athletes during the Tour de France. Complete relaxation, normalization of adrenaline levels, beneficial warmth in the legs, and longer respiratory phases in a very short time as a result of RTF. Highly positive RTF experience both while preparing for and during the Tour de France.

Apart from osteopathy and manual lymphatic drainage, the professionals would not want to be without RTF. I have the full support of the team physician.

31.4

Diseases of the Digestive Tract

31.4.1 Diverticulitis

General experience with four patients: all four had stomach and back pain, flatulence, diarrhea, and bloating. In all four the symptoms had already eased significantly after the first RTF session.

Treated zones: The entire digestive tract, head, neck, lower spine, and pelvic ligaments were always greatly affected. Frequent stabilizing grips. Duration of individual treatment changed.

Result: Symptoms largely disappeared in all four patients. The symptoms were usually triggered by psychological problems. RTF for each patient was always accompanied by a change of diet.

31.4.2 Hemorrhoids and Constipation

A 40-year-old male patient presented to us at the hospital with hemorrhoids and constipation.

Treatment process: Treatment of the intestinal zones was unpleasant for him and also changed nothing. As the patient was subject to a heavy workload, I treated the zones of his head ("digestion" is not simply a physical process!)

Reactions: The patient heaved a sigh of relief during the very first RTF session, his digestion began working, and the symptoms of his hemorrhoids eased. A subsequent return to the zones of the digestive organs was of no benefit to him either, and so I mainly focused on the zones of the head and stabilizing grips.

31.4.3 Digestive Complaints

A 24-year-old female patient had had only one bowel movement a week since childhood, despite a healthy diet. Started RTF 4 months after the birth of her child.

First RTF: Cautious tonifying of the zones of the digestive organs and frequent stabilizing grips. Two days later: from then on, regular bowel movements every day. **Second RTF** 1 week later somewhat more vigorous.

Reaction: Bilious attack—the first in her life—with elimination of a stone of which she had been completely unaware. A medical examination revealed more gall stones, an operation was recommended but she declined as she was still nursing.

Personal observation: To my great relief, the patient did not view the bilious attack in a negative light but as the solution to her long-standing bowel movement issues.

31.5

Diseases of the Urinary Tract

31.5.1 Recurrent Bladder Infections, Backache

Active 75-year-old woman had had bladder infections at intervals for 20 years. Appeared tense, unable to settle down. Scars on left hip, operation in the lower abdomen. Hemorrhoids. Had treatment every 7 to 14 days for 9 months, also for other complaints.

Treated zones: Lymphatic system, urinary tract, lower spine, intestine, all sphincters. RTF scar treatment.

Reactions: Physical: temporary sensations of stimuli in bladder, stomach, rectum, and back. Eyes and nose "start streaming," more restful sleep. Emotional: grief, crying, rage, sometimes talks a lot during the treatment sessions. During lymphatic RTF she calms down completely; she finds that sphincter treatment clearly invigorates her.

Result: "I finally have the strength to clear up my house, my desk, and my life." The bladder makes its presence known from time to time in an attenuated form, back problems significantly improved.

31.5.2 Urethral Calculus on Right Side

A 51-year-old widow, depressed since her husband's death, very attached to her only son. Came for treatment because of renal gravel and urethral calculus.

Initial findings: Very tense overall, but feet feel as though they have "no energy." Extremely painful: bladder, ureter, right kidney, organs of the lesser pelvis.

Treated zones: Frequent stabilizing grips, lower spine. Frequent, vigorous stroking of ureter in the direction of the bladder. Pelvic ligaments. Subsequently the head, endocrine system, and parts of RTF lymphatic treatment.

Reactions: Urine becomes darker. Painless elimination of the urethral calculus after second RTF session. Patient is much more stable and relaxed since then, she continues to come for treatment at long intervals and says: "I simply need it."

31.6

Respiratory Disorders

31.6.1 Status after Pneumonia

A 65-year-old female patient presented with respiratory problems after severe pneumonia. She was listless and weak. High blood pressure. On cortisone and cardiovascular medication.

Initial findings and treated zones: Thorax, including the shoulder girdle, neck and stomach, pancreas, hips, sacroiliac joint, pelvic ligaments and left knee. Frequent stabilizing grips. Patient needs to talk a lot as she lives alone.

Reactions: Lung problems have become more acute with coughing and yellow-green expectoration. Profuse sweating, diarrhea. After third RTF, temporary earache; after seventh RTF, tooth 43 becomes painful and patient undergoes root canal treatment. Nine RTF sessions, once a week initially and then every 14 days.

Result: After the fourth RTF session the lung complaints had resolved, her blood pressure was normal at the end of the course and she was able to stop taking cortisone after consulting her doctor.

Personal observation: The patient was sent by her daughter and was highly skeptical initially but the course of treatment and the results of RTF convinced her.

31.6.2 Chronically Blocked Nose

For years a 58-year-old female neighbor had had a blocked nose with an extremely nasal voice for hours every morning. As a result of RTF training I learned that the nose could be cleared by tonifying the lymphatics of the neck.

Treated zones the very next day: Repeated gentle tonifying of the lateral lymphatics, intestine, lung, spleen, heart, lesser pelvis and spine. Stabilizing grips.

Reactions and outcome: During the first RTF session the woman was already able to breathe more easily. Copious secretion of mucus from the nose the following morning. Four further treatment sessions followed, after which the cervical lymph nodes were no longer painful and the nose remained clear—this has been stable for 3 years.

31.7

Headaches

31.7.1 Headaches since Childhood

A 22-year- old female patient, pale, lifeless facial expression, dull eyes.

Affected zones: All the areas of the head, in particular the base of the skull, neck, shoulder girdle, spine and sacrum/sacroiliac joint, pelvic floor and pelvic ligaments.

Begin treatment sedatingly from the pelvis (counterpart) in the direction of the head, RTF lymphatic treatments. Additional zones of the head–neck area later.

Reactions: After first RTF session significant relaxation; after second RTF session, 2 days without headaches, loosening of the neck and shoulder muscles. Localization of the headache changes. Fifth RTF: posture and gait are full of vigor, the eyes sparkle. After eighth treatment session, hissing and "peeping" in the head due to stress at work which eased significantly with sedation of the head–neck zone.

Result: After 11 RTF sessions, symptoms almost gone. The patient would like another course of treatment in a few months' time. Feldenkrais recommended to compensate for the imbalance in the musculoskeletal system.

Personal observation: I am extremely irritated that patients with headaches are only given medication usually, despite there being so many alternatives.

31.7.2 Migraine

A 53-year-old male patient had weekly migraines, pain from the eye to the neck, accompanied by vomiting. Problems in the cervical and lumbar spine, sensitive stomach with heartburn and diarrhea. Various small scars.

Treated zones: Head sedated, stomach/intestine, spleen and lumbar spine tonified. Two lymph treatments. Sphincters. Frequent stabilizing grips; in particular, solar plexus.

Reactions: Headaches become more acute briefly, digestion of more solid consistency. Bouts of coughing with mucus, streaming eyes. Increased stomach complaints "as if the heart is beating into the stomach."

Result: After the first treatment sessions hardly any more migraine attacks and after the sixth RTF session they have stopped completely. No further heartburn and diarrhea. Lower spine and shoulder-neck pain-free, patient feels "well all-round."

31.8

Gynecology

31.8.1 Hot flushes

A 66-year-old female patient had been suffering from severe hot flushes several times a day for 15 years, so severe that beads of sweat appeared on her skin. Usually had cold feet.

Treated zones: Twelve treatments involving excretory organs, endocrine system, shoulder girdle, head (in particular, the end phalanges of the toes) and RTF lymphatic treatment.

Result: After only the fourth RTF session, fewer hot flushes—at the end of the course of treatment they had stopped completely.

31.8.2 Amenorrhea

A 26-year-old patient had not had menstrual periods for 6 years despite taking the "pill" regularly.

Initial findings, treated zones: Organs of the lesser pelvis, colon, pancreas. Fifth metatarsal dorsal (pathway of bladder meridian). Second to fourth toes. Eutonic grips on the sacrum.

Reactions: Directly after the initial treatment, menstruation starts, coincidentally it occurs during the "pill break." Severe tension in the temporomandibular joint, neck ache, increased diuresis. Intense itching of the ears, symptoms of a cold, she is clearly aware of her wisdom teeth. Eight RTF sessions.

Result: Patient feels fine and would like to stop taking the "pill" after this course of treatment as she wishes to start a family. Six months later, and following another course of RTF, she is pregnant.

31.8.3 Cyst on the Left Ovary

My 26-year-old friend came to me because her gynecologist had found a 6-cm cyst during an ultrasound scan, which had to be surgically removed immediately. I offered her RTF in preparation for the operation.

Treated zones: A lot of stabilizing grips. Tonifying of the spine, heart, spleen, and intestine. In the left ovarian zone I palpated a small nodule of approximately 3 to 4 mm in size. As the site was very painful, I treated the pelvic ligaments thoroughly. During the lymphatic grips, tears came into her eyes, her stomach felt quite warm, and she fell asleep.

Reactions: During the night she had a temperature and pain similar to that during menstruation. She felt as if all her energy was focusing on one point. The next morning, the day of the operation, her mother firmly insisted on another ultrasound scan. The gynecologist consented reluctantly only to then quickly ascertain to his surprise that the cyst was no longer visible. As a precaution, he repeated the scan and obtained the same result.

Pregnancy and Birth

31.9.1 Preparation for the Birth

A 29-year-old primipara was expecting twins. She came to me as her midwife in the 25th week of pregnancy in a state of considerable anxiety because the ultrasound scan had revealed that one of the twins was not receiving an adequate supply of nutrients. Severe back pain, pulling in the abdomen, lacking sleep.

Treated zones: Initially only stabilizing grips—in particular, solar plexus—in order to stabilize the autonomic nervous system. Later: spine, sacroiliac joint, digestive organs, heart, thymus, and endocrine glands.

Reactions: During the first three treatments the woman fell asleep each time. In the course of further treatment all of her symptoms improved significantly. Another ultrasound scan revealed that the second baby was continuing to develop well according to dates. The petite woman already feels heavily pregnant and everything is becoming more difficult.

Water retention in the 31st week of pregnancy. Comprehensive RTF lymphatic treatments alternating with "merima" (= treatment of the meridians in the microsystem of the foot) twice a week until the birth results in good diuresis.

In the 35th week of pregnancy, stagnation of weight gain in the second twin. In the 37th week of pregnancy gynecologist recommends delivering the babies by cesarian section because the smaller twin was lying lower in the pelvis and would therefore be the first to have to undertake the intensive work of birth.

Finally: The babies were well and did not have to go to the pediatric clinic. They were allowed to go home with their mother on the third day (unusual). They were fully breast-fed, not something which is taken for granted with cesarian deliveries.

31.9.2 Urinary Retention in 9th Week of Pregnancy

A primiparous 39-year-old woman was admitted to hospital because of urinary retention; she already had a urinary catheter. The patient was to stay in hospital for 2 to 3 days only, if possible. Our doctor agreed with the decision to try RTF.

Patient details: Afraid to go to the toilet, thinks the baby might fall out. No bowel movements for several days, seems "normal" for her.

Treated zones: Frequent stabilizing grips, in particular, the solar plexus. Gentle tonifying of pituitary gland, urinary tract, intestine, and finally, lymphatic grips. The patient relaxed well, became more open during the treatment and was able to talk about her fears.

Reactions: The woman lay in bed without a catheter the next day after being able to pass water freely; she had already had a bowel movement on the day of RTF and requested a second treatment of her feet. The focus was on the zones of the urinary tract, intestine and, for somewhat longer, the lymphatic regions. The next day she was discharged free of symptoms.

31.9.3 Induction of Labor via the Feet

A 27-year-old friend's baby was thought to be three days overdue. The doctor recommended a cesarian section as her pelvis was too narrow. At the second clinic a decision was taken that labor was to be induced the following day and she was only to have a cesarian section in an emergency.

This friend asked for RTF in preparation. She was slightly nervous as it was her first delivery. Had quite "virginal," soft feet, which quickly become moist. Reacted very well to the heel stretching grip for the autonomic nervous system.

Treated zones: Gentle tonifying grips on abdominal muscles. Sedation on the solar plexus and pelvic floor very pleasant. Tonifying of the spine, sacrum, symphysis, hip joints, shoulder girdle, endocrine system, intestine, and uterus. Particularly painful in the pelvic ligaments: the genitofemoral nerve and posterior sacroiliac ligament. Duration of treatment, including a lot of stabilizing grips, around one hour.

Result: The next day I am delighted to hear that it was possible for Timo to be delivered naturally during the night.

31.10

Treatment of Infants

31.10.1 Experiences in the Premature Baby Intensive Care Unit

Midwife's report: In our unit we look after premature babies from the 28th week of pregnancy onward, usual birth weight approx. 1,160 g, including neonates with respiratory problems. Some require mechanical respiratory support. After the basic RTF course, I started treating these babies with RTF in addition to orthodox medical care.

- **Respiratory problems:** The most important zones are the thorax, small intestine, and solar plexus—gently tonify these zones for a few minutes several times a day. In some babies, mechanical respiratory support could be stopped within 12 hours of this and the additional oxygen in the incubator reduced or stopped completely.
- **Eructation after drinking:** If babies have difficulties with eructation, the sedating grip in the zone of the cardia has proved very effective.
- **Lymphatic swelling of the legs:** After the lymphatic course, I gave an infant a brief but complete RTF lymphatic treatment for 2 days, which he very much enjoyed. The swelling subsided considerably after the first RTF session. I was unable to observe the boy's progress thereafter as he was returned to his mother.
- **Stabilizing grips:** I was very impressed that it was possible to use stabilizing grips highly effectively even with the smallest of feet (the baby weighed 1,160g). A girl literally extended her feet toward me as I employed Yin-Yang stroking.

I am delighted that I can incorporate RTF into my work to such good effect.

31.10.2 Intestinal Colic, Torticollis

A 9-week-old boy (delivered at 35 weeks) had severe abdominal problems immediately after being bottle-fed: colic, dark-green bowel movement only every 2 to 3 days with a lot of whining. The doctor diagnosed lactose intolerance and prescribed special formula whereupon the situation grew worse: extremely bloated abdomen, bowel movement only every 5 days, and bouts of crying lasting for hours. In addition, the baby was found to have torticollis, which had been overlooked postpartum.

Initial findings, treated zones: The baby has clammy skin, wriggles, and screams. Red-bluish distended abdomen. Cautious treatment of the intestine, upper abdomen, diaphragm, and pelvic floor. Frequent stabilizing/harmonizing grips. Sternocleidomastoid muscle and temporomandibular joint gently sedated.

Reactions: One hour after first RTF session much more solid, partly bloody feces; once more during the night. Sleep without bouts of crying, distension of abdomen decreased, skin became pinker. Interesting point: The baby began to smell like pungent cheese in the folds of its skin and on its hands and feet.

Progress and results: Within 10 RTF sessions, the smell had vanished completely. The boy liked putting his little feet in my hands and enjoyed the contact. Daily bowel movements since third RTF session, severe flatulence declined. The torticollis corrected itself completely and the baby is now contented and "crows" happily to himself.

31.10.3   Congested Tear Duct

A 3-month-old boy was fully breastfed. Left eye red and sticky. The left half of the face was also red with deep-red blotches. Overall impression: a listless, unhappy baby.

Treatment: Frequent stabilizing grips, in particular, the Yin-Yang grip. Gentle tonifying of the zones of the face and tear duct, which was distinctly palpable. The three diaphragms (floor of the mouth, diaphragm, and pelvic floor). The small intestine and colon: strikingly high tone. The urinary tract and, specifically, the urethra (similar in anatomical structure to tear duct) also gently tonified.

Reactions: Clearly becoming more acute initially. However, the yellowish, viscous lacrimal fluid soon became clearer and more liquid. Malodorous stool twice, strong-smelling urine, rash over whole body, weeping in places.

Result: After six RTF sessions each lasting 10 to 15 minutes the boy was radiant, highly curious, and alert.

31.11

Treatment of Children

31.11.1   Spasmodic Torticollis, Acute

A 12-year-old boy suddenly developed a stiff neck in the middle of a school lesson and could not turn and tilt his head to the left any longer. His mother, my friend, asked me to treat him with manual therapy. As I was unable to provide the treatment in situ because of the boy's intense pain, I proposed RTF, despite having only attended Course I.

Treatment: It was very helpful that Jan (the patient) was able to tell me precisely where, how intensively, and for how long I could work on each specific zone: sedation of the neck, left side of cervical spine, middle phalanges of second to fourth toes (base of the skull) on both sides, coccyx including the rectum, all regions three times in total. In the last session, I included a cautious neck massage in situ.

Reactions and outcome: While I was performing the palm-to-sole stabilizing grip during the first RTF session, he suddenly shouted: "Look, I can turn my head again!" After 2 days the zones were scarcely noticeable anymore and on the third day Jan was completely free of symptoms again.

Personal observation: After working as a physical therapist for many years, in RTF I am happy to have discovered a treatment which addresses the **whole person**.

31.11.2   Tics Presenting as Blinking of the Eyelids

A 4-year-old boy was brought for treatment for tics that he had had for 9 months. The trigger was an insect in his eye. A doctor removed the insect against fierce resistance from the boy—several people had to restrain him for this. The tics got worse when the boy was under stress, for example, while watching television or when not being allowed to play with his older brother's toys. The psychologist was also unable to reach him emotionally.

Initial and further treatment: The boy can barely lie still and has a constant urge to move. Zones of the eyes sedated, likewise head/neck, lymphatics (skin folds between toes), thorax, lesser pelvis laterally as they were very sensitive. Intestine, spleen, and liver tonified.

Interesting reactions: The boy really appreciated some of the stabilizing grips, for example, Yin-Yang and palm-to-sole grips, while some made him restless, for example, heel stretching. He had to pass wind frequently during RTF. After the first RTF session, the tics grew worse for a day and he was noticeably tired. Then the tics declined from one RTF session to the next and since the fifth session they have disappeared.

Result: The intervals between treatment sessions were up to 4 weeks—the boy is much calmer and fidgets less.

31.11.3   Constipation, Lack of Peristalsis

The mother of a 6-year-old girl was concerned because the child's intestine was evacuated under anesthesia at a pediatric hospital a week previously. She found this experience traumatic for the child and wanted to avoid further manual evacuation. The child had had all the standard childhood vaccinations.

Treated zones: Tonifying head, teeth (= all toes), all the digestive organs and sphincters, lumbar spine, and abdominal wall. Heel stretching grip for autonomic balance.

Result: The girl had a bowel movement the very same evening.

Advice for the mother: Avoid sweets as far as possible, more fruit and vegetables, increase fluid intake. Massage of the zones of the lumbar spine and buttocks with olive oil every day, giving the girl more attention as a result.

The treatment was performed every 3 days for 3 weeks and since then the girl has been able to go to the toilet regularly.

31.12

Treatment of the Elderly

31.12.1 Hardness of Hearing at 101 Years Old

At the request of a colleague, I treated a 101-year-old man who had been invited to be interviewed on television but was very hard of hearing despite hearing aids. He was very uncertain as to whether he would understand the moderator's questions sufficiently.

Treated zones: In addition to the symptoms, lymphatics of the head/neck, eustachian tubes, wisdom teeth (energetically associated with the ear), intestine, urinary tract, pelvic organs, stabilizing grips.

Reactions: The patient was astonishingly relaxed and visibly enjoyed RTF.

Result: He was able to hear better immediately afterward. Naturally, I watched the television program: the elderly man answered every question spontaneously and substantively and was very warmly applauded for his account of his long and eventful life. Not even the moderator had noticed his hardness of hearing. For the next 2 years he came for RTF once a month until half a year before his death.

Personal observation: Although with a shoe size of 44 he gave me plenty to do, to my surprise and delight I ascertained that the human power of regeneration is retained into advanced old age.

31.12.2 Condition after a Complex Fracture of the Radius and Mastectomy on the Left Side

Six months ago the 79-year-old female patient had a complex fracture of the radius on the left side involving a stay in hospital. Very frail generally, mastectomy 5 years previously, after which the left shoulder had restricted mobility. Paresthesia

in the left hand. Her great wish was to have recovered sufficiently in 3 months' time to be able to celebrate her 80th birthday.

Initial findings, treated zones: Feet very tense overall. Gently tonified: shoulder girdle, organs of the lesser pelvis, spine, upper abdomen, and ileocecal valve. **Scar treatment:** first fracture collaterally and contralaterally on the right wrist and left ankle. Scar on the breast from second operation which looked alarming: approximately 10 cm of hard, nodular tissue around the scar, very painful.

Reactions: Paresthesia in the hand and restricted movement in the shoulder only became less painful as a result of RTF scar treatment in the zone of the breast. The patient had a pressing need to talk about her many fears. Initially, she was unable to rub scar ointment into the scar on her breast herself, as I had suggested, because she found it hideous and repugnant. Later she was able to do so and was very relieved about this.

Result: After 15 RTF sessions, her wrist and shoulder were significantly better, bowel movements were normal and her general health very good for her age. Fortunately, she was able to celebrate her birthday almost free from pain, as she had wished.

Personal observation: I worked as a surgical nurse for some years but I had never seen such a neglected scar before and I am very impressed by what RTF can achieve with scars. As a result, the woman allowed herself to become aware of past experiences and feelings which had manifested themselves physically. She was then able to let go of them. With her, in particular, I realized how important talking can sometimes be during treatment.

31.13

Self-Treatment

31.13.1 Positive Gynecological Results

Self-reporting: I am 44 years old. Mucosal changes were ascertained in the cervix. A repetition of the smear test was scheduled in 4 to 6 weeks.

Treatment: Every second or third day, 5 to 10 minutes, approximately 12 times the zones of the pituitary gland, the suprarenals, thyroid gland, and spleen were well tonified, and now and then the zone of the uterus too.

Result: The next smear test 6 weeks later was negative, likewise the next screening examination. I was very glad that no further treatment or even an operation was now necessary.

31.13.2 Scar Treatment—Transferred from the Microsystem to the Macrosystem

I have symptoms from scars on the inside of both malleoli and also externally on the right foot as well as on the tibia. As these scars represent zone assignments at the same time, on the course I was advised to

- treat the scars collaterally and contralaterally and
- transfer the corresponding points to the "seated person" in large format and to vigorously massage them in the muscles there.

I followed this advice. In addition, I had had knee and sciatica-like pain for a long time. During the course I became aware of a scar on my thigh at the same time (a fall from a bike during childhood), which I had forgotten. I also treated this scar collaterally and contralaterally (upper **arm** on the same side and **thigh** on the opposite side) myself.

Result: I have been completely free of symptoms for 3 weeks now and hope that it will stay this way.

31.13.3 Cyst on Right Ovary

When I was 43 years old, I had a 4 × 5 cm cyst pervaded by septa and with internal bleeding diagnosed on my right ovary using ultrasound. An operation was the only option because with this finding it was not possible to hope for a spontaneous regression. I was to be admitted to hospital 24 days later.

As I had already done a course in RTF and had read in the course book that cysts can be influenced positively, I decided to give myself intensive treatment.

I obtained initial results and treated myself daily for approximately 20 to 30 minutes for 23 days.

Results, treated zones: Initially the symptomatic zone of the ovary was extremely painful but the pain eased during the course of treatment and a few days before the hospital appointment it had gone completely. In addition, I treated the zones of the uterus, fallopian tubes, hip, shoulder girdle, and part of the lymphatic system. Furthermore, I rubbed an ointment good for scars into the zone of the right ovary daily and treated the corresponding zones of the hands at the same time.

Result: The professor and the senior physician did not find any cysts in the next ultrasound scan. Thus, I had spared myself an operation thanks to treating myself with RTF.

31.14 Lymphatic Disorders

31.14.1 Chronic Suppurative Otitis Media, Bronchitis and Sinusitis

Treatment of a 5-year-old boy for acute otitis media.

Treated zones: Ears, nasopharyngeal space, eustachian tubes sedated. Lymphatics of head–neck. Genital area, intestine, appendix, spleen, heart, and kidneys gently tonified.

Reactions and outcome: After a few grips, the pinna of the affected ear became bright red. The pain eased shortly afterward. Increased mucus secretion from the throat during and after RTF.

In the next RTF session, his mother reported that the previously very querulous and agitated boy was a changed person immediately after treatment. Three RTF sessions in total, the last one only as lymphatic RTF. I showed the mother some grips, which she continued to use at home.

After a 2-week vacation in the sun, the boy returned hale and hearty, no doubt also thanks to his parents' treatments. Since then, no further otitis media and only rare colds of short duration.

31.14.2 Glandular Fever

Personal experience: I am a pediatric nurse. A year ago I had glandular fever and had to stay in bed for several weeks, extreme fatigue, a lot of headaches, for months I felt sometimes better and sometimes worse. Nonetheless, I decided to attend Course III on the Lymphatic System.

Reactions: On the last day, when we were practicing the whole lymphatic treatment on each other, while I myself was carrying out the treatment, sweat ran down my chest and back, and my trousers were completely soaked in the inguinal region. While I was **receiving** treatment, I felt very well, remarkably well in fact. Afterward, I immediately had to pass a lot of water but was no longer perspiring.

Result: That was **the** treatment which brought about the turning point in my illness. Now I am able to work again like I used to.

NB: This experience cannot be repeated at will but is still encouraging.

31.14.3 Lymphedema of Both Legs

A 52-year old woman had already been treated using Manual Lymphatic Drainage for a long time but without significant improvement. The patient came to me as a result of a change of therapist.

Treated zones: Intestine badly afflicted, upon inquiry the patient reported a severe intestinal infection on holiday involving a long stay in hospital. Lymphatic RTF with associated organs.

Result: No intestinal problems any more after a few treatment sessions; the edema decreased significantly, she lost 10 kg in weight. The patient now gets more exercise and has a greater lust for life.

Therapeutic homework: She continues to treat the intestine and pelvic organs in the zones of the hands by herself for some time afterward.

31.15

Allergies, Skin Diseases

31.15.1 Allergic Rhinitis

A 27-year-old female colleague developed an allergy 8 years ago; her hay fever and itchy eyes grew worse with every season. In appearance: slim, athletic, fair skin with a tendency to blemishes.

Initial findings and treated zones: Nasopharyngeal space, small intestine and colon, spleen, appendix, pelvic organs, spine and shoulder girdle, stabilizing grips.

Reactions: After the treatment sessions her feet were noticeably warm and she felt very tired, but in the evenings she was full of energy. She passed water less frequently, but in greater amounts. She had a cold and tonsillitis when nearing the end of the course of treatment but both abated quickly. Seven RTF sessions in 6 weeks.

Result: Eyes no longer itchy, sneezing attacks very rare, fewer blemishes on the skin. I have the impression that all the mucosa and the skin have benefited.

31.15.2 Allergic Cough

A 30-year-old woman had had violent coughing bouts with fear of asphyxiation every evening before going to bed for around 15 years. Mild allergy to grasses and house dust. Had only one bowel movement a week.

Initial findings, treated zones: Remarkably calloused feet. Nasopharyngeal space, head, pelvic ligaments, lymphatics, thorax, spine and knee tonified. Intestine was affected surprisingly little.

Reactions: Increased irritation of the throat initially, extremely tired. After fifth RTF session, extensive herpes below the nose, severe pain at tooth 25 (assignment, inter alia, to the lung, thymus, and colon), given emergency dental treatment.

Result: After 12 RTF sessions no further coughing bouts, regular bowel movements every 2 days, calloused skin almost completely gone, patient feels well.

NB: The patient had a change of address during the course of treatment. Observation: perhaps she had been exposed to allergenic substances in the old apartment, in addition to her personal underlying medical history?

31.15.3 Condition after Herpes Zoster, Allergies

A large, robust-looking 34-year-old woman had pain in the rib and thoracic spine region, was allergic to various substances, and had food intolerances. Clammy hands and feet. "Embryonic fold" (embryonic inversion of a tissue fold in the knee joint) in the left knee corrected by surgery.

Initial findings: The zones of the stomach, including the cardia and pylorus, hepatic and splenic flexure of the colon, organs of the lesser pelvis, all the wisdom teeth and tooth 34, shoulder/upper arm are affected.

Treatment: Initially, almost exclusively stabilizing grips as intense autonomic overreactions even with slight contact. Later, cautious treatment of the zones of the intestine, spleen, gall bladder, and urinary tract. Scar RTF for scar on knee.

Reactions: During brief treatment of the zones of the pelvic ligaments, severe autonomic dysfunction, facial allergy, burning eyes, but the strong, burning pain in the region of the herpes zoster had gone. The patient feels extremely tired, yawns and sleeps a lot. Is very hungry and thirsty. The facial allergy eases as a result of lymphatic RTF. Talks a lot about her mother having cancer.

Result: After 12 RTF sessions the pain of herpes zoster has vanished, the patient feels much better but continues to need a lot of sleep.

31.16

Neurological Diseases

31.16.1 Stroke with Cerebral Hemorrhage

A 71-year-old male patient suffered respiratory arrest after a week in hospital and was subsequently on a ventilator for 3 months. Heavy perspiration, restlessness, great difficulties with breathing every night. Various visits to the doctor brought only minimal relief.

Appearance: So short of breath that he could barely speak. Beads of sweat on his forehead. Thorax and stomach extremely tense during each inhalation, 32 to 35 inhalations per minute.

Treated zones: Elevated position. Very frequent stabilizing grips. Light tonifying of the intestine and head. Eutonic grips. Later, in addition: heart, thorax including the bronchial tubes, spine, expansion of the diaphragm, scar cream for intubation scar. "Merima," lymphatic treatments.

Reactions: After the second RTF session, breathing returned to normal at 17 times per minute. In the third RTF session more acute: respiration rate accelerated significantly again. Since the fourth RTF session, the crisis has been overcome. Twelve RTF sessions in total.

Result: Inhalations remain normal, no nocturnal perspiration any more, sleep peaceful and without fear. Patient is radiant during each treatment. His wife also has treatment to recover from the many sleepless nights.

Personal observation: I think the patient lost his own rhythm as a result of long-term use of the ventilator and had to rediscover it gradually. I was very pleased by how quickly Mr. B. recovered.

31.16.2 Restless Legs

A 55-year-old female patient had had this complaint since her husband died approximately 2 years previously.

Treatment: At first, only stabilizing holding and neutral mobilizing of the feet, stabilizing grips which give her the feeling of having "the earth under her feet" again.

Treated zones: Shoulder girdle, spine, pelvic ligaments, and intestine. The head including the brain stem and spinal cord are sedated.

Result: Although the patient felt exhausted after the first RTF session, she is relieved. She does not need the medication prescribed for Parkinson's disease any more. She comes for treatment every 3 weeks for an extended period and feels stable.

31.16.3 Multiple Sclerosis, Granuloma of the Right Maxilla

A 54-year-old female patient had had the aforementioned disease for 18 years. She had minor relapses every 2 to 3 weeks which resolved themselves. Cold, clammy feet.

Treated zones: Head and spine treated cautiously. Gastrointestinal and tracts, lesser pelvis, and right hip. The teeth on the upper right greatly affected. Frequent stabilizing grips.

Reactions: After a few RTF sessions, the general overtension eased, reflexive twitching decreased. No nighttime urination any more.

Result: After 12 RTF sessions she was able to walk two kilometers without a walking aid, general health significantly better but minor relapses as before.

Later: I had advised her to go to a holistic dentist because of the affected tooth zones. She hesitated because the corresponding teeth had crowns fitted only a year before. She later reported on the telephone that at breakfast one day a crown broke off and she had very severe toothache. A granuloma between tooth 17 and 18 was removed by means of partial resection and healing took several weeks. Since then she has had **no further relapses**.

31.17
Cancer

31.17.1 End-Stage Lung Cancer

A 68-year-old male patient, with whom I had been doing breathing exercises two to three times a week for an extended period, was lying in bed at home turning blue due to severe breathing problems. He looked at me fearfully. Emergency spray had brought no relief.

Treated zones: Stabilizing grips, in particular heel stretching and diaphragm extending in the direction of the intestinal tract. Gentle tonifying of the lungs and intercostal muscles.

Result: The patient soon regained his normal color, the inhalations grew slower and deeper. After this positive experience he asked me for RTF time and again. He lived another 3 months.

31.17.2 Acute Bladder Infection after Surgery for Breast Cancer

The 40-year old female patient had been treated by me for a long time following surgery, chemotherapy, and radiation. Fortunately, my working relationship with the physicians in the surrounding area was good and patients were able to be treated with RTF whenever they liked.

Acute treatment: Surprisingly, the affected zones did not become completely pain-free as in earlier reflexotherapy treatment. I therefore made inquiries. The trigger for the acute bladder infection was a cold, which the woman had caught when she had let an acquaintance persuade her to help with work outdoors.

Result: Reviewing the situation, she recognized that once again she had done what **others** expected of her and not what **she** wanted to do. When she realized this the zones were pain-free within minutes.

Personal observation: I have long observed that many problems on the emotional level can be solved and/or processed through RTF.

31.17.3 Condition after Breast Cancer, Left Side

A 67-year old female patient had pronounced lymphedema in the left breast, almost twice as large as the right breast. Chemotherapy. After radiotherapy, second-degree burns, skin brown, fibrotic, large-pored.

Treatment process: The patient comes for Manual Lymphatic Drainage. I combine it with lymph RTF. Good preliminary treatment including the zones of the kidneys, intestine, liver, and spleen. Then lymph RTF of the head/neck and thorax, the axilla on both sides particularly thoroughly. Solar plexus grip as autonomic compensation is especially beneficial for her.

Doctor's statement: "Nothing more can be done, what is burned is burned." I continue to receive prescriptions, however.

Reactions: The patient feels very well, is able to relax easily after having experienced a great deal of pain in the past. She comes for treatment twice a week for 6 months.

Result: The major edema slowly recedes, after 6 months it is significantly smaller. After a year the swelling has gone down completely and the condition of the skin at the burn site is very good.

The patient has now been coming once a week for 3 years, has had no relapses, and is happy about her good condition.

31.18

Palliative Care, Terminal Care

31.18.1 A Special Good Bye

A 38-year-old female patient with end-stage breast cancer following surgery on the left side. Multiple metastases, pulmonary heart failure, emotional instability, and attempted suicide. I looked after her during the daytime for 2 months as a "charity nurse" and treated her feet daily.

Treatment process: Initially only for 10 minutes on each occasion with stabilizing grips, often solar plexus. Later gentle tonifying of the zones of the

diaphragm, intestine, and endocrine system. RTF sphincter sedation, "Small energy cycle" (**see Fig. 6.7**), lymph RTF, scar treatment also in situ.

Reactions: Frequently clammy hands, sometimes the patient fell asleep during RTF. After lymph treatments (four sessions) she cried and felt weak. Warm feet during sphincter treatment. Increased diuresis. As a result of scar treatment better expectoration of mucus, respiration easier.

Result: After several RTF sessions, the patient became significantly calmer, no further suicidal thoughts. Lymphatic congestion in the left arm decreased.

Personal observation: After orthodox medical care had failed to have any effect, I was able to help the patient through her extremely difficult final stage of life with RTF. I combined the treatment sessions with spiritual talks whenever the patient asked for them, and with periods of active silence. Empathy and support were particularly important for her and her family.

31.18.2 Experiences with In-patients

As a nurse, I belong to a group of specialist physicians, pain therapists, physical therapists and music therapists, psycho-oncologists, spiritual counsellors and social workers. Our patients are treated consistently according to their needs.

Frequent afflictions: Pain, nausea, vomiting, digestive problems, pyrexia, edema, circulatory problems, fears, emotional state.

Choice of treatment: For a great many patients **RTF lymph treatment**, with the emphasis on the lymphatic vessels. Many stabilizing grips, excretory organs. The treatment alternates between lymph RTF and supporting the excretory organs.

Always including movement of the entire foot, stretching of the interdigital skinfolds, often treatment of the start and end points of the meridians. Caution is generally advised with regard to the symptomatic zone, which can only be touched lightly usually.

- **Sphincter treatment:** In patients with abdominal tumors, ascites, nausea, and vomiting and peritoneal carcinomatosis, it provides at least temporary relief.
- **In edema patients** (e.g., pleural effusions, lymphatic congestion in the inguinal region as a result of a tumor) always good fluid excretion but a **good balance** (in terms of time and intensity) is important in order to avoid overreactions.
- **General reactions:** The patients' faces relax, wrinkles on the forehead due to pain are

smoothed out, they become calm and sometimes fall asleep. Fears subside.

- **RTF for the dying?** If the dying process has started, sometimes direct contact with the feet is no longer appropriate. Usually patients help by signaling their needs. Relatives are always included and supported as well.
- **Personal observation:** I am grateful to find that treatment sessions involve give and take because "no one can touch without being touched themselves."

31.19

Teeth as Interference Fields

31.19.1 Sacroiliac Joint/Lumbar Spine Complaints

A 28-year-old female formation dancer had to give up dancing because of severe lower back pain. Analgesics brought no relief. Temporary improvement with osteopathy.

Medical history: Whiplash injury involving cervical vertebrae and allergic asthma since pneumonia as a child. Chronic cracking of the jaw, dysmenorrhea, very healthy teeth.

Findings, treated zones: Spine, in particular, sacroiliac joint, shoulder girdle, intestine, urinary tract, lesser pelvis, solar plexus, Eutonic sacrum grip. The wisdom teeth on the top right and left were the most painful. RTF of these teeth and their associations in accordance with Voll did not result in any lasting freedom from pain.

Energetic measurement by a holistic dentist revealed that the upper wisdom teeth produce significant interference because the jaw is too small. To avoid healthy teeth having to be extracted, a bionator after Prof. Balters was fitted.

Result: In the last RTF session, the patient commented that "everything is on the move." Her backache has decreased considerably and the zones of the teeth are also significantly less sensitive. If bionator therapy fails to produce the desired result, the patient will have her wisdom teeth extracted and then have follow-up treatment.

31.19.2 Knee Complaints

A 61-year-old female patient after breast cancer and breast-conserving operation 4 years previously now coming for treatment because of knee complaints.

Course of treatment: I treat the whole foot neutrally but emphasize the zones of the knee, spine, and shoulder girdle. Breast gently.

Reactions: After the second RTF session she catches a "cold." Upon my advice that it is a reaction, she does not treat it with symptom-suppressing measures. Surprisingly, the knee pain has gone. But after the third RTF session, she has severe toothache under her crowns. The dentist cannot find anything initially but removes the crown a few days later and has to extract teeth 44 and 45 (energetic relationship with the knee) because of root decay.

Result: Since the seventh RTF session, the remaining five sessions have been a real pleasure for the patient. She feels well, her new teeth have been fitted, and her mouth and knee are calm.

31.20

Scars as Interference Fields

31.20.1 Clavicle Scar as Interference Field with Pain in Lumbar Spine and Sacroiliac Joint

A 53-year-old male patient, athletic, creative, had been in severe pain for 6 months. Two fractures of the clavicle and both elbows, appendectomy, and tonsillectomy. Stomach problems.

Preliminary treatment: Five visits to orthopaedists, acupuncture several times without any improvement.

Affected and treated zones: Upper abdominal organs, intestine, upper and lower spine, appendix scar, shoulder/elbow, and left hip.

Reactions and outcome: Brief reduction in pain after treatment of the appendix scar and the tooth associations in accordance with Voll. The C7 to T1 transition remains very painful. After treatment of the **clavicle scar** in the seventh RTF session, the back was immediately and permanently free from pain, the lumbar spine/sacroiliac joint blockages resolved themselves permanently.

31.20.2 Status after Gall Bladder Operation, Diarrhea

A 63-year-old woman had suffered six to eight episodes of burning, watery diarrhea daily for 7 years. Surprisingly, no tissue desiccation.

Initial findings: Zones of the intestine not noticeable. However, cervical vertebrae, neck lymphatics, both hips, and abdominal wall.

Treated zones: Intestine overall, initially sedating, pelvic ligaments, sphincters, examination of tooth associations, lymph RTF.

Reactions: Although the zones of the intestine did not appear to be affected, episodes of diarrhea decreased and bowel movements were better formed. Perspiration with a penetrating smell. **Scar RTF** (in part very painful) as the diarrhea began after a gall bladder operation. Scar in situ, which was very thin and white at first, became elevated, red and burned "like fire" in the lower third in the course of three scar RTF sessions.

Result: Defecation returned to normal completely after 12 RTF sessions—the patient is happy.

31.20.3 Uterine Fibroid Surgery

A 41-year-old patient has suffered from severe paresthesia in the abdominal region since the operation.

Initial findings, treated zones: Scar RTF, frequent stabilizing grips, thoracic spine, lumbar spine, abdominal wall, organs of the lesser pelvis, stomach, hips, and thigh. Later pelvic ligaments. Three RTF lymph sessions.

Reactions: Aggression, diarrhea, binge eating. After the third RTF session the scar was inconspicuous, increased sensation in the abdominal region, then improved bowel movement, earlier start of period. After treatment of pelvic ligaments, elimination of clear, liquid mucus from lower abdomen.

Result: Sensitivity almost completely restored. The course of treatment was interrupted by a fracture of the lateral malleolus. The patient later reported that her sensitivity in the abdominal region is completely normal again.

In addition, there was virtually no swelling of the ankle after the fracture, which the patient attributed to the preceding RTF.

31.21

Postoperative Treatment

31.21.1 Status after Total Endoprothesis, Right Knee

An 84-year-old female patient, good general health, mentally alert. Medical history: coronary vascular disease, aortic valve replacement, hypertension, varicosis.

Start of treatment on first day after the operation: Tonifying of the acupuncture points on the toes as these meridians all supply the knee. Short RTF lymph treatment with emphasis on the upper abdomen and urinary tract. Knee collaterally and contralaterally, at first only with gentle touch to "convey information," later tonifying as well. Frequent stabilizing grips.

Further course of treatment: RTF scar treatment during and after rehabilitation as well as application of a suitable ointment to scar in situ. The patient had virtually no swelling on her knee and could already take alternating steps in hospital using a walking aid without great pain.

Result: In the view of the physicians and nursing staff, healing progressed remarkably well. She was already able to walk without a walking aid during rehabilitation but used it now and then for safety reasons.

31.21.2 Status after Sigma Resection 2007

A 74-year-old highly skeptical pharmacist still had severe flatulence and strikingly loud borborygmus 2 years after surgery and self-medication. He only came for treatment because his wife sent him.

Initial findings and treated zones: Muscles of the feet extremely tense. Gastrointestinal tract including the liver/gall bladder, thoracic spine, lumbar spine, plantar side of head (similarity in shape: the intestine and brain), frequent stabilizing grips, in particular, solar plexus. Ten RTF sessions once or twice a week.

Reactions: Patient feels better from one RTF session to the next. After the sixth session the flatulence has significantly improved and there is less borborygmus.

Result: At the end of the course of treatment he is completely free of symptoms. His initial skepticism has vanished and now he comes for a course of treatment once a year to keep himself in good condition.

31.22

Combination Treatments

31.22.1 Condition after Operation for Pleural Empyema and Effusions

I have the good fortune to be able to work in the interdisciplinary intensive care department of a hospital using a combination of psychotonic **respiratory and craniosacral therapy and RTF**.

A 66-year-old female patient came to our intensive care ward after several operations (partial rib resection, evacuation of empyema, and skin graft).

Treatment: I treated her, as I often do, using the aforementioned combination. From RTF I selected lymphatic treatment to heal the thigh wound (after a skin graft) and for overall relaxation, which was particularly beneficial for the patient.

Additional selection of zones and result: Sedating grips in the thorax reduced the intense pain in and around the wound. Tonifying of the **hepatic flexure of the colon** and parts of the RTF lymph treatment resulted in a normal bowel movement the very next day—previously this was as hard as "concrete marbles." Tonifying of the **small intestine and gall bladder**, sedation of the sternocleidomastoid muscle made her headache disappear.

31.22.2 ADHD, Hyperactivity

General experiences: Although I mostly work **osteopathically,** my hands **must** also go to the feet in every session. Often the findings mutually corroborate each other. With these children, grips on the feet are very often the only kind of touch that is tolerated initially.

Important zones: Children often dislike their heads being touched. If so, I work in the **zones** which I could not treat osteopathically in situ. Solar plexus and other stabilizing grips. Mobilization of the toes and metatarsals, and widening the space between the toes.

Frequent change of the child's position to take account of the need for movement. **Important note:** At the end of treatment I tonify the entire spine, resulting in stability. After three or four treatment sessions parents come to the practice more contented because their child is becoming calmer. We cannot turn little rascals into angels, of course!

Personal observation: The practice also reveals a **sad trend**, however—nearly every bright, vivacious, active child is "pigeonholed" under medication, a change of school or overstretched parents while often it is "only" a dysfunction of the skull stemming from pregnancy/birth which has failed to correct itself of its own accord.

31.22.3 Multiple Myogeloses

Self-reporting: I attended the refresher course with a lot of very painful myogeloses between my right scapula and spine. Radiation of pain into the right shoulder joint and upper arm.

On the first day of the course as **acute treatment:** Eutonic shoulder–arm grip, zones of the spine and lymphatic system, axilla. When discussing **meridian relationships**, it occurred to me that I had bruised the fourth toe on my right foot

in the summer. Then it dawned on me and the whole group: the **gall bladder meridian** ends on the fourth toe and also supplies the shoulder with its energy. Treatment of the **left** fourth toe and the right ring finger.

Result: The next day the symptoms had improved by 80% and the acute pain had vanished completely.

31.23

Miscellaneous and Special Issues

31.23.1 "Heel Spur"—Chronic Constipation

A 35-year-old woman diagnosed with a heel spur described pain on the plantar side (in the zones of the intestine) of both feet and was able to walk only with difficulty. Bowel movement every 2 days, very hard consistency. Abdominal pain with heartburn since pregnancy.

Treated zones: Intestine, cardia and pylorus, pelvis, lumbar spine, shoulder girdle including the cervical spine and mastoid process, thorax.

Reactions: After the first treatment session loud borborygmus and tingling in the feet. She felt "quite different." Since the third RTF session, daily bowel movement, less pain in the feet but briefly in the neck.

Result: After six RTF sessions twice a week, soles of the feet completely painless, hardly any heartburn anymore, sleeps through the night now, digestion remains regular.

Personal observation: Since then I have been fully alert when someone comes to me with a diagnosis of "heel spur."

31.23.2 Pelvic Ligaments and Belly Dancing

I have noticed that unlike my other female patients, the zones of the **pelvic ligaments are not afflicted at all** in many female Turkish acquaintances who do belly-dancing.

31.23.3 Piercing

Self-reporting by a therapist: For approximately 10 years I had had a piercing in my lower lip. I had got so used to it that it did not occur to me that various complaints that I had might be related to it.

Treatment: During the practical exercises in the course I was bothered by tingling in my feet and legs and at night; my feet and legs were very restless too. After that, I removed the piercing.

Result: Immediately afterward the symptoms improved significantly and in addition, my vision grew sharper and my hearing better.

31.23.4   Astigmatism, Inflamed Tonsils

In October I treated my 8-year old son because his tonsils were greatly enlarged and inflamed and he had a permanent cold.

Treated zones: Tonsils and appendix with sedating grips. Ears including the eustachian tubes, gastrointestinal tract, kidneys, joints and heart with tonifying grips. Six RTF sessions in total.

Result: At the beginning of November, I took my son for his annual eye check-up as he is nearsighted and astigmatic and has worn glasses for 2 years. To our great surprise, the ophthalmologist can de-tect **no nearsightedness** any more and only a very slight squint still.

Personal observation: My son's vision may have improved because I also treated the zones of the eyes "incidentally" by way of the lymphatic system, eustachian tubes, and stomach (inter alia, the stomach meridian supplies the eye with its energy).

31.23.5   Symptoms on the Foot

This fall I had an emergency operation: a ruptured ovarian cyst that was initially diagnosed as a tumor caused internal bleeding—it was a close call!

Interesting point: Two days before this, my foot had suddenly been painful in precisely the region of the ovary. I could hardly walk on it and at first thought I had twisted it unknowingly but the pain disappeared just as quickly as it had started—after the operation.

32 Summary of the Method

1. In its practical application, from a theoretical perspective and as a result of the similarity in shape between the foot and a seated person, reflexotherapy of the feet (RTF) is easily understandable and can easily be learned.
2. It is more than a local foot massage because, as a microsystem, the feet are in constant interaction with the whole person.
3. It enables personal access to the patient through work with the hands and hence conveys the important "remedy of touch."
4. It can be combined with all the other methods from the medical–therapeutic sector and, in particular, trains the eye with regard to the effectiveness of simplicity.
5. Its results are convincing as the effects and changes can be experienced both spontaneously during treatment and in the outcome of a course of treatment.
6. It directly addresses the regenerative and vital forces of the sick because it avoids technical aids and substitutes.
7. It is cost-saving and economical in use as it does not suppress the symptom but also includes the background causes.
8. It conveys the realistic experience that pain does not have to be fought like an enemy but can also offer the opportunity for change.
9. Depending on the occupational profile, it can be used as a therapeutic tool and/or for health care and maintenance, and, depending on the profession, as an aid to diagnosis.
10. It can be offered to all age groups for many acute and chronic diseases, on its own or as an adjunctive therapy.
11. It subordinates itself to important laws of life because it employs the principles of rhythm and dynamism in the therapeutic grip.
12. It creates contented patients and therapists as the shared experience of treatment results directly in substantial and constructive life contexts.

Special Topics and Further Developments

Part IV
Appendix

33 Authorized RTF Schools and Further Information

Since 1977 a number of scientific and evidence-based studies have been published on Reflexotherapy of the Foot as it is taught in our RTF centers.

A list of training schools in Germany and in other European countries can be found on our internet homepage www.fussreflex.de, along with more detailed information.

These courses are taught in the native language of the host country. All our training courses, including those outside Germany, are intended to provide additional specialization to those already qualified in the medical-therapeutic profession. They cannot however, be interpreted as leading to an independent professional profile as may be understood by the term "Reflexology" as it is used in various other countries.

Postal address of German school:

Ausbildungszentrum
Hanne Marquardt GmbH
Prof. Domagk-Weg 15
78126 Königsfeld-Burgberg
Germany
Tel.: 0049 (0)7725 7117
Fax: 0049 (0)7725 7080
info@fussreflex.de

RTF literature in English and other languages and further information:

www.verlaghannemarquardt.de
info@verlaghannemarquardt.de
Postal address: see above

By Hanne Marquardt:

- Translation of the original German textbook into 14 languages (some with addresses of book suppliers).
- Autobiography "Unterm Dach der Füße" (Under the Roof of the Feet) [German]
- Color charts of reflex zones of the feet in various languages (different sizes available)
- Brochures on the topic in various languages
- Information on English-language 2-day courses in other countries

34 Figure Sources

Fig. 1.2: from FitzGerald WH, Bowers EF. Zone Therapy or Relieving Pain at Home. 1917

Fig. 1.3: from Ingham E. Stories the Feet Can Tell. New York; 1938

Fig. 21.1: from Schünke M, Schulte E, Schumacher U. Thieme Atlas of Anatomy, General Anatomy and Musculoskeletal System. 2nd ed. © Thieme 2014, illustrations by Markus Voll and Karl Wesker

Figs. 21.5 and 22.2:
from Mees LFC. Das menschliche Skelett. Form und Metamorphose. Stuttgart: Urachhaus; 1981

Fig. 27.1: modified from Rossaint A. Medizinische Kinesiologie, Physio-Energetik und Ganzheitliche (Zahn-) Heilkunde. Das Hand buch für Therapeuten. Kirchzarten: VAK; 2005

Illustrations: Christiane Schott, Rottweil

All other illustrations by the author

35 Technical Terms

Analogy	similarity
Bilateral	on both sides
Caudal	at or near the posterior part of the body
Cranial	relating to the skull or cranium
Distal	situated away from the center of the body or from the point of attachment
Dorsal	on or relating to the upper side or back
In situ	in the natural location in the body
Kyphosis	excessive outward curvature of the spine, causing hunching of the back
Lateral	of, at, toward, or from the side or sides
Lisfranc line	connection between the base of the five metatarsal bones and the sphenoid bones and the cuboid bone
Malleolus	ankle
Medial	pertaining to the middle
Palliative	alleviating of symptoms
Phalange	individual digital bone of the fingers and toes
Plantar	on the sole of the foot
Plantar flexion	movement of the foot in which the foot or toes flex downward toward the sole
Pronation	inward rotation
RTF	Reflexotherapy of the feet
Supination	outward rotation (e.g., of the hand)
Unilateral	on one side

36 Bibliography

Bossy J. Morphological Data Concerning the Acupuncture Point and Channel Network. Acupunct Electrother Res 1984;9:79-106

Chancellor PM. Handbook of the Bach-Flower Remedies. Ashingdon, Essex: C.W. Daniel; 1979

Feldenkrais M. Awareness through Movement. Health Exercises for Personal Growth. Reprint. San Francisco, CA: Harper; 1990

FitzGerald WH, Bowers EF. Zone Therapy or Relieving Pain at Home. Columbus, OH: I.W. Long Publishers; 1917

Kramer F. Lehrbuch der Elektroakupunktur. Heidelberg, Germany: Haug; 1999

Marquardt H. Reflex Zone Therapy of the Feet. A Comprehensive Guide for Health Professionals. 2nd ed. Rochester, VT: Inner Traditions – Bear & Company; 2010

Mees LF. Secrets of the Skeleton. Form in Metamorphosis. Great Barrington, MA: Steiner Books; 1984

Nogier P. From Auriculotherapy to Auriculomedicine [in French]. Moulins-les-Metz: Maisonneuve; 1983

Nogier P. A Practical Introduction to Auriculotherapy [in French]. Moulins-les-Metz: Maisonneuve; 1977

Pischinger A. The Extracellular Matrix and Ground Regulation. Basis for a Holistic Biological Medicine. Berkley, CA: North Atlantic Books; 2007

Rauch E. Health through Inner Body Cleansing. The Famous F. X. Mayr Intestinal Therapy from Europe. 6th ed. Stuttgart: Thieme; 2008

Voll R. Topographic Positions of the Measurement Points in Electro-Acupuncture. Vol 3. Kulmbach, Germany: Medizinisch-Literarische Verl.-Ges.; 1977

Zhang Y. ECIWO biology and medicine: a new theory of conquering cancer and a completely new acupuncture therapy. People's Republic of China: Neimenggu People's Press; 1987

37 Index

Page numbers in *italics* refer to illustrations